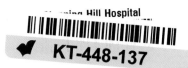

Handbook of Women's Health

Second Edition

Handbook of Women's Health

Second Edition

Edited by

Jo Ann Rosenfeld MD

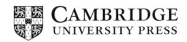

CAMBRIDGE UNIVERSITY PRESS
Cambridge, New York, Melbourne, Madrid, Cape Town, Singapore,
São Paulo, Delhi

Cambridge University Press
The Edinburgh Building, Cambridge CB2 8RU, UK

Published in the United States of America by
Cambridge University Press, New York

www.cambridge.org
Information on this title: www.cambridge.org/9780521695251

First published 2009

Printed in the United Kingdom at the University Press, Cambridge

A catalogue record for this publication is available from the British Library

Library of Congress Cataloging-in-Publication Data

Handbook of women's health / edited by Jo Ann Rosenfeld. – 2nd ed.
    p. ; cm.
  Includes bibliographical references and index.
  ISBN 978-0-521-69525-1 (pbk.)
1. Women–Health and hygiene–Handbooks, manuals, etc.
2. Evidence-based medicine–Handbooks, manuals, etc. I. Rosenfeld,
Jo Ann. II. Title.
  [DNLM: 1. Women's Health–Handbooks. 2. Evidence-Based
Medicine–Handbooks. WA 39 H2365 2009]

  RC48.6.H365 2009
  613′.04244–dc22
                                                          2009030225

ISBN 978-0-521-69525-1 Paperback

Dedicated to Jennifer and Robyn

Contents

Contributors

Kathryn Andolsek MD MPH
Professor, Community and Family Medicine,
Duke University School of Medicine;
Associate Director, Graduate Medical Education,
Duke University Hospital,
Durham, NC, USA

Barbara S. Apgar MD MS
Chelsea Medical System,
Chelsea Michigan
Ann Arbor, MI, USA

Deborah Bostock MD
Medical Operations Squadron Commander,
Langley AFB, VA, Adjunct Assistant Professor
of Family Medicine, Uniformed University
of the Health Sciences,
Bethesda, MD, USA

Kay Bauman MD MPH
Department of Public Safety, Wahiawa Hospital,
University of Hawaii,
Mililani, HI, USA

Abenaa Brewster MD
Johns Hopkins Oncology Center,
Baltimore, MD, USA

Sandra K. Burge PhD
Professor, Department of Family
and Community Medicine,
University of Texas Health Science Center at
San Antonio, TX, USA

Nancy Davidson MD
Johns Hopkins Oncology Center,
Baltimore, MD, USA

Mary-Anne Enoch MD MRCGP
Laboratory of Neurogenetics, National Institute
on Alcohol Abuse and Alcoholism, NIH,
Bethesda, MD, USA

Margaret Gradison MD MHS-CL
Associate Professor, Department of Community and
Family Medicine, Duke University Medical Center,
Durham, NC, USA

Cathrine Hoyo MPH PhD
Assistant Professor, Department of Community and
Family Medicine, Duke University Medical Center,
Durham, NC, USA

William J. Hueston MD
Professor and Chair,
Department of Family Medicine,
Medical University of South Carolina,
Charleston, SC, USA

Victoria S. Kaprielian MD
Professor, Department of Community
and Family Medicine,
Duke University Medical Center,
Durham, NC, USA

Connie Marsh
Kansas School of Medicine
Wichita KS, USA

Diana McNeill
Professor of Medicine, Internal Medicine Residency
Program Director, Vice Chair Medical Education,
Department of Medicine, Division of Endocrinology
and Metabolism, Duke University Medical Center,
Durham, NC, USA

Phillippa J. Miranda MD
Medical Instructor, Department of Medicine,
Division of Endocrinology and Metabolism,
Duke University Medical Center,
Durham, NC, USA

Tanya A. Miszko EdD CSCS Lic.Ac.
Prescriptive Health, Inc.,
Watertown, MA, USA

Cathleen Morrow MD
University of Maine School of Medicine
Fairfield,
ME, USA

Gwendolyn Murphy MS PhD RD LDN
Assistant Consulting Professor,
Department of Community and Family Medicine,
Duke University Medical Center,
Durham, NC, USA

Jo Ann Rosenfeld MD
Assistant Professor of Medicine,
Johns Hopkins School of Medicine,
Baltimore, MD, USA

Ellen L. Sakornbut MD
Family Health Center of Waterloo,
Waterloo, IA, USA

Jeannette E. South-Paul MD
Andrew W. Mathieson Professor and Chair,
Department of Family Medicine, University of
Pittsburgh School of Medicine, PA, USA

Valerie Ulstad MD MPH MPA
Hennepin County Medical Center,
Minneapolis, MN, USA

Meghan Walsh MD MPH
Hennepin Hospital,
Minneapolis, MN, USA

Cheryl E. Woodson MD FACP AGSF
Director, Woodson Center for Adult HealthCare,
Chicago Heights, IL, USA

Introduction

Jo Ann Rosenfeld

Women's health concerns have been considered, examined, and researched differently by the medical establishment than those of men. Their concerns and diseases have often been considered unusual and abnormal when compared to those of men. Yet, the differences between women and men, discovered and noted in medicine and research, may be more a creation of society and its expectations than that of nature.[1] Women are more similar to men than they are different.

Research
Extension, exclusion, and marginalization

Historically, researchers and clinicians who read the results have assumed that the data and conclusions on men, often middle-aged white men, could be applied to women of all ages, the elderly, children, and different ethnicities.[2] The American Medical Association (AMA) concluded that "Medical treatments for women are based on a male model, regardless of the fact that women may react differently to treatments than men or that some diseases manifest themselves differently in women than men. The results of medical research on men are generalized to women without sufficient evidence of applicability to women."[3]

Exclusion

Women, children, ethnic minorities and the elderly were historically excluded from research protocols. Justification for this behavior was either that women's differences would affect the results, or that the differences did not matter, that women were just smaller men.[4]

For example, research into and concerning acquired immune deficiency syndrome (AIDS) was almost completely androcentric. Until 1993, the Center for Disease Control (CDC) did not recognize that the symptoms of AIDS in women might be different than those in men; its criteria for the disease did not include pelvic inflammatory disease (PID), candidal vaginal infections, and cervical cancer. This occurred while the percentage of women with AIDS is increasing; women are at least twice as susceptible to being infected by the human immunodeficiency virus as men.[5] Research into AIDS in developing countries has not highlighted women, although more women are becoming infected. In five eastern African countries, the prevalence of AIDS in urban women is 17 to 32%, while 1.5 million women in India are infected by HIV.[6]

Marginalization

Much of the research on women's health concerns has emphasized women's genitourinary organs and diseases and childbearing diseases. This impacts both men and women. There is extensive research on women's contraceptive methods, but little on men's.[2] A report on women's mental health research stated:

> . . . the women's health field has moved beyond an exclusive emphasis on women's reproductive function to one that defines health as a scientific enterprise to identify clinically important sex and gender differences in prevalence, etiology, course, and treatment of illnesses affecting men and women in the population as well as conditions specific to women. Nonetheless, for mental disorders, women's reproductive function and its impact on mental health conditions is still understudied.[7]

Trends in research

In 1994, the National Institutes of Health (NIH) issued new guidelines for research funding, insisting on the inclusion of women and minority groups in all research it funded. It stipulated the following.

- Women and minorities should be included in all human research, and "women of childbearing potential should not be routinely excluded."[8]
- Women and minorities must be included in phase III trials.
- Cost is not a reason to exclude these groups.
- NIH must make a positive plan and effort to include women and minorities in research.

In the last 15 years since these disparities were first noted, some changes have been made specifically to include women, the elderly, the young, and minorities into research studies, and to report the results of the studies by gender, age, and ethnicity. It does little good to have 25% women in a study, and not be able to compare women's results to those of men. A US government accounting office (GAO) report in 2000 commended NIH for including women in their research trials, but stated that fewer trials reported data by gender.[9]

Despite recruiting efforts, still, fewer women and minorities are participating in NIH cancer treatment trials. Fewer women than men enrolled in lung cancer trials and colorectal cancer trials, although the rate of colon cancer is similar in men and women and the rate of lung cancer in women is increasing.

In the past decade, there has been a concerted effort to define differences and similarities in the diagnosis and treatment of women, as compared to men. Many studies specifically report results by gender. However, whether the study concerns treatment of hypercholesterolemia or the effects of exposure to metals, most studies conclude that they are only at the beginning in defining differences that concern women's health. With women's diseases, researchers are often just starting to define the problems. For example, a great deal of literature has been written on men's sexual dysfunction. The literature on women's sexual dysfunction is still trying to create definitions.

For example, a study found that women are more likely than men to develop nickel-induced allergy and hand eczema,[10] but the reasons for this can only be imagined. One study concluded that women were less likely to be screened for hypercholesterolemia than men,[11] while another study questions even what levels are important for women, and concludes that other studies are not examining the most important levels for women.[12]

Population studies (Table 1.1)

Few large, long-term population studies included women from their inception. The Framingham Study included 2200 women, primarily to be a control group, in the study of the development of heart disease in men.

The Baltimore Longitudinal Study of Aging of the National Institute of Aging did not include women at its inception in 1951; however, it added women to its study in 1979. The reports from this study often compare differences by age, race and gender.

The Nurses' Health Study (NHS) enrolled 120,000 women between the ages of 30 and 55 to examine the effect of lifestyle and behaviors on health. Participants, now age 55 to 80, have been followed for more than 25 years. Every two years, the group has been reexamined about their health and lifestyles.

The Women's Health Initiative (WHI) was a prospective observational study started in 1991 that investigated the most common causes of morbidity and mortality in women, including breast and colorectal cancer, cardiovascular disease, and osteoporosis, involving 161,808 women. It investigated the effects of hormone replacement therapy, vitamin D and calcium supplements, and diet on these diseases.[13]

There were two arms of the study, one looked at the effect of estrogen alone in women without a uterus, and the other looked at the effect of estrogen and progesterone. The study was ended early because of striking increases in morbidity and mortality in the study group. Further evaluation is now being considered.

Societal differences between men and women that affect health

Men and women often live different lives within society and the way they live affects their health.

Living circumstances

Circumstances for women may be different than those for men and this may impact disease and treatment. These differences must be taken into account in the care of women.

For example, men with chronic obstructive pulmonary disease (COPD) are very likely to be in their 60s, covered by Medicare (in the USA), be married, and have a wife who is able to help with their care and the activities of daily living (ADL). Women with COPD are more likely to be in their 50s, living alone, and uninsured.

Table 1.1 Population studies focused on women's health

Authors	Title	Comments
Colditz, Stampf and others	Nurses' Health Study	Prospective study of 121,701 registered women nurses (98%) white, age 30–55 on initiation in 1976, followed 12 years or more.
Buring	Women's Health Study	Started in 1992. More than 38,000 health care women professionals, studying the effect of aspirin on heart disease.
NIH	Women's Health Initiative	Prospective study started in 1991, examining the effects of diet, calcium and hormone replacement therapy on morbidity and mortality. Stopped in 2002–2003.
	Framingham Study	Prospective long-term study included 2200 women used as controls to study the factors that affect heart disease in men.
	Postmenopausal Estrogen/ Progestin Intervention (PEPI) Trial	Started 1987, a prospective long-term study to determine how hormonal therapy affected HDL cholesterol and heart disease in 875 women.
Clay	Royal College of General Practitioners Oral Contraception Study	1400 general practitioners examining more than 46,000 women for effects of oral contraceptives.
NIH	NIAID Women's Interagency HIV Study (WIHS)	Started in 1993 examining more than 2500 women with AIDS, "collaborative, multi-site, natural history study designed to investigate the biological and psychological impact of HIV infection on U.S. women." More than 80% of the women are from minority populations.[a]

Note: [a]Women's Interagency HIV Health Study, NIH, http://www.niaid.nih.gov/reposit/wihs.htm, accessed 10/1/06.

When they need help, they will have to contact other family members or community agencies.

Similarly, for adults who return home after a stroke, women are more likely to live alone, need help with ADLs, and use community support (56% versus 23%). In one study, 80% of women with strokes lived alone. Elderly women are more likely to be the caregivers for stroke victims than men.[14]

Women with drug abuse problems are more likely than men to be multiply addicted, homeless, and have children. In caring for the woman with addiction, dealing with her individual circumstances is very important.

Women are more likely to smoke at home while men smoke during breaks at work. Women are less likely to use smoking cessation programs, especially work-related programs, and are less likely to quit.

Caregiving

Women are more likely to be the caregivers of their spouse, children, and elderly family members. This puts them at risk of increased stress and depression. Twenty five percent of women working full time also care for a relative.

Long-term care for relatives usually devolves upon the woman. Lower income women bear a disproportionate burden in caring for elderly relatives.[15]

Caregivers are more likely to suffer anxiety, depression, and role stress.

Insurance

Women are more likely to be uninsured or underinsured. They may work in part-time jobs or in jobs that do not provide insurance. If they are divorced or single, they may not be eligible for spouse or family insurance.

Elderly women who have insurance are more likely to see their physicians, use preventive care, and comply with medication regimes than women without insurance.[16]

Elderly women

Among the elderly, more men are married and more women are living alone (two-thirds of women versus one-half of men, see Figure 1.1).

Women are more likely to be widowed and live alone a longer time than men. Many men are less

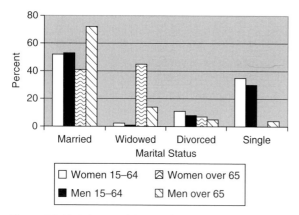

Figure 1.1 Marital status of the population 15 years and over by age and sex, March 2000. Source: US Census Bureau, Internet Release date March 15, 2001, http://www.census.gov/population/socdemo/gender/ppl-121/tab13.txt.

prepared to experience loss. Women have more years to adapt to their loss.

More elderly men have an adequate income and more perceive their health status as excellent than women do. Fewer men have activity restrictions and very few men have trouble with ADLs. Women are more likely to be disabled.[17]

The average elderly woman takes eight drugs daily.[18] Women and the elderly are more likely to have comorbid disease processes and to be taking more medication that affects other drugs.

Older women have a lower blood volume, decreased gastric acid production, and reduced intestinal motility, affecting the levels of drugs required.

Older women are more likely to suffer central nervous system side effects such as confusion, disorientation, delirium, and hallucinations from drugs.

Inherent physical and medical differences between women and men

Immunology

Women are usually less likely to become infected (except with AIDS) and more likely to develop autoimmune diseases.

Drug use and metabolism

Drug studies have historically been performed on white middle-aged men. Some drug studies, such as those of heart disease and antibiotic medications, used men primarily.

Drug use, distribution, and toxicities may be fundamentally different in women and in the elderly.

Women are more likely to receive drugs during a physician's visit, are more likely to receive a prescription for a psychotropic drug, and to spend more money on prescription and non-prescription drugs. Older women spend 17% more on drugs than older men.[19]

Women have longer gastric emptying times and less gastric acid. They have a slower intestinal transit time and these differences are independent of hormone use and menstrual status. Women metabolize some common substances, such as alcohol, differently from men. In women, alcohol levels are higher with the same amount of alcohol.

Women have a larger percentage of fat and a lower total body water value, except when they are pregnant. Antidepressant levels, for example, are dependent on body size and fat levels. Thus, their side effects and therapeutic effects may occur at lower doses than they do in men.

Age affects pharmokinectics. Older individuals have decreased renal function.

Men have different renal functions with higher serum urinary creatinine levels and higher creatinine clearance values. This affects the clearance of drugs such as antibiotics.

Individual differences, such as size or muscle mass, may affect pharmacokinetics and health. While not all women are the same size, more women are likely to be smaller and have smaller muscle mass than most men.

There are particularly "female" concerns involved with pharmacokinetics in women. These include the influence of the cycling menstrual hormones on drug pharmokinetics, the effect of menopausal status, and the influence of hormone replacement therapy or oral contraceptives on drug clearance (see Table 1.2).

Pregnant women have larger volumes of distribution and total body water and fat levels. They may need higher doses of drugs such as antibiotics to reach therapeutic levels. Pregnancy induces a decrease in pepsin activity and gastric acid secretion. There is a slower gastric emptying time in later trimesters, although intestinal motility is greater.

Specific examples

Drugs, especially those that are metabolized in the liver, in the cytochrome P450 system, are affected by estrogen, oral contraceptives (OCPs), and hormone replacement therapy (HRT) (Table 1.2).

Table 1.2 Interaction of oral contraceptives with other drugs

Causes decreased clearance

Imipramine

Diazepam

Chlordiazepoxide

Phenytoin

Caffeine

Cyclosporine

Increases clearance

Acetaminophen

Aspirin

Morphine

Lorazepam

Temazepam

Reduces the effectiveness of OCPs

Carbamazepine

Phenytoin

Rifamipin

Ampicillin

Source: Data from Department of Health and Human Services. Food and Drug Administration. Guidelines for the study and evaluation of gender differences in the clinical evaluation of drugs, Washington, DC: FDA, 1993.

1. **Seizure medications**
   a. Most drugs for seizures are metabolized in the liver. Estrogen-containing OCPs affect the metabolism of most of these drugs, while the drugs reduce the effectiveness of OCPs.
   b. Women on anti-seizure medications often have reduced fertility and hormone levels and abnormal menstrual cycles, including disturbance in luteinizing hormone (LH), growth hormone, prolactin, and androgen levels.
   c. Epileptic women are more likely to have OCPs fail. The failure rate of OCPs in epileptic women is more than four times that in non-epileptic women.[20]
   d. Some epileptic drugs have no reported interactions with OCPs, including valproate, benzodiasepams, and ethosuximide. Phenytoin, barbiturates, and carbamazepine should be avoided in women on OCPs.[21]

   e. In double-blind randomized controlled trials, women have responded better to gabapentin than men, both as a first line and as an additional drug for seizures.[22]
   f. Some women with epilepsy experience sexual dysfunction that may be improved with effective monotherapy and worsened by serotonin-related antiepileptic drugs.[23]
   g. Antiepileptic drugs, especially phenytoin, phenobarbital, and carbamezine, have been known to affect bone metabolism and induce hypocalcemia and these effects occur more often in women.

2. **Antidepressants** Studies have suggested that antidepressant levels vary during the menstrual cycle; a constant level of drug may require varying the dose.

3. **Antipsychotic drugs** Antipsychotic drugs are more often prescribed for women than men. Side effects including sexual dysfunction, anorgasmia, and menstrual abnormalities occur in women. Levels of lithium may differ with the same dose in women and in men.

4. **Cardiovascular drugs** Although more women than men use antihypertensive medications, most recommendations have been made from studies performed on men younger than age 65 years. Calcium channel blockers and nitrates may be better choices for angina in women, because women usually have smaller coronary arteries in which artery tone is a more important determinant of flow. High blood pressure levels in women may be more responsive to calcium channel blockers and diuretics.

5. Side effect profiles may be different. Women who use beta-blockers may have more side effects, including Raynaud's phenomenon and alterations of diabetic responses. Women who take hydralazine are more likely than men to develop drug-induced lupus.

Conclusions

Women's health care has been ignored or marginalized. Recent changes have attempted to mainstream women's concerns into research. Women are more likely to be caregivers, elderly, poor, alone and uninsured, making their health care needs and treatment different than those of men. Women's immunology, drug use and metabolism may differ and may affect the treatment of diseases. However, there are more differences among women, making easy conclusions difficult.

References

1. Nelson H. L. Cultural values affecting women's place in medical care. In Rosenfeld J. A. ed., *Women's Health in Primary Care*, Baltimore, MD: Williams and Wilkins, 1997, pp. 9–18.

2. Mann C. Women's health research blossoms. *Science* 1995; **269**, 766–770.

3. Council on Ethical and Judicial Affairs, American Medical Association. Gender disparities in clinical decision making. *J Am Med Assoc* 1991; **266**, 599–662.

4. Vagero, D. Health inequities in women and men. *Br Med J* 2000; **320**, 1286–1287.

5. Cohen J. Women: absent term in AIDS research equation. *Science* 1995; **269**, 777–780.

6. Joint United Nations Programme on HIV/AIDS (UNAIDS). *Report on the Global HIV/AIDS Epidemic*, Geneva: UNAIDS, 2002.

7. Blehar M. C. Public health context of women's mental health research. *Psychiatr Clin North Am* 2003; **26**(3), 781–799.

8. National Insitutes of Health. *Guidelines on the Inclusion of Women and Minorities as Subjects in Clinical Research*. Bethesda, MD: NIH, 1994.

9. Murthy V. H., Krumholz H. M., Gross C. P. Participation in cancer clinical trials: race-, sex-, and age-based disparities. *J Am Med Assoc* 2004; **291**(22), 2720–2726.

10. Vahter M., Akesson A., Liden C., Ceccatelli S., Berglund M. Gender differences in the disposition and toxicity of metals. *Environ Res* 2007; **104**(1), 85–95.

11. Persell S. D., Maviglia S. M., Bates D. W., Ayanian J. Z. Ambulatory hypercholesterolemia management in patients with atherosclerosis. Gender and race differences in processes and outcomes. *J Gen Intern Med* 2005; **20**(2), 123–130.

12. Kim C., Kerr E. A., Bernstein S. J., Krein S. L. Gender disparities in lipid management: the presence of disparities depends on the quality measure. *Am J Manag Care* 2006; **12**(3), 133–136.

13. National Institutes of Health. *National Women's Health Initiative*. http://www.nhlbi.nih.gov/whi/, updated 4/13/06, accessed 10/1/06.

14. Gosman-Hedstrom G., Claesson L. Gender perspective on informal care for elderly people one year after acute stroke. *Aging Clin Exp Res* 2005; **17**(6), 479–485.

15. Ward D. H., Carney P. A. Caregiving women and the US welfare state. The case of elder kin care by low-income women. *Holistic Nurse Pract* 1994; **8**, 44–58.

16. Schoen C., Simantov E., Gross R., Brammli S., Leiman J. Disparities in women's health and health care experiences in the United States and Israel: findings from 1998 National Women's Health Surveys. *Women's Health* 2003; **37**(1), 49–70.

17. Barer B. M. Men and women aging differently. *Int J Aging Hum Dev* 1994; **38**, 29–40.

18. Fletcher C. V., Acosta E. P., Sryrykowski J. M. Gender differences in human pharmacokinetics and pharmacodynamics. *J Adolesc Health* 1994; **15**, 619–629.

19. Correa-de-Araujo R., Miller G. E., Banthin J. S., Trinh Y. Gender differences in drug use and expenditures in a privately insured population of older adults. *J Womens Health (Larchmt)* 2005; **14**(1), 73–81.

20. Morrell M. J. Maximizing the health of women with epilepsy: science and ethics in new drug development. *Epilepsia* 1997; **38**, S32–S41.

21. Crawford P. Best practice guidelines for the management of women with epilepsy. *Epilepsia* 2005; **46**(Suppl 9), 117–124.

22. Morrell M. J. The new antiepileptic drugs and women: efficacy, reproductive health, pregnancy and fetal outcome. *Epilepsia* 1996; **37**(Suppl 6), S34–S44.

23. Harden C. L. Sexuality in women with epilepsy. *Epilepsy Behav* 2005: 7(Suppl 2):S2–S6. Epub 2005.

Chapter 2

Preventive health care for older women

Jeannette E. South-Paul, Deborah Bostock and Cheryl E. Woodson

Primary preventive measures for women must be accomplished early in life to make an impact later in life. Prevention for the older person includes maintaining quality of life, preserving function, preventing collapse of family support systems, and maintaining independence in the community.

> Primary preventive measures are optimally accomplished early in life to make an impact later in life.

Goals of preventive care for the older woman

1. The percentage of US adults older than age 65 years is growing rapidly and is expected to almost double between 1995 and 2030 (12.8% to 20%).[1]
2. Life expectancy for women is longer than that of men, at all ages older than 65 years. By age 85, only 45 men will be alive for every 100 women.[2] This significantly changes the social environment in which older women live. Understanding the specific needs and circumstances of an individual woman helps to guide preventive health decisions.
3. The annual physical examination encompasses screening and preventive counseling. Both primary preventive measures (i.e. interventions targeted at preventing specific conditions in asymptomatic persons) and secondary preventive measures (i.e. screening for early detection and treatment of modifiable risk factors or preclinical disease) are described.

General assessment
Well-being/living situation/independence

1. Health status assessment and primary and secondary prevention encompass more than a periodic physical examination. A multidimensional assessment focusing on mental health, physical health, basic functioning, social functioning, and economic well-being provides a complete picture of the older woman (Table 2.1).
2. Early in the evaluation, establishing the older woman's marital status, her current living arrangements and household partners, and whether she has experienced the loss of a spouse or long-time friend is important. Is she currently working or active in group activities outside the home?
3. The accuracy of the history depends on adequate mental and affective functioning of the patient. The accuracy of historical information gathered from the older woman, family member or friend, and the consistency of the information between sources, provide clues regarding the older woman's cognitive function and whether she can remain independent.

Caregiver responsibilities

1. Older women often have substantial responsibilities caring for spouses, siblings, children, and grandchildren. More than 15 million adults currently provide care to relatives.[3] Of all caregivers for disabled elders, 70% are women and 30% of these are older than age 74 years.[4]
2. Caregiving taxes physical, social, emotional, and financial resources, and can significantly affect the health and functional status of the caregiver. The combination of loss, prolonged distress and the physical demands of caregiving increase the caregiver's risk for physical and emotional health problems.[3]
3. Caregivers who provide support to their spouses and report caregiving strain are 63% more

Handbook of Women's Health, second edition, ed. Jo Ann Rosenfeld. Published by Cambridge University Press.
© Cambridge University Press 2009.

Table 2.1 Checklist of assessment areas for maintaining healthy geriatric patients

Injury prevention

Use of safety belts or helmets

Smoke detectors (in place and working)

Hot water temperature at ≤48.8 °C (120 °F)

Smoking near bed or upholstery

Poor lighting

Obtrusive furniture

Slippery floors and loose rugs

Handrails and grab bars

One-leg balance (5 seconds)

"Get Up and Go" test*
   *The patient rises from a sitting position, walks 3 m (~10 feet), turns and returns to the chair to sit. The test is positive if these activities take more than 16 seconds.

Sensorium

Snellen eye chart

Ophthalmology examination

Hearing Handicapped Inventory for the Elder – Screening version

Pure tone audiometry

Nutrition

Nutritional health screen

Tooth brushing, flossing and dental visits

Immunizations

Tetanus and diphtheria toxoid

Influenza vaccine

Pneumococcal vaccine

Sexuality

Review of chronic conditions and medications

Initiation of discussion about sexuality

Continence

Review of chronic conditions and medications

Initiation of discussion about incontinence

Focused physical examination (pelvis, rectum)

Mental status (consider one of the following)

Mini-Mental State

Clock Test

Informant Questionnaire on Cognitive Decline in Elderly

Geriatric Depression Scale

Yale Depression Screen

Questioning about suicide

Social issues

Changes in living arrangements, finances, or activities

Caregiver support or burnout

Advance directives

Family training in cardiopulmonary resuscitation

Activities of daily living

Instrumental activities of daily living

Performance test of activities of daily living

likely to die within four years than non-caregivers.[3]

4. Significant levels of depression are seen in caregivers of Alzheimer's patients. Assistance is available through support groups and information accessible through the Internet: www.alz.org and www.alzheimers.com.

5. Reducing caregiving demands by providing respite care or other relief for the caregiver may mitigate the strain so that the caregiver and cared for family member can remain independent longer.

> Caregiving taxes physical, social, emotional, and financial resources, and can significantly affect the health and functional status of the caregiver.

Presence of chronic disease

1. With aging, the older woman becomes more susceptible to chronic illness and disease. For example, the incidence of degenerative joint disease is increased in older women. This causes an increased incidence of knee pain, which is associated with diminished quality of life.[5]

2. There is a higher incidence of all chronic diseases, especially diabetes mellitus and hypertension, in minority groups.[6]

3. The presence of common chronic health problems is associated with lower levels of cancer screening – presumably because of the time commitment required by the clinician to care for

these chronic illnesses, negatively impacting on preventive services.[7]

Access to care

Insurance coverage/underinsurance

1. In the USA, underinsurance is the inability to pay out-of-pocket expenses despite having insurance, and usually implies inability to use preventive services also. Medicare-eligible citizens may be unable to afford medical expenses not covered by Medicare. Many elderly recently joined Medicare Health Maintenance Organizations (HMOs) to obtain added benefits, including prescription benefits, and have been confused and abandoned by the failure and break-up of these Medicare HMOs.

2. The underinsured category also includes unemployed persons age 55 to 64 and those not provided with coverage through their jobs. They are not yet eligible for Medicare and must pay high individual health premiums when they can obtain some form of group coverage. Women are more likely to be underinsured because they are more likely to be divorced and no longer covered by a husband's insurance, or underemployed in a part-time job that does not provide medical insurance. Lack of health insurance is associated with delayed health care and increased mortality.

3. Underinsurance may also result in adverse health consequences.[8] There is a dose-response relationship between the level of insurance coverage and receipt of preventive services.

4. Women access the health care system more frequently than do men. They receive more health services and prescriptions, undergo more examinations, laboratory tests, and blood pressure checks than men.

5. However, when US physicians were surveyed recently regarding making the diagnosis of coronary artery disease and recommending coronary angiography and/or revascularization procedures, they were significantly less likely to make these recommendations for women and minority groups.[9]

> Lack of health insurance is associated with delayed health care and increased mortality.

Mobility

1. Those women most likely to get screening and preventive services have a usual source of care and no limitations on mobility.[10]

2. This is evident in the higher risk for delayed diagnosis of breast and cervical cancer in disabled women.[11]

> Those women most likely to get screening and preventive services have a usual source of care and no limitations in mobility.

Language/acculturation

1. A low level of acculturation results in a lower likelihood of receipt of preventive services.[12] Cultural explanatory models are important in describing the woman's willingness to receive care. Eliciting this information is easier when the clinician and the older woman have a comfortable relationship. Otherwise, the clinician may be unaware of why therapies prescribed are unsuccessful or why the woman fails to follow advice.

2. Religion is a significant part of the culture of racial and ethnic communities representing a range of socioeconomic status. Physical health, depressive symptoms, and hypertension improved, and tobacco and alcohol use decreased as a woman's religious involvement increased in ethnic communities.[13]

Emotional/mental status/cognitive functioning

1. **Depression**

   Depression is the most commonly diagnosed mental illness in older adults in the primary care setting, although it often goes unnoticed.[14] Major depression is seen in 1–5% and significant depressive symptoms in up to 25% of community-dwelling older people. Older women receive more antidepressants every year than men, though this difference decreases as they get older.[15]

   a. Older adults with major depression who are seeing primary care physicians have significantly higher medical costs (reflecting more outpatient visits, laboratory tests, X-rays, inpatient days, and specialty medical visits)

Table 2.2 Laboratory testing for cognitive dysfunction

Basic metabolic testing

Thyroid function

Electrolyte levels

Complete blood count

When suggested by history or examination

Erythrocyte sedimentation rate

Testing for syphilis

Imaging studies

Magnetic resonance imaging

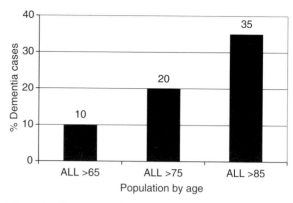

Figure 2.1 Percentage of elderly with dementia, by age.

than controls matched for age, gender, and chronic mental illness.[16]

b. Older caregivers demonstrate significantly higher levels of depressive symptoms, anxiety, and lower levels of perceived health than do their non-caregiving counterparts.[16]

c. In addition to depression, stress-related symptoms are common in older adults. Lower stress levels are evident in retirees compared with those approaching retirement,[17] or working.

2. **Cognitive dysfunction**

a. Cognitive decline in the very old has been underestimated and must be assessed carefully and regularly (Table 2.2).[18]

b. A complete mental status examination includes an evaluation of level of consciousness, attention, language capabilities, memory, proverb interpretation, comparisons, calculations, writing, and constructional ability.

> Older adults with major depression who are seeing primary care physicians have significantly higher medical costs.

c. Condensed mental status screening tools can substitute for the complete mental status examination and detect cognitive deficits that are often seen in dementia syndromes.

d. Deficits often occur without a change in level of consciousness, are significantly different from the patient's baseline results, and always result in some impairment of function.[19]

e. The average age of onset of dementia is 69 years (Figure 2.1).

f. Dementia imposes heavy responsibilities on family and resources and must be distinguished from delirium (reversible cognitive deficits).

g. Brief mental status tests may evaluate intellectual functioning only or also include a functional assessment. Two commonly used tests are the Pfeiffer Short Portable Mental Status Questionnaire and the Folstein Mini Mental State Examination.[20] None of these tools has complete diagnostic accuracy and they may fail to identify subtle changes in highly functioning elderly. Basic testing is included in Table 2.1.

h. When there are negative results in both the metabolic work-up and the mental status examination for patients with functional impairment, formal neuropsychological testing is necessary. The results can also assist in care coordination by suggesting beneficial environmental adaptations.

> Dementia imposes heavy responsibilities on family and resources and must be distinguished from delirium.

3. **Family support**

a. The caregiving ability and availability of family and friends must be determined to identify who could help the elder in the event of an illness, accident, or other acute event that would limit self-care ability.

b. Caregivers can also provide valuable information regarding subtle changes in functioning or cognition.

4. **Social network**

    The older woman's involvement in the community reflects her ability to make and sustain relationships and also defines a support system outside the family. The active woman is unlikely to be severely handicapped by mental and emotional conditions.

5. **Religious involvement**

    a. After adjusting for physical and mental health conditions, social connections, and health practices, older women who attend church at least once weekly had a better chance of survival.[21]

    b. The positive effects of religion have been seen in all age groups. Fewer depressive symptoms occur in women who have a denominational affiliation, whereas women with no or low frequency of church attendance have more current smoking and daily drinking.[13]

    c. Religious participation has short- and long-term influence on functioning in the elderly, especially those who are disabled, including the following.

        i. Attendance at services is a strong predictor of better functioning.

        ii. Health practices, social ties, and indicators of well-being reduce, but do not eliminate, these effects; disability has minimal effects on subsequent attendance.

    d. Older adults who reside in deteriorated neighborhoods experience more physical health problems than older people who dwell in more favorable living environments.[22] Data from a nationwide longitudinal survey of older people suggest that the noxious impact of living in a dilapidated neighborhood on changes in self-rated health over time is offset completely for older adults who are deeply religious.

6. **Sexuality**

    a. Like younger adults, older adults are sexual beings. Assumptions of sexual activities or lack thereof based upon age alone are unwarranted. Even in the presence of significant ongoing health problems, appropriate sexual history questioning of all older women is helpful.

    > Older women who attend church at least once weekly had a better chance of survival.

    b. Issues include lack of availability of partners (widows or spouses with significant health problems), physiological changes associated with age (mucosal dryness in postmenopausal women) and changes in relationships with aging. As with younger patients, discussions of sexual activity include inquiries and education on risky sexual behaviors.

    > Older adults who reside in deteriorated neighborhoods experience more physical health problems than do older people who dwell in more favorable living environments.

Functional assessment
Activities of daily living/instrumental activities of daily living

1. Periodic health examination provides an opportunity to detect functional problems that can decrease life expectancy. Classifying the older woman by functional ability is more helpful than classifying her by age (Table 2.3).

2. Instrumental activities of daily living (IADLs) are those that require the patient to use integrative thought processes and complex musculoskeletal coordination to perform the necessary daily tasks of life (e.g. working, shopping, cooking, managing money, driving or arranging transportation, using the telephone) (Table 2.4).

3. Basic activities of daily living (ADLs) are those that are necessary to maintain personal care (e.g. bathing, dressing, maintaining continence, transferring or walking, toileting, eating).

4. Multiple instruments exist for research and social service purposes, but the most commonly used clinical instrument is the Katz Index of Activities of Daily Living.[23]

Ambulation/activity patterns

1. More than 40% of women older than age 65 report a sedentary lifestyle that is associated with many chronic illnesses.[24] Maintenance of regular leisure-time activity results in lower lipid levels, coronary artery disease, diabetes mellitus, and hypertension.

2. Regular exercise improves neurobehavioral function.[25]

Table 2.3 Index of activities of daily living

Name:

Date of evaluation:

For each area of functioning listed below, check the description that applies. (The word "assistance" applies to supervision, direction or personal assistance.)

Bathing (sponge bath, tub bath or shower)

Receives no assistance (gets in and out of bathtub by self if tub is usual means of bathing)	Receives assistance in bathing only one part of the body (such as back or legs)	Receives assistance in bathing more than one part of the body (or is not bathed)

Dressing (gets clothes from closets and drawers, including underclothes and outer garments, and uses fasteners, including braces, if worn)

Gets clothes and gets completely dressed without assistance	Gets clothes and gets dressed without assistance, except for assistance in tying shoes	Receives assistance in getting clothes or in getting dressed, or stays partly or completely undressed

Toileting (going to "toilet room" for bowel and urine elimination, cleaning self after elimination and arranging clothes)

Goes to "toilet room," cleans self and arranges clothes without assistance (may use object for support, such as cane, walker or wheelchair, and may manage night bedpan or commode, emptying in morning)	Receives assistance in going to "toilet room," in cleaning self or in arranging clothes after elimination, or in using night bedpan or commode	Does not go to "toilet room" for the elimination process

Transfer Moves in and out of a bed and chair without assistance (may use object for support, such as cane or walker)

	Moves in and out of a bed and chair with assistance	Does not get out of bed

3. Strength training is important for maintenance of strength, physical function, bone integrity and psychosocial health.[26]

Diet/nutrition

1. Approximately 21–45% of women between ages 65 and 74 years are overweight.[31] Diet affects the development of most chronic diseases that are also impacted by exercise patterns. In addition, stroke, constipation, and diverticular and dental disease are all influenced by diet.

2. This may be the appropriate time in the history to ask about the use of vitamins and nutritional supplements. They serve as a potential source of symptoms and drug interactions.

3. Accurate weights at the clinical visit are important, rather than relying on the stated weight. Unfortunately the national norms do not include data on older people.

4. Significant weight loss (1–2% of body weight in one week, 5% in one month, or 10% in six months) may reflect many diseases (Table 2.5), poor dentition, cognitive impairment, respiratory dysfunction, poor hand-to-mouth coordination, a need for assistance in purchasing or preparing foods or other factors affecting the amount of food consumed (such as elder abuse).

Risk assessment
Risk of elder abuse

1. As many as 2.5 million older adult persons are abused each year and the number of cases is likely to increase as this population grows. Elder abuse

Table 2.4 Instrumental activities of daily living (self-rated version)

For each question, circle the points for the answer that best applies to your situation

1. *Can you use the telephone?*
   Without help — 3
   With some help — 2
   Completely unable to use telephone — 1

2. *Can you get to places that are out of walking distance?*
   Without help — 3
   With some help — 2
   Completely unable to travel unless special arrangements are made — 1

3. *Can you go shopping for groceries?*
   Without help — 3
   With some help — 2
   Completely unable to do any shopping — 1

4. *Can you prepare your own meals?*
   Without help — 3
   With some help — 2
   Completely unable to prepare any meals — 1

5. *Can you do your own housework?*
   Without help — 3
   With some help — 2
   Completely unable to do any housework — 1

6. *Can you do your own handyman work?*
   Without help — 3
   With some help — 2
   Completely unable to do any handyman work — 1

7. *Can you do your own laundry?*
   Without help — 3
   With some help — 2
   Completely unable to do any laundry at all — 1

8a. *Do you take any medicines or use any medications?*
   Yes (if "yes", answer question 8b) — 1
   No (if "no" answer question 8c) — 2

8b. *Do you take your own medicine?*
   Without help (in the right doses at the right time) — 3
   With some help (take medicine if someone prepares it for you and/or reminds you to take it) — 2
   Completely unable to take own medicine — 1

8c. *If you had to take medicine, could you do it?*
   Without help (in the right doses at the right time) — 3
   With some help (take medicine if someone prepares it for you and/or reminds you to take it) — 2
   Completely unable to take own medicine — 1

9. *Can you manage your money?*
   Without help — 3
   With some help — 2
   Completely unable to handle money — 1

Note: Adapted with permission from Lawton M. P., Brody E. M. Assessment of older people: self-maintaining and instrumental activities of daily living. *Gerontologist* 1969; **9**, 279–285.

Table 2.5 Causes of significant weight loss

Chronic diseases
Chronic infections
Diabetes
Cancer
Poor dentition
Cognitive impairment
Respiratory dysfunction
Poor hand-to-mouth coordination
A need for assistance in purchasing or preparing food
Other factors affecting the amount of food consumed (such as elder abuse)

Note: Data from Bignotti D. D., Evans J. M., Fleming K. C. *The Geriatric Patient*, 7th edition, ABFP Reference Guides, Lexington, KN: American Board of Family Practice, 1999.

exists in many forms: physical, emotional, financial, and sexual; neglect and self-neglect.

2. Most states have mandatory reporting; however, this may infringe on the autonomy of competent geriatric individuals. Supportive assessment and

management focuses on both the patient and the caregiver for problem solving.

3. Physicians infrequently report elder abuse. This may be caused by unfamiliarity with reporting laws, fear of offending patients, concern about time limitations, and the belief that they do not have appropriate evaluation skills. In the USA, reporting suspected abuse directly to the appropriate state agency facilitates the coordination of thorough long-term assessment and management.

4. Older women and men have similar abuse rates. Abuse is best correlated with the emotional and financial dependence of the caregivers on the geriatric victims. Relatives, usually spouses, most commonly abuse older patients.

5. No specific screening tools have been found to be clearly effective in identifying elder abuse victims. A few direct questions in the course of routine history taking may provide the physician with insight into those patients at risk (US Preventive Services Task Force (USPSTF) class C). Helpful questions include, "Are you afraid of anyone at home?", "Have you been struck, slapped, or kicked?" or "Do you ever feel alone?"[28]

> Elder abuse is best correlated with the emotional and financial dependence of the caregivers on the geriatric victims, and relatives, usually spouses, most commonly abuse older patients.

Risk for substance abuse

1. Substance abuse, including alcohol and tobacco abuse, afflicts the older patient as well as the young. The periodic examination is the logical time to screen for substance abuse and provide appropriate counseling. Emphasizing the relatively short-term rewards of smoking cessation, such as decreasing the risk of stroke, can be persuasive for the older person struggling with tobacco abuse.

2. Referral to a specific program is more helpful for the patient than merely suggesting she discontinue tobacco use. However, more women and more elderly quit smoking "cold-turkey" and on their own than using a program. The multiple ways other than cigarettes (snuff, pipes, etc.) that an older woman can use tobacco should be recognized.

3. The four-question CAGE instrument (see Chapter 27) can be very helpful in identifying alcohol abuse or dependence. It is less sensitive for early problem drinking, heavy drinking or drinking in any woman or the elderly than it is with men.

> More women and more elderly quit smoking "cold-turkey" and on their own than using a program.

Risk of injury

1. **Safety belts**

   Older adult persons are less likely to be involved in a motor vehicle accident (caused by decreased driving distances and lower speeds). Older women and their passengers still benefit from the use of lap/shoulder belts at all times even in the presence of air bags (USPSTF class A).[29] For some small, frail women, air bags can pose a potential risk of injury.

2. **Falls**

   Falling is a common, serious problem in older individuals. Falls are the leading cause of non-fatal injuries and unintentional injury deaths in older persons in the USA. Screening for falls may include asking the patient whether she has fallen in the past year or whether she is afraid of falling. Gait assessment and rehabilitation can be offered to such women. These measures have been shown to reduce the risk of falling and subsequent injuries.[28]

Periodic medical care
Examination frequency

All elders benefit from a periodic examination that focuses on prevention. However, with accurate record keeping, this evaluation can be accomplished through serial visits as the older woman is monitored for chronic diseases. This approach is consistent with the current USPSTF guidelines (Table 2.6).

Immunizations

1. Older adults are often inadequately immunized. Formal documentation of remote vaccine history is often unavailable. A review of immunization history and documentation can be performed during the periodic examination (Table 2.7).

Table 2.6 Ten-minute screen for geriatric conditions

Problem	Screening measure	Positive screen
Vision	Ask this question: "Because of your eyesight, do you have trouble driving a car, watching television, reading or doing any of your daily activities?" If the patient answers "yes," test each eye with the Snellen eye chart while the patient wears corrective lenses (if applicable).	"Yes" to question and inability to read greater than 20/40 on the Snellen eye chart
Hearing	Use an audioscope set at 40 dB. Test the patient's hearing using 1000 and 2000 Hz.	Inability to hear 1000 or 2000 Hz in both ears or inability to hear frequencies in either ear
Leg mobility	Time the patient after giving these directions: "Rise from the chair. Then walk 6 m (20 feet) briskly, turn, walk back to the chair and sit down."	Unable to complete task in 15 seconds
Urinary incontinence	Ask this question: "In the past year, have you ever lost your urine and gotten wet?" If the patient answers "yes," ask this question: "Have you lost urine on at least 6 separate days?"	"Yes" to both questions
Nutrition and weight loss	Ask this question: "Have you lost 4.5 kg (10 lb) over the past six months without trying to do so?" If the patient answers "yes," weigh the patient.	"Yes" to the question or a weight of less than 45.5 kg (100 lb)
Memory	Three-item recall.	Unable to remember all 3 items after 1 minute
Depression	Ask this question: "Do you often feel sad or depressed?"	"Yes" to the question
Physical disability	Ask the patient these six questions: "Are you unable to do strenuous activities, like fast walking or bicycling?" "Are you unable to do heavy work around the house, like washing windows, walls, or floors?" "Are you unable to go shopping for groceries or clothes?" "Are you unable to get places that are out of walking distance?" "Are you unable to bathe – sponge bath, tub bath, or shower?" "Are you unable to dress, like put on a shirt, button and zip your clothes, or put on your shoes?"	"Yes" to any of the questions

Note: Adapted with permission from Moore A., Siu A. L. Screening for common problems in ambulatory elderly: clinical confirmation of a screen instrument. *Am J Med* 1996; **100**, 438–443. Copyright 1996, with permission from Excerpta Medica Inc.

Table 2.7 Recommended immunizations for older women

Influenza vaccine annually

Pneumococcal polysaccharide vaccine once after age 65 years for all immunocompetent adults

Tetanus-diphtheria vaccine every 10 years or a single booster at age 65 years

Adacel as a single dose in persons up to 64 years of age

2. **Influenza vaccine**

Annual influenza vaccine is recommended for all older adults, particularly those who are chronically ill or at high risk of contracting influenza, such as those patients in institutions (assisted living centers, nursing homes, boarding and daycare homes) (USPSTF class B). The vaccine is effective in reducing hospitalizations, deaths, associated complications and health care costs from influenza.

15

3. **Pneumococcal polysaccharide vaccine**

   A single immunization is recommended for all immunocompetent adults age 65 years and older (USPSTF class B). Universal revaccination is unnecessary as the protection afforded by the vaccine persists for up to nine years or more. The American College of Physicians does recommend revaccination for patients who have received the vaccine before age 65 years and for whom more than six years have passed since the initial vaccine.

4. **Tetanus**

   Although tetanus is an uncommon disease in developed nations, more than 60% of cases occur in patients older than 60 years. The standard recommendation is a combined tetanus-diphtheria (Td) given every 10 years for all patients (USPSTF class A).

   A single Td booster at age 65 years may be a cost-effective alternative, given current compliance with the 10-year guideline. A complete primary series of three toxoid doses over 6 to 12 months is necessary for those patients who have never been vaccinated. Adacel vaccine, similar to DTaP but with reduced quantities of d and detoxified PT, provides active booster immunization for the prevention of tetanus, diphtheria and pertussis as a one-time shot to patients up to 64 years.

Screening (Table 2.8)

1. **Hypertension**

   a. **Impact**

      Elevated blood pressure occurs in 60% of non-Hispanic whites, 71% of non-Hispanic African-Americans, and 61% of Mexican-Americans older than age 60 years. There is a 90% lifetime risk of becoming hypertensive in normotensive population at 55 years of age. Prehypertensive individuals (systolic BP 120–139 mmHg or diastolic BP 80–89 mmHg) require lifestyle modifications to prevent the progressive rise in blood pressure and cardiovascular disease.

   b. Systolic rather than diastolic blood pressure is a better predictor of coronary artery disease, cardiovascular disease, heart failure, stroke, end-stage renal disease, and all-cause mortality than diastolic blood pressure in the elderly. Primary hypertension is the most common form of hypertension in older persons.[30]

   c. Blood pressure measurements at least every two years for adults with diastolic blood pressures less than 80 mmHg and systolic blood pressures below 120 mmHg are recommended.[30]

   d. Annual blood pressure managements are recommended for persons with diastolic blood pressures 80 to 89 mmHg or systolic blood pressures 120 to 139 mmHg. Persons with higher blood pressure require more frequent measurements.

   e. Older individuals are more likely than younger individuals to exhibit an orthostatic fall in blood pressure and hypotension. Therefore, blood pressure should be measured in both the standing and sitting positions in older individuals.

   > Systolic rather than diastolic blood pressure is a better predictor of coronary artery disease, cardiovascular disease, heart failure, stroke, end-stage renal disease, and all-cause mortality than diastolic blood pressure in the elderly.

   f. Treating hypertension in the elderly is important and does decrease their risk of morbidity and mortality. Effects of non-pharmacological first-line therapy (i.e. weight reduction, increased physical activity, sodium restriction, decreased alcohol intake) on cardiovascular morbidity and mortality are less well studied.[29]

   g. For individuals 40–70 years of age with BP in the range of 115/75 to 185/115 mmHg, each increase of 20 mmHg in systolic BP or 10 mmHg in diastolic BP, doubles the risk of cardiovascular disease. The benefit of treatment of hypertension was demonstrated even in patients aged above 80.[29]

   > Treating hypertension in the elderly is important and does decrease their risk of morbidity and mortality.

2. **Breast cancer**

   a. The USPSTF recommends routine screening every 1–2 years with mammography and annual clinical breast examination (CBE) for women aged 50 to 69 years.[29]

   b. There is insufficient evidence to recommend for or against routine mammography and CBE

Table 2.8 Recommended screening for older women

Disease	Recommended screening	Comments
Hypertension	BP measurements every 2 years for BP < 120/80	Measure blood pressure both standing and sitting to assess for orthostatic changes
	BP measurements annually for BP 120–139/80–89	
Breast cancer	Encourage monthly self breast examination	
	Clinical breast examination annually	
	Mammography every 1–2 years	
Cervical cancer	Pap smears every 1–3 years	Consider discontinuing screening if repeated Pap smears are normal
Colon cancer	Annual fecal occult blood test	
	Flexible sigmoidoscopy every 3–5 years	
Depression	Mini Mental Status Examination	5-item version reduces administration time
Cognitive impairment	Screening of asymptomatic women not recommended	Especially women with symptoms of cognitive or affective deficits
Hyperlipidemias	TSH	
	May consider screening otherwise healthy women with major risk factors for CHD	
Thyroid disease		
Incontinence	Direct questioning	
Osteoporosis	Dual energy X-ray absorptiometry for high risk women	
Hearing loss	Periodic direct questioning about potential hearing loss	Handheld audioscopes may be more sensitive
Vision loss	Periodic Snellen acuity testing	

for women age 70 years or older, although recommendations for healthy women older than age 70 may be made on other grounds (e.g. those with a past history of malignancy). Women who have had one mammogram after age 70 years are much less likely to die of breast cancer. With higher risk of breast cancer, women older than 70 years of age, whose life expectancy is not compromised by other co-morbidities (i.e. dementia, life expectancy less than five years) may benefit from routine mammography as younger women do.[31,32,33]

c. Older women with low bone mineral density have a lower risk of breast cancer (presumably caused by decreased exposure to estrogen) and may benefit less from continued screening.[34]

d. Data regarding the sensitivity of monthly breast self-examination (BSE) in detecting breast cancer are extremely limited. Sensitivity may be approximately 15%. Sensitivity for detecting breast cancer rises to 26% if the women are also screened by CBE and mammography.[35]

e. Factors that have been associated with inadequate screening are advanced age, poor cognitive function, and nursing home residence.[36]

> The USPSTF recommends routine screening every 1–2 years with mammography and annual clinical breast examination for women aged 50 to 69 years.

3. **Cervical cancer**

a. For those older women in whom repeated Pap smears have been normal, further screening does not appear to be beneficial. Those women with no prior screening, previously inadequate screening or for those women engaging in high-risk sexual behaviors, screening with Pap smears every 1–3 years is recommended.

b. Women who have undergone hysterectomy for non-cervical cancer diagnoses, with complete removal of the cervix do not benefit from Pap smear screening.[29]

c. There is insufficient evidence to provide for or against an upper age limit to Pap smear screening. The USPSTF and the American College of Physicians offer guidelines to cease screenings after age 65 years, while the Canadian Task Force recommends ceasing after age 69 if prior screening has been normal (USPTFP class C).[29]

> For those older women in whom repeated Pap smears have been normal, further screening does not appear to be beneficial.

4. **Colon cancer**

a. Colon cancer is the second most common form of cancer in the USA and the second highest cause of cancer mortality. Although its peak incidence is between ages 70 and 80 years, none of the available studies focuses on the geriatric population.

b. Digital rectal examination (DRE) is of little value in screening for colon cancer, since fewer than 10% of colorectal cancers can be palpated.

c. Annual fecal occult blood testing (FOBT) in asymptomatic patients has a high rate of false-positives. The positive predictive value is only 2–11% for carcinomas and 20–30% for adenomas in patients older than age 50 years. The predictive value may be higher in older patients caused by the higher prevalence of colorectal cancers in these age groups. Two recent studies have shown reductions in mortality in patients offered FOBT every one to two years.[37] Traditional three-card FOBT is more sensitive than office fecal occult after DRE.[33] All positive results need to be further evaluated with appropriate testing (colonoscopy, air contrast barium enema).

d. Screening with sigmoidoscopy, with or without FOBT, is recommended every three to five years by most authorities, although intervals of 10 years may also be adequate (USPSTF class B).[29]

e. Sigmoidoscopy with longer (60 cm) flexible sigmoidoscopes has been shown to have greater sensitivity and is better tolerated by the patient than rigid sigmoidoscopy.

f. The American Cancer Society recommended colonoscopy every 10 years as one way of screening for colon cancer. One study showed that colonoscopy is slightly more sensitive at screening and follow up of the rate of polyp progression.[33] But it also has more serious complications compared to other screening methods.

> Screening for colon cancer with sigmoidoscopy, with or without fecal occult blood testing, is recommended every three to five years.

5. **Depression/cognitive impairment**

a. The ideal depression-screening tool for older persons is both accurate and easy to administer. The original 30-item Geriatric Depression Scale (GDS) was developed by Brink and Yesavage in 1982 and condensed to a 15-item version by Sheikh in 1986 with improved efficiency and no loss of accuracy.[38] Most recently, a five-item version of GDS has been developed, resulting in a marked reduction in administration time (Table 2.9).[39]

b. Education and cultural background moderate Mini Mental Status Examination (MMSE) results. College-educated women perform better on these examinations and racial and ethnic minorities do more poorly, almost entirely related to lower socioeconomic status and poorer educational attainment.[40]

6. **Hyperlipidemias**

a. Current recommendations for screening of asymptomatic women older than age 65 years are conflicting. Although hyperlipidemia is strongly associated with atherosclerotic heart disease, little correlation has been shown between elevated total or low-density lipoprotein (LDL) cholesterol and long-term heart disease risk or mortality in women older than age 65 years.

b. Currently the American College of Physicians and USPSTF do not recommend cholesterol

Table 2.9 Geriatric Depression Scale (short form)

For each question, choose the best answer for how you felt over the past week

1. Are you basically satisfied with your life?	Yes/NO
2. Have you dropped many of your activities and interests?	YES/No
3. Do you feel that your life is empty?	YES/No
4. Do you often get bored?	YES/No
5. Are you in good spirits most of the time?	Yes/NO
6. Are you afraid that something bad is going to happen to you?	YES/No
7. Do you feel happy most of the time?	Yes/NO
8. Do you often feel helpless?	YES/No
9. Do you prefer to stay at home, rather than going out and doing new things?	YES/No
10. Do you feel you have more problems with memory than most?	YES/No
11. Do you think it is wonderful to be alive now?	Yes/NO
12. Do you feel pretty worthless the way you are now?	YES/No
13. Do you feel full of energy?	Yes/NO
14. Do you feel that your situation is hopeless?	YES/No
15. Do you think most people are better off than you are?	YES/No

Note: The scale is scored as follows: 1 point for each response in capital letters. A score of 0 to 5 is normal; a score above 5 suggests depression. Adapted with permission from Sheikh J. I., Yasagave J. A. Geriatric Depression Scale (GDS): Recent evidence and development of a shorter version. *Clin Gerontol* 1986; **5**, 165–172.

screening in asymptomatic women older than age 65. Individualized screening of otherwise healthy women with major risk factors for CHD (smoking, hypertension, and diabetes) is a class C recommendation.[29] Screening with fasting or non-fasting samples is appropriate. The ratio of total to high density lipoprotein (HDL) cholesterol appears to be the best predictor of coronary risk in older patients.[41] Data showed that lipid lowering is as or more effective in older patients than in younger ones, and with the higher risk of CHD events in older patients,[42] the decision of screening

of cholesterol and appropriate treatment needs to be made based on each case. Patients with life expectancy sufficient to benefit from treatment may benefit from screening.

> The ratio of total to high density lipoprotein cholesterol appears to be the best predictor of coronary risk in older patients.

7. **Thyroid disease**

   a. Although there is a high prevalence of thyroid disorders in older patients, especially women, no benefits of thyroid screenings have been shown in clinical trials.

   b. Asymptomatic elevations in thyroid-stimulating hormone (TSH) or low thyroxine (T_4) levels have been found in up to 15% of women older than age 60 years.[43] Subclinical thyroid disease is also described, especially in patients with cognitive and affective deficits.

   c. With reasonable assay costs, screening for mild thyroid failure at the periodic health examination may be cost effective. The US and Canadian Task Forces agreed that it might be reasonable to test high risk patients, especially women, and those with possible symptoms (class C recommendation).[29]

   d. A TSH assay alone is a reasonable test, with a subsequent follow-up of abnormal values.

   e. Screening every five years has been suggested as an appropriate interval.

8. **Incontinence**

   a. Urinary incontinence is a common, disruptive, and potentially disabling condition. Women, more commonly than men, experience urinary incontinence with increasing frequency with age and level of institutionalized care. Significant problems with incontinence may lead to social isolation, with resultant decline in physical well-being and quality of life (see Chapter 18).

   b. Simply, direct questioning in the routine history taking will often reveal symptomatic urinary incontinence. Because urinary incontinence is curable or treatable in many elderly women, it is essential that specific questions be included in the periodic examination.

9. Osteoporosis

(see also Chapter 28)

a. Approximately 1.3 million osteoporosis-related fractures occur each year in the USA. Seventy percent of fractures in those 45 years or older are types related to osteoporosis.

b. Osteoporosis is defined as a bone mineral density 2.5 standard deviations (SD) below the normal mean.[44] However, it is not necessary to obtain such measurements in order to initiate treatment (see Chapter 28).

c. Dual-energy X-ray absorptiometry (DEXA) is recognized as the safest, most accurate, and more precise modality for measuring bone density in the clinical setting and is the gold standard. If the patient already has evidence of vertebral fracture, the diagnosis of osteoporosis is present and treatment is indicated.

d. Randomized trials show that estrogen and calcium supplementation is effective in preserving bone density in postmenopausal women. Postmenopausal women who have discontinued HRT within the past five years have a risk for hip fracture that is at least as high as that in women who have never used HRT.[45]

e. Benefits of hormonal prophylaxis on bone mass and fracture risk appear greatest when treatment is begun close to menopause (before the period of rapid bone loss) and continued for longer periods (more than five years) (Table 2.10).[29] But the use of HRT has decreased due to the increased risks of breast cancer, ovarian cancer, strokes and CHD.

f. Prevention, diagnosis and screening methods are listed in Table 2.11.

10. Sensory impairment

a. Hearing loss

Hearing impairment occurs with increasing prevalence as patients age. Presbycusis is the most common cause, with approximately 33% of patients aged 65 years and older suffering objective hearing loss. Periodic questioning about potential hearing loss is a rapid and inexpensive screen for hearing impairment. Handheld devices (audioscopes) may be more sensitive but there is inconclusive evidence to support routine audiometry testing (USPSTF class B).[29]

Table 2.10 Risk factors and indications for bone density screening

Age
Smoking
Estrogen deficient status
Low body weight
Calcium deficient diet
Nulliparity
Family history of osteoporosis
Caucasian or Asian race
Sedentary lifestyle/immobility
Excessive alcohol intake
Long-term medications (e.g. glucocorticoids, phenytoin, excessive thyroxine)

Source: Data taken from AACE clinical practice guidelines for the prevention and treatment of postmenopausal osteoporosis. *Endrocrine Pract* 1996; **2**, 157–171.

b. Vision loss

Visual impairment is a common problem among older patients, with potentially serious complications in general health and quality of life. Presbyopia, cataracts, age-related macular degeneration (ARMD) and glaucoma are the most common causes of visual impairment. Routine screening with Snellen acuity testing is recommended for older women (USPSTF class B).[29] Screening asymptomatic patients with ophthalmoscopy by the primary care physician is a class C[29] recommendation. No specific frequency for screening is recommended.

11. Polypharmacy

a. Polypharmacy is the rule rather than the exception for older patients. Multiple chronic illnesses, self-medication, and the physiopharmocological changes with aging can lead to adverse reactions and drug interactions that may go unrecognized in the older patient.

b. Incorporating a medication review into the periodic health examination and then again frequently in follow-up visits can help to avoid adverse drug reactions. Inquiring

Table 2.11 Prevention, diagnosis and treatment of osteoporosis

Prevention is achieved by maintaining the following

Balanced, calcium-rich diet from adolescence onward

Regular, weight-bearing exercise

Stable estrogen levels

Avoidance of tobacco, alcohol, certain medications

Chemoprophylaxis (bisphosphonates, alendronate) if at risk

Diagnosis

History and assessment of risk factors are the most important elements of diagnosis

Clinical manifestations

Early: upper- or mid-thoracic back pain associated with activity, aggravated by long periods of sitting or standing, easily relieved by rest in the recumbent position

Late: common osteoporadic fracture sites: vertebrae, forearm, femoral neck, proximal humerus, dorsal kyphosis (dowager's hump)

Bone density screening: DEXA preferred, quantified computed tomography (much more expensive and greater radiation exposure), plain films (if positive, consistent with 50% bone loss)

Treatment

All women should receive calcium unless specifically contraindicated. Other therapies available include weight-bearing exercise, balanced nutrition, as well as consideration of the following:

Antiresorptive agents – estrogen (only for high risk of fracture after risks and benefits analysis), bisphosphonates, raloxifene, calcium, calcitonin

Bone forming agents – sodium fluoride

Miscellaneous – vitamin D metabolite (especially in those with limited sun exposure)

DEXA, dual energy X-ray absorptiometry

about all medications taken, including over-the-counter medications, vitamins, herbals and alternative/complementary therapies is helpful. Asking the patient to bring in the entire content of her medicine cabinet can be illuminating. Expired drugs, medications for illnesses no longer requiring treatment and prescriptions from multiple providers are frequently noted.

c. Encouraging the patient to use a pharmacy with database capability can help to reduce the likelihood of drug–drug interactions or adverse effects of multiple drug regimens. A good relationship between the physician and pharmacist can also be beneficial in avoiding adverse reactions or drug–drug interactions.

12. **Abdominal aortic aneurysm (AAA)**

a. An AAA is present when the infrarenal aortic diameter exceeds 3 cm. USPSTF recommends one-time US screening of AAA in men with risk factors: age (being 65 or older), male sex, a history of ever smoking (at least 100 cigarettes lifetime), and a first-degree family history of AAA.[46,47]

b. USPSTF recommends against routine screening of AAA in women (class D). This is based on the lower prevalence of AAA in women (about 15% of that in men) and late onset in the 80s. But certain risk groups in female patients may also benefit from AAA screening.[46,47]

c. The Society for Vascular Surgery and the Society for Vascular Medicine and Biology recommend screening all men aged 60 to 85, women aged 60 to 85 with cardiovascular risk factors, and men and women aged 50 and older with a family history of AAA.

d. Beginning in January 2007, Medicare will provide coverage for a one-time ultrasonography screen for AAA in men with risk factors, and in men and women 65 to 74 years of age with a family history of AAA.

Chemoprophylaxis

Aspirin

Aspirin prophylaxis for stroke and myocardial infarction prevention has been well studied in men. There is, as yet, inconclusive evidence to recommend for or against aspirin prophylaxis in older women. Individual patients may benefit from such intervention but potential risks (gastrointestinal bleeding or cerebral hemorrhage) must be weighed (USPSTF class C).[29]

21

Postmenopausal therapies

1. Osteoporosis prevention

(see also Chapter 28)

   a. HRT, alendronate, and raloxifene are all efficacious, but individual risk profiles determine which is best for a given patient.[48] Weight-bearing exercise is very important for maintaining adequate bone density.

   b. HRT in women with high risk of postmenopausal osteoporotic fracture can be considered an option. A lower dose of estrogen (i.e. 0.3 mg conjugated estrogen orally, or 0.025 mg transdermal patch) may provide nearly equivalent vasomotor and vulvovaginal symptom relief and bone density preservation.[49]

   c. Calcium supplementation produces beneficial effects on bone mass throughout postmenopausal life and may reduce fracture rates by as much as 50%.[50]

   d. Bisphophonates (alendronate, risedronate, and ibandronate) are effective for preventing bone loss associated with estrogen deficiency, glucocorticoid treatment, and immobilization.[51]

2. Coronary artery disease prevention

(see also Chapter 24)

   a. HRT was once recommended for CAD prevention in postmenopausal women without contraindications.[48] The conclusions of early observational studies are challenged by later randomized controlled trials, such as the Women's Health Initiative (WHI), showing increased fatal and non-fatal myocardial infarctions shortly after the start of HRT.[52] In 2005, The US Preventive Services Task Force (USPSTF) released a recommendation statement against the routine use of combined estrogen and progestin for the prevention of chronic conditions in postmenopausal women (class D).[52]

   b. Secondary analysis of WHI trials by Rossouw and Prentice et al.,[53] found a non-significant reduction of CHD in women starting hormone therapy within 10 years of menopause and increased risk thereafter. This finding supports the current recommendation of HRT for moderate to severe vasomotor symptoms for a short period of time.

3. Alzheimer's disease prevention

The impact of estrogen replacement therapy on cognitive functioning over time is unclear. Current and past users of HRT performed better on initial MMSE in one prospective cohort study, but not in randomized controlled trials.[54] Recent data showed that HRT started after 65 years may increase the risk of dementia. The evidence is insufficient to recommend for or against routine screening for dementia in older adults (I) according to USPSTF.

Conclusion

By attending to the differing risk factors of older women and following a systematic periodic evaluation (not necessarily at one visit), physicians can assist older women in maintaining their health and functional status. Secondary prevention issues can also be addressed and the appropriate preventive or therapeutic interventions highlighted.

References

1. Desai M., Hennessy C. Surveillance for morbidity and mortality among older adults – United States 1995–1996. *MMWR Morb Mortal Wkly Rep* 1999; **48**, 7–25.

2. Speroff L. Preventative healthcare for older women. *Int J Fertility Menopausal Study* 1996; **41**, 64–68.

3. Schulz R. Caregiving for children and adults with chronic conditions. *Health Psychol* 1998; **17**, 107–111.

4. Ineichen B. Measuring the rising tide: how many dementia cases will there be by 2001? *Br J Psychiatry* 1987; **150**, 193–200.

5. Andersen R. Prevalence of significant knee pain among older Americans. *J Am Geriatric Soc* 1999; **47**, 1435–1438.

6. Caspar M., *et al.* Blood pressure, diabetes, and body mass index among Chippewa and Menominee Indians. *Public Health Rep* 1996; **111**, 37–39.

7. Fontana S., Helberg C., Love R. The delivery of preventative services in primary care practices according to chronic disease status. *Am J Public Health* 1997; **87**, 1190–1196.

8. Faulkner L., Schauffler, H. The effect of health insurance coverage on the appropriate use of recommended clinical preventative services. *Am J Prev Med* 1997; **13**, 453–458.

9. Schulman K., Berlin J., Harless W. The effect of race and sex on physician's recommendations for cardiac catheterization. *N Engl J Med* 1999; **340**, 618–626.

10. Caplan L., Haynes S. Breast cancer screening in older women. *Public Health Rev (Israel)* 1996; **24**, 193–204.

11. Nosek M., Holand C. Breast and cervical cancer screening among women with physical disabilities. *Arch Phys Med Rehabil* 1997; **27**, 37–57.

12. Harmon M. Acculturation and cervical cancer: knowledge, beliefs, and behaviors of Hispanic women. *Women's Health*, 1996; **24**, 37–57.

13. Matthew D., McCullough M., Larson D. Religious commitment and health status: a review of the research and implications for family medicine. *Arch Fam Med* 1998; **7**, 118–124.

14. Wooley D. Geriatric psychiatry in primary care: a focus on ambulatory settings. *Geriatric Psychiatry* 1997; **20**, 241–260.

15. Mamdani M., Herrmann N., Austin P. Prevalence of antidepressant use among older people: populations based on observations. *J Am Geriatric Soc* 1999; **47**, 1350–1353.

16. Unutzer J., Patrick D., Simon G. Depressive symptoms and the cost of health serivices in HMO patients age 65 and older: a 4 year prospective study. *J Am Med Assoc* 1997; **277**, 1618–1623.

17. Midanik L., *et al.*, The effect of retirement on mental health and health behaviors. *J Geronto Ser B Psychol Sci Social Sci* 1995; **50**, S59–S61.

18. Brayne C., Spiegelhalter D., Dufouil C. Estimating the true extent of cognitive decline in the old. *J Am Geriatric Soc* 1999; **47**, 1283–1288.

19. South-Paul J., Woodson C. Optimal care of older women. *Postgraduate Med* 1992; **91**, 439–458.

20. Gallo J., Anderson L. *Handbook of Geriatric Assessment*, Rockville, MD: Aspen, 1988.

21. Koenig H., Hays J., Larson D. Does religious attendance prolong survivial? A six year follow up study of 3968 older adults. *J Gerontol Ser A Biol Sci Med Sci* 1999; **54**, 370–376.

22. Krause N. Neighborhood deterioration, religious coping, and change in health during late life. *Gerontologist* 1998; **38**, 653–664.

23. Katz S., Moskowitz R., Vignos P. A standardized measure of biological and psychological function. *J Am Med Assoc* 1963; **185**, 914–919.

24. Caspersen C., Christenson G., Pollard R. Status of the 1990 physical fitness and exercise objectives: evidence from NHIS 1985. *Public Health Rep* 1985; **101**, 587–592.

25. Okumiya K., *et al.* Effects of exercise on neurobehavioral function in community dwelling older people more than 75 years of age. *J Am Geriatric Soc* 1996; **44**, 569–572.

26. Tauton J., *et al.* Exercise for the older woman: choosing the right prescription. *Br J Sports Med* 1997; **31**, 5–10.

27. Kamimoto L., *et al.* Surveillance for five health risks among older adults – United States 1993–1997. *MMWR Morb Mort Wkly Rep* 1999; **48**, 89–130.

28. Bignotti D., Evans J., Fleming K., eds. *The Geriatric Patient*, 7th edition, ABFP Reference Guides, Lexington, KY: American Board of Family Medicine, 1999.

29. USPST Force, ed. *Guide to Clinical Preventative Services*, 2nd edition, Baltimore, MD: Williams and Wilkins, 1996.

30. NIH. *The Sixth Report of the Joint National Committee on the Prevention, Detection, Evaluation, and Treatment of High Blood Pressure*, Bethesda, MD: National Institutes of Health, 1997.

31. Mandelblatt J., *et al.* The cost-effectiveness of screening mammography beyond 65: a systematic review for the US preventative services task force. *Ann Inter Med* 2003; **139**, 835–842.

32. Pignone M., *et al.* Screening for colorectal cancer in adults at average risk: summary of the evidence for the US preventative services task force. *Ann Inter Med* 2002; **137**, 132–141.

33. USPST Force, ed. *Screening for Colorectal Cancer: Recommedations and Rationale*, Rockville, MD: Agency for Healthcare Research and Quality, 2002.

34. Zhang Y., Kiel D., Kreger B. Bone mass and the risk of breast cancer among post menopausal women. *N Engl J Med* 1997; **336**, 611–617.

35. O'Malley M. Screening for breast cancer with breast self examination. *J Am Med Assoc* 1987; **257**, 2197–2203.

36. Marwill S., Barry P. Patient factors associated with breast cancer screening among older women. *J Am Geriatric Soc* 1996; **44**, 1210–1214.

37. Mandel J., Bond J., Church T. Reducing mortality from colorectal cancers by screening for fecal occult blood. *N Engl J Med* 1993; **328**, 1365–1371.

38. Sheikh J. I., Yesavage J. A., Brooks J. O. III, *et al.* Proposed factor structure of the geriatric depression scale. *Int Psychogeriatric* 1991; **2**, 23–28.

39. Hoyl M., Alessi C., Harker J. Development and testing of a five item verson of the geriatric depression scale. *J Am Geriatric Soc* 1999; **47**, 873–878.

40. Butler S., Ashford J. W., Snowdon D. Age, education, and changes in the mini mental status exam scores of

23

older women: findings from the Nun Study. *J Am Geriatric Soc* 1996; **44**, 657–681.

41. Kinosian B., Glick H., Garland G. Cholesterol and health disease: predicating risks by level and ratios. *Ann Intern Med* 1994; **121**, 641–647.

42. Pignone M., *et al.* Screening and treating adults for lipid disorders. *Am J Prev Med* 2001; **20**(3s), 77–89.

43. Rosenthal M., *et al.* Thyroid failure in the elderly: microsomal antibodies as discriminant for therapy. *J Am Med Assoc* 1987; **258**, 209–213.

44. Kanis J. A., Melton L. J. III, Christiansen C., *et al.* The diagnosis of osteoporosis. *J Bone Miner Res* 1994; **8**, 1137–1141.

45. Yates J., *et al.* Rapid loss of hip fracture protection after estrogen cessation: evidence from the national osteoporosis risk assessment. *J Obstetr Gynecol* 2004; **103**, 440–446.

46. Screening and management of abdominal aortic aneurysm: the best evidence. *Am Fam Physician* 2006; **73**, 1198.

47. Chobianian A., Bakris G. The seventh report of the joint national committee on prevention, detection, evaluation, and treatment of high blood pressure: the JNC 7 report. *J Am Med Assoc* 2003; **289**, 2560.

48. Col N., Pauker P., Goldberg, R. Individualizing therapy to prevent long term consequences of estrogen deficiency in post menopausal women. *Arch Intern Med* 1999; **59**, 1458–1466.

49. Hart L. The minimum effective dose of estrogen for prevention of postmenopausal bone loss. *Obsetr Gynecol* 1984; **63**, 759–763.

50. Aloia J., Vaswani A., Yeh J. Calcium supplementation with and without hormone replacement therapy to prevent postmenopausal bone loss. *Ann Intern Med* 1994; **120**, 419–439.

51. Watts N. Treatment of osteoporosis with bisphosphonates. *Endocrinol Metabolism Clin N Am* 1998; **27**, 419–439.

52. USPST Force. *Hormone Therapy for the Prevention of Chronic Conditions in Postmenopausal Women: Recommendation Statement*, Rockville, MD: Agency for Healthcare Research and Quality, 2005.

53. Roussow J., Prentice R. Postmenopausal hormone therapy and risk of cardiovascular disease by age and years since menopause. *J Am Med Assoc* 2007; **297**, 1465–1477.

54. Matthews K., *et al.* Estrogen replacement therapy and cognitive decline in older community women. *J Am Geriatric Soc* 1999; **47**, 518–523.

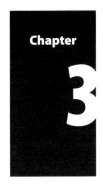

Nutrition

Gwendolyn Murphy, Victoria S. Kaprielian and Cathrine Hoyo

Normal healthy diet

> M. J. is a 57-year-old woman who is overweight and comes in for her yearly physical. She has a family history of heart disease and diabetes, and her older sister just had a heart attack, so she wants to know what she should do with her diet to stay healthy.

A healthy diet is a concern for people of all ages. Having traditionally been in charge of feeding the family, women tend to be even more interested. Current dietary recommendations for women focus in three main areas: caloric balance, fat intake, and calcium.

Balancing caloric intake and output

The most important characteristic of a healthy diet is balance – of food types, and of intake and output. To maintain a stable weight, one must burn off as much as one has taken in. Therefore a healthy diet is always closely connected with healthy levels of activity (see Chapter 4).

Two useful models regarding the proper balance of food types are the Food Pyramid and the New American Plate. The Food Pyramid, developed by the US Department of Agriculture (USDA), illustrates the healthy diet as based on a foundation of plant-based foods, including whole grain complex carbohydrates and substantial amounts of vegetables and fruits. Meat and dairy products make up a smaller proportion, with fats and sweets to be used sparingly.[1]

The New American Plate, developed by the American Institute for Cancer Research, shows a model meal in which two-thirds or more of a dinner plate consists of vegetables, fruits, whole grains and beans, while one-third or less is animal protein.[2] Both the Food Pyramid and the New American Plate encourage a diet that is high in fiber, vitamins and minerals, adequate essential amino acids, mono- and polyunsaturated fats. However, it limits refined sugars, saturated fats and calories. This type of diet helps to prevent obesity, diabetes, heart disease, and cancer.

While there is no one diet that constitutes the "Mediterranean" diet, when people refer to this they generally mean a diet that is high in fruits, vegetables, whole grain breads and cereals, beans, nuts, and seeds. Olive oil is the main fat that is added to foods. Small portions of dairy products, fish, eggs and poultry are eaten, but not much red meat. Wine is used in moderation. This type of diet is high in fiber and antioxidants, carotenoids, phytochemicals, and adequate in protein. While it is high in fat, most of the fat comes from monounsaturated olive oil. Europeans who adhere to a Mediterranean diet have lower rates of heart diseases and overall death rates, but diet may not be the only factor[3,4] (Table 3.1).

Protein intake

Most Americans get more protein than is necessary in their diets. However, as people age, they may not get adequate protein for a variety of reasons including lack of money, inability to purchase or prepare food, and isolation or depression making them less interested in food. Women who have severely low intakes of protein can become malnourished to the point where serum albumin falls.

Low protein intake is associated with a higher risk of bone fracture.[5] There is controversy about whether high animal protein intake increases the risk of fractures in women.[6] It appears that a high protein intake with low dietary calcium increases urinary calcium losses.[5]

Handbook of Women's Health, second edition, ed. Jo Ann Rosenfeld. Published by Cambridge University Press.
© Cambridge University Press 2009.

Table 3.1 Useful resources

USDA My Pyramid: http://www.mypyramid.gov/
New American Plate: http://aicr.convio.net/site/PageServer?pagename=pub_nap_index_21
The Harvard School of Public Health has developed a different pyramid. For the Harvard Pyramid and a discussion of concerns about the USDA My Pyramid see: http://www.hsph.harvard.edu/nutritionsource/pyramids.html

Table 3.2 Good ways to increase fiber

Replace refined grains such as white flour and white rice with whole grains.
Substitute legumes for meat 2–3 times per week
Eat whole fruits instead of drinking juice
Include raw vegetables as snacks or side dishes

Fiber intake

Fiber is important in the prevention of a number of medical conditions, including heart disease,[3,7] insulin resistance,[8] type 2 diabetes and constipation. There is good evidence that a high fiber diet reduces heart disease and insulin resistance.[9,10]

Whole grain intake, particularly cereal grain fiber, is inversely associated with lipid levels, insulin resistance and metabolic syndrome.[11] Fiber also assists in relieving constipation, wheat or oat bran being more efficacious than fruit or vegetable fiber (Table 3.2). However, fiber intake is no longer considered to be correlated with colon cancer.[3]

Refined sugar

The average American calorie intake has risen steadily over the past 50 years. This may in part be due to the availability of high fructose corn syrup and other refined sugars, but there is no research to support a sinister role of refined sugars other than their contribution of calories.[12]

Fat intake

In the "average" American diet, approximately 36% of calories come from fat. To control cholesterol levels and lower the risk of heart disease, a reduction in trans and saturated fat while increasing unsaturated oil intake is recommended.

When considering both heart disease and cancer risk, fewer than 10% of total calories per day should come from each category of fat (saturated, monounsaturated, polyunsaturated).[13] Some say that both saturated and trans fats should be as low as possible and combined should be less than 7% of calories (grade: imperative, strong).[14]

Providers should recommend the use of low-fat dairy products, limited amounts of lean meats, and avoidance of added fats. For cooking, high monounsaturated oils (olive, canola) are preferable. Education including 2–6 registered dietitian visits has been shown to reduce LDL cholesterol by 7–16% (grade: strong, conditional).[14]

Calcium and vitamin D

One serving of calcium equals a cup of milk, a cup of yogurt, or one ounce of cheese.

Menopausal women are at increased risk for osteoporosis, especially if they are Caucasian and/or thin. Cigarette smoking and a positive family history increase risk. While taking adequate calcium during the bone-building years (before age 30) is essential, calcium intake in later years is still important to slow the bone mineral loss that inevitably happens after menopause.

The best calcium source is dairy products. Three servings provide the recommended daily allowance of 1000 mg. Some people feel that an even higher intake of calcium (up to 1500 mg/day) is essential after the age of 50.[15] Use of low-fat or fat-free dairy products enables one to reach these amounts of calcium without exceeding fat goals.

Many adults have some degree of lactose intolerance, and are thus unable to take in this quantity of dairy products without abdominal discomfort, increased gas, nausea and/or diarrhea. Individuals may need to experiment with different foods to assess their own level of tolerance. While a cup of milk has 11 grams of lactose, a cup of yogurt has only 5 grams. Cheese and cottage cheese have high levels of calcium, but are much lower in lactose than milk; they are often tolerated by those who are lactose intolerant. Other options for lactose intolerant individuals are listed in Table 3.3.

Calcium is absorbed better from food than from tablets. Taking supplements with meals can help increase absorption.

Vitamin D is needed for optimal calcium absorption and utilization. Milk in the USA is fortified with vitamin D; those who get their calcium from dairy products generally have an adequate vitamin D

Table 3.3 Options for lactose intolerant individuals

Taking lactase supplements with ordinary dairy products

Using lactose-reduced or lactose-free dairy products

Using substitutes such as calcium-fortified orange juice or soy milk

intake. Individuals with limited dairy intake who do not get year-round sun exposure may benefit from vitamin D supplementation. Many calcium supplements now contain vitamin D as well.

Cancer risk

Many patients are interested in the possibility of reducing cancer risk through diet. The relationship between diet and cancer is controversial and an area of active research. A number of factors are worth considering.

Dietary factors that may increase risk

Alcohol has been associated with cancer of the mouth, pharynx, larynx,[16] breast,[17] esophagus,[18] and liver.[19] The combination of alcohol and tobacco use appears to increase risk far more than either one alone.[20] Women should limit intake of alcohol to no more than one drink per day (12 oz beer, 5 oz wine, 1 oz 100 proof spirits), although some studies find a lower risk of esophageal and gastric cancers among red wine drinkers.[21] Women who are at high risk for breast cancer may consider not drinking any alcohol.

Obesity is associated with increased risk of colon,[22] breast,[23] esophageal,[24,25,26,27] and endometrial cancers.[28] Avoidance of excessive calorie intake and maintenance of normal body weight reduces this risk.

Other caroteinoids such as lycopene, lutein and zeaxanthin (found in egg yolk and a variety of fruit and vegetables) are thought to provide health benefits due to their role as antioxidants. However, randomized clinical trails show high dose beta-carotene supplements increase the risk of lung cancer in smokers.[29] Therefore, rather than taking supplements, eating naturally occurring sources of caroteinoids should be encouraged.

Red meat is associated with colon cancer according to well-designed and conducted cohort studies.[30] Thus, one should avoid excessive consumption of red meats.

Broiled or grilled meats contain heterocyclic amines. Rather than cooking at high temperatures for long periods, meats should be braised, steamed, poached, stewed, or microwaved.

Nitrates found in preserved meats are associated with colorectal, esophageal, and stomach cancer. One should reduce the intake of meats preserved by smoke or salt. If preserved meats are eaten, the meal should also contain vegetables and fruits that contain vitamin C and phytochemicals that retard the conversion of nitrates to carcinogenic nitrosamines in the stomach.[31]

Pickled and salty foods have been associated with stomach, nasopharyngeal, and throat cancer. The best advice is to avoid excessive salt and pickled foods.

Many foods that were once thought to be associated are now seen as safe. These include aspartame, bioengineered foods, food additives, irradiated foods, and saccharin.[32]

Dietary factors that may decrease risk

Case control and cohort studies show an association between fruit and vegetable consumption and decreased incidence of lung, oral, esophageal, gastric, and colon cancer.[33] One should eat five or more servings per day. Food sources are superior to supplements. Tomatoes in particular (with a small amount of added fat) are thought to aid in cancer prevention because of their ability to interrupt lipid oxidation and to neutralize peroxyl radicals.[34]

Previous controlled trials reported that foods high in calcium help prevent colorectal cancer. However, studies from the last three years have not confirmed this association.[35] Nonetheless, because preneoplastic adenomas can be prevented with calcium,[36] women over 50 years of age should consider consuming at least 1200 mg/day.

Folate deficiency is associated with cancer of the colon, rectum, cervix and breast. In the USA, many grain products are now fortified with folate. A diet that includes fruits, vegetables, and enriched grains should provide sufficient intake.

Selenium deficiency, according to animal studies and one human study, is associated with lung, colon, and prostate cancer. Selenium is especially high in mushrooms and fish; it is also found in meats and grains. If selenium supplements are taken, the maximum dose should be 200 micrograms per day.[33]

Insufficient water intake is associated with bladder cancer. One should drink eight or more glasses per day to dilute bladder carcinogens.

Omega-3 fatty acids (found in fish oils and flax seeds) have been shown to suppress cancer formation in animals; it is theorized that they would do the same in humans, but as yet there are no human studies that support this.

While in the past fiber was thought to be protective against colon cancer, more recent studies have shown that this is not the case.[3]

There is insufficient evidence to support the following foods/supplements for reduction of cancer risk: antioxidant supplements (including vitamins A, C, E), garlic, lycopene supplements, olive oil, organic foods, phytochemical supplements, soy products, tea.[33]

Diet as therapy

S. K. is a generally healthy 49-year-old woman who presents with the complaint of hot flashes and asks what she can do about them without taking hormones. She does not want to take hormones because her mother died of breast cancer. She would also like any information you can give her about how to prevent cancer.

Menopausal symptom control

With fewer women taking hormone replacement therapy, more women are looking for alternatives to control menopausal symptoms, particularly hot flashes. Several possibilities have been promoted for this, with limited evidence.

The type of natural product most commonly used for menopausal symptoms are phytoestrogens or "plant estrogens." The most potent and common of these, isoflavones, are found in soy products. They are converted in the liver to substances similar to selective estrogen receptor modulators (SERMs), and have both agonist and antagonist activity at estrogen receptors. Intake of 20–60 grams/day of soy protein may be helpful in the short-term (2 years or less) treatment of hot flashes associated with menopause (evidence level B).[37,38,39] Soy intake does not improve lipid levels or bone mineral density when begun at age 60 or older (evidence level A).[40] Dietary soy intake may differ in biological activity from that of isoflavones in supplements.

Red clover contains isoflavones similar to those in soy products, but is much less well studied. There is conflicting evidence as to whether red clover has any effectiveness in reducing menopausal symptoms, and its safety is less clear.[37,38,41]

Less frequently mentioned is flaxseed, a rich source of lignan phytoestrogens. Some have suggested that dietary flaxseed (40 grams/day) may be effective for mild menopausal symptoms, but evidence is not consistent.[38,42] The high fat and calorie content of flaxseed may limit its ease of use.

Black cohosh, one of the top-selling herbs in the USA, is sometimes referred to as a phytoestrogen but recent evidence suggests it may not affect estrogen receptors. Black cohosh appears to relieve menopausal symptoms in some women. The American College of Obstetricians and Gynecologists supports short-term (less than 6 months) use for relief of vasomotor symptoms (evidence level B), while the North American Menopause Society concluded that evidence is insufficient.[40,43] The long-term safety of black cohosh is unknown.[37]

Vitamin E has been suggested as an option for women with a history of estrogen-dependent cancers who must avoid use of estrogenic substances. Evidence is inconsistent as to whether vitamin E (up to 1200 IU/day) might have a benefit for reducing hot flashes in breast cancer survivors.[37,38] Because of its safety and low cost, it is one of three non-prescription remedies suggested by the North American Menopause Society (along with isoflavones and black cohosh).[44]

Chasteberry (aka vitex), evening primrose oil, dong quai, ginseng, and wild yams have not been shown to have significant effect in reducing menopausal symptoms. They should not be recommended for this purpose.[37,38]

Weight concerns

M. B. is a 51-year-old woman who presents asking for advice on how to lose weight. She is 5 feet, 4 inches tall and weighs 190 pounds (BMI = 33). She's been overweight all her life; everyone in her family is heavy. She's tried Weight Watchers, the Atkins diet, and several others. Sometimes she loses weight, but she always gains it back. She wonders if there's a way for her to really lose weight, or if it is hopeless at this point in her life.

Obesity is one of the most important public health problems in the USA. The combined prevalence of overweight and obesity (defined as BMI greater or equal to 25) in American adults is 65.1%.[45] The prevalence of obesity (defined as BMI greater than or equal to 30)

Table 3.4 Conditions in which weight loss is recommended

To lower blood pressure in overweight and obese persons with high blood pressure

To improve plasma lipid levels in overweight and obese persons with dislipidemia

To lower blood glucose levels in overweight and obese persons with type 2 diabetes

increased 61% between 1991 and 2000. According to the latest figures, 30.4% of adults are obese.[45]

Strong evidence supports an association between obesity and increased morbidity and mortality. Research has linked excessive weight and body fat to metabolic syndrome, which includes diabetes, hypertension, and coronary artery disease.[46]

A recent review of the literature examined the relative risk of obesity in older Americans.[47] Assessment of 32 longitudinal analyses of weight-related health concluded that obesity increases risk for cardiovascular disease, some cancers and impaired mobility, but protects against hip fracture.

As people age, the association between obesity and mortality declines. Nonetheless, in developing evidence-based guidelines for the treatment of obesity, a National Heart Lung and Blood Institute (NHLBI) expert panel assumed that for most adults, the beneficial effects of weight loss exceed potential risks.[48] Weight loss is specifically recommended in the circumstances listed in Table 3.4 (all evidence level A).

The NHLBI guidelines recommend a two-step process of assessment and management. Treatment is recommended for patients with a BMI of 25–29.9 or a high waist circumference, if they have two or more risk factors. Patients with a BMI of 30 or more should receive treatment regardless of risk factors. The initial goal for weight loss should be to reduce body weight by 10% from baseline (evidence level A). With success, further loss can be attempted if warranted. A combined intervention including caloric reduction, increased physical activity, and behavior therapy is recommended as most effective.[49]

The key to weight control lies in the first concept of the normal healthy diet: balancing intake and output. In order to lose weight, one must burn off more calories than are taken in. If calories in (i.e. dietary intake) are less than calories out (energy expenditure), then the result will be weight loss. As long as the body's minimal requirements are met for protein, water, vitamins, and minerals, reducing calories below maintenance level should allow for safe weight reduction.

This again raises the unbreakable link with activity levels: the less active a person is, the less they can eat without gaining weight. Physical activity is recommended as part of a comprehensive weight control program because it contributes to weight loss (evidence level A), may decrease abdominal fat (evidence level B), increases cardiorespiratory fitness (evidence level A), and may help with maintenance of weight loss (evidence level C).[49] Encouraging patients to be physically active to become as healthy as they can be (no matter what their weight) is more effective than telling them to exercise in order to lose weight.

The simplest approach to caloric reduction is reducing portion size. Caloric deficits are additive over time; decreasing intake by only 100 calories per day (the equivalent of half a large cookie) will result in loss of 10 pounds over a year. The NHLBI panel recommended a deficit of 500–1000 kcal/day to achieve a weight loss of 1–2 pounds per week (evidence level A). Simply taking in less at each meal can make a significant impact over time. Combining this with an increase in activity amplifies the effect.

Reducing excessive dietary fat can also help. Fat has more than twice the number of calories per gram of either protein or carbohydrate. By replacing fatty foods with less fatty ones, the amount of calories is decreased even without decreasing the portion size. For example, half a cup of potatoes with 1 teaspoon of butter or margarine has about 110 calories; without the added fat (butter or margarine) the potatoes have only 65 calories. Reducing dietary fat alone, without reducing total caloric intake, is not sufficient to create weight loss (evidence category A).

There is fair evidence that eating breakfast aids in weight management by helping to control appetite and reducing overall caloric intake. Thus, one recommendation to patients could be to eat a small breakfast every morning to help them control and reduce overall appetite. The prevalence of skipping breakfast ranges from 3.6 to 25%[50,51,52] and is associated with both higher BMI and increased risk of obesity, even though patients report lower energy intakes.[53] Two randomized controlled trials show that those who eat breakfast have less impulsive snacking and less consumption later in the day.[54,55] People at normal weight and those who maintain weight loss usually eat a breakfast of high-fiber cereal with about 20% of their daily energy intake.[3,56] However, high calorie breakfasts are associated with higher BMI.[1,57]

In addition, there have been many studies on low glycemic index diets versus low calorie diets that are high in glycemic index. Glycemic index is the term used for the relative rise in glucose following the intake of 100 grams of carbohydrate from different types of food (e.g. processed mashed potatoes (a high glycemic food) versus high fiber, natural rolled oats). In general, there are no consistent differences between high- and low-glycemic diets, but some studies have found that there are differences in the patient's appetite and/or reduction in abdominal obesity (Grade III).[58,59]

Special diets for weight loss

There are many other approaches to weight loss that are promoted widely, many promising dramatic results in a short time. Some of the most well known include the following.

The Atkins Diet

This is a severely restricted carbohydrate, high-protein, high-fat diet. This diet takes advantage of the ketosis that develops during starvation; the resulting anorexia reduces appetite. However, ketosis can also cause fatigue, constipation, and vomiting. Potential long-term side effects include heart disease, bone loss, and kidney damage. In addition, high-protein, low-carbohydrate diets tend to be low in calcium, fiber, and antioxidants. The proponents of this diet advise taking vitamin-mineral supplements to replace lost nutrients. This type of diet has been found to result in greater initial weight loss than a low-fat diet; however, after six months there is no appreciable difference between weight lost with the two approaches (Table 3.5).

The Pritikin Diet

This is a very low fat (15% of calories), high fiber, vegetarian (or nearly vegetarian) diet combined with exercise. It claims to reduce serum cholesterol and prevent or reverse cardiovascular disease.

The Dean Ornish Diet

This carries low fat even further, with only 10% of calories from fat. Again, it claims reduction of serum cholesterol and prevention of heart disease.

Diet pills

According to NHLBI guidelines, pharmacotherapy may be considered for those with a BMI of 30 or more, or BMI between 27 and 29.9 with comorbidity.[49] Women are significantly more likely to use diet pills than men.[60,61] A discussion of the available agents and

Table 3.5 Ways to improve the diet of patients with cancer

1. If immune function is compromised, avoid uncooked meats, unpasteurized dairy products, raw vegetables, and herbal nutrient supplements.

2. Because fever expends considerable energy, adequate intake of carbohydrates, fats, and vitamins should be encouraged, especially during episodes of infection.

3. During chemotherapy treatments, meat often has a very bad taste and smell. Using fruit or fruit juice when preparing or serving meat may help.

4. Dry mouth symptoms can be alleviated by rinsing with a saline mouthwash (one teaspoon salt and one teaspoon baking soda added to a quart of water) before meals. Commercial mouthwash, alcoholic and acidic beverages can aggravate an irritated mouth.

5. For patients with mouth or throat soreness, bland, lukewarm, or cool foods can be soothing. Acidic, spicy, or salty foods may be irritating.

6. Drinking enough fluids will help counteract the constipation often caused by analgesics. If the GI tract is not too tender, constipation may be alleviated by high fiber foods such as whole grain breads, raw fruit and vegetables, dried fruit, seeds and nuts.

7. Diarrhea due to chemotherapy or radiation may be alleviated by a soft diet and avoidance of whole grains, legumes, dried fruit, raw fruit and vegetables. Limiting intake of high-fat foods may also help.

8. Patients reporting difficulty swallowing solids should be advised to drink thick fluids such as soups, high-calorie or protein drinks, yogurt, ice cream, and milk shakes to meet nutritional needs.

9. The primary concern in vomiting patients is dehydration. Frequent fluid intake should be advised. Clear, light, and cool drinks may be better tolerated than icy or hot drinks.

10. If chemotherapy causes an immediate negative GI reaction (nausea, vomiting, or diarrhea), food eaten just prior to treatment may cause an aversion reaction thereafter. It is best not to eat a favorite food just prior to chemotherapy.

their use is beyond the scope of this chapter. Numerous combined dietary supplements are marketed as helping weight loss. None have been shown to be effective, and side effects can be significant.

Weight reduction diets alone (with or without medication) usually do not result in maintenance of weight lost. Lifestyle changes which include nutritional, behavioral, and exercise components can reduce weight by 5–7% long term. Reduced fat and calories, regular physical activity, and provider contact and support are recommended (evidence level A).[49] A program consisting of dietary therapy, physical activity, and behavior therapy should be continued indefinitely (evidence level B).[49]

Low Carb Diets

Consumption of *ad libitum* low carbohydrate diets and reduced calorie diets both result in lower caloric intake. While low carbohydrate diets resulted in greater body weight loss in the first six months, after one year, these differences were no longer significant[62] (evidence fair).[63]

Meal replacement diets

Meal replacement diets such as Slimfast, Nutrisystem, or the Zone diet take the worry out of planning what you are going to eat. A company will sell low calorie balanced meals. The consumer pays dearly for this service, but if the patient sticks to the plan, she will likely lose weight. Several studies comparing isocaloric diets have shown an equivalent or greater weight loss efficacy with structured meal replacement plans, compared to reduced calorie diet treatments. One or two daily vitamin- and mineral-fortified meal replacements, supplemented with self-selected meals and snacks, may be a successful weight loss and weight maintenance strategy for overweight and obese adults who have difficulty with self-selection of food and portion control (evidence good).[64]

Eating disorders

Eating disorders are most commonly associated with younger women – teenagers and young adults. Follow-up studies on women who had anorexia when they were adolescents show that approximately 50% of them achieve a relatively normal weight as adults, and less than 10% are overweight.[65] With regard to eating patterns at follow-up, one-third are found to eat normally. Half avoid high calorie foods, and between 14% and 50% of them continue to have bulimic problems with binge eating, vomiting and laxative abuse. Menstrual function had returned in 70–90% despite weight and eating irregularities.

For psychosocial functioning, there is a wide range of findings with many patients showing psychiatric comorbidities and/or psychological dysfunction. When anorexia does last into mid-life, serious health consequences can arise due to prolonged malnutrition. These include heart failure, liver damage, and hypokalemia-induced arrythmias. Mortality in long-term studies shows rates of 15%.[65]

Data for bulimia nervosa are scarce, but are thought to be similar to those for anorexia.[65] As with adolescents, bulimia and binge eating in mature women may be associated with obesity. Purging is less common in mature women than in adolescents, and may take different forms. Self-induced vomiting is unlikely to be continued into mid-life, and would likely result in severe dental damage. Laxative and diuretic abuse may be more likely in this age group.

Underweight patients are easy to identify and question further about eating habits. Because many bulimics are normal weight or heavier, they are more difficult to recognize. Routine questions may be helpful in identifying patients for more targeted assessment:

- Are you concerned about your weight?
- Do you ever binge or feel out of control when eating?

A positive response should trigger further assessment of intake, purging, exercise, and use of laxatives or diuretics.

Patients with eating disorders can often benefit from counseling, whether or not they are willing to attempt to "cure" their problem. True anorexia nervosa generally requires a multidisciplinary team approach to management. Some women, while not meeting strict criteria for anorexia, maintain an unhealthy fixation on weight and may over-restrict their intake. Providers can work with these patients to identify a healthy body weight, and encourage a balanced, varied diet.

Diet and medical problems
Diabetes

> *A. P. is a 47-year-old woman diagnosed with diabetes 5 years ago. She recently started on metformin and is tolerating it well. The need to start medication has motivated her to really work on losing weight and controlling her disease. She wants to know what she should and should not eat.*

The recommended diet for people with diabetes follows the same guidelines as a normal healthy diet.[66] It should contain carbohydrate, protein, and fat in reasonable proportions. Calories should be at a level that promotes a healthy weight, and the diet should be based on a variety of foods. People with diabetes should receive individualized medical nutrition therapy (MNT), preferably with a registered dietitian, as needed to reach their treatment goals (evidence level B).

The major nutrient that affects blood sugar levels is carbohydrate in the form of sugar and starch, as found in grains, fruits, vegetables, sweets, and milk. The total amount of carbohydrate consumed is more important than the source or type (evidence level A).

Sucrose, or table sugar, does not increase blood sugar any more than the same amount of starch, so sucrose can be substituted for other carbohydrates in the diet. There is no evidence to support the avoidance of concentrated sweets as long as total energy and carbohydrate levels are maintained. Non-nutritive sweeteners such as aspartame, saccharin, acesulfame potassium, and sucralose appear to be safe at normal levels of intake (evidence level A). Low carbohydrate diets (<130 grams/day) are not recommended for patients with diabetes (evidence level E).

Protein, while an insulin stimulant, does not increase blood sugar in the amounts usually eaten. Hyperglycemia can contribute to increased protein turnover. However, since most adults eat much more protein than is required, there is no need for diabetics to increase protein intake beyond usual levels (evidence level B). For those with any degree of chronic kidney disease, protein intake should be limited to 0.8 grams per kg body weight (evidence level B).

Whereas dietary fat helps to modulate the absorption of glucose, saturated fat, trans fat and cholesterol should be limited in the diet. Saturated and trans fats in the diet stimulate LDL cholesterol production, and persons with diabetes are more sensitive to dietary cholesterol than the general public. Less than 7% of calories should come from saturated fats (evidence level A); trans fats should be minimized (evidence level E).[66]

Weight loss is recommended for all adults with BMI ≥ 25 who have or are at risk for developing diabetes (evidence level E). Both reduced energy consumption and weight loss improve insulin resistance and blood glucose levels. In patients with impaired glucose tolerance, weight loss of 10–15% may be sufficient to hold off frank diabetes.

Supplementation with antioxidants (vitamins E, C and beta-carotene) is not advised due to lack of evidence of efficacy and concern about long-term safety (evidence level A). Chromium supplementation in people with diabetes and obesity has not been shown to be of benefit (evidence level E).

Treatment of hypoglycemia is best accomplished with oral glucose or glucose-containing food. The addition of fat should be avoided, as it retards the absorption of the glucose. Ten grams of oral glucose will raise blood sugar levels by ~40 mg/dL over 30 minutes, and 20 grams will raise blood sugar levels by ~60 mg/dL over 45 minutes.[67]

The New American Plate may be a helpful model. Sometimes having the patient eat on a smaller plate helps in portion control. Patients should be encouraged to eat more fruits and vegetables, but restrict juice and sweetened drinks to no more than 4–6 ounces per day. Monounsaturated fats (such as olive or canola oil) should be used to replace saturated fats in cooking.

Heart disease

C. B. is a 58-year-old woman who presents for hospital follow-up. She is now 4 weeks post MI, and still stunned that this happened to her. At hospital discharge she declined cholesterol-lowering medication, saying she really doesn't want more drugs. She asks what she can do with her diet to reduce her risk of another heart attack.

Weight maintenance/reduction

Encourage weight maintenance or reduction through balance of caloric intake, physical activity, and behavioral programs. The goal is to keep BMI below 25 and waist circumference less than 35 inches (effective, level B).[68]

Diet

Encourage overall healthy eating including fruits, vegetables, whole grains, low-fat dairy products, fish, legumes, and lean meats.[68]

Fat

What has become clear with 20 years follow-up from the Nurses' Health Study is that the type of fat is more important than the total fat in the diet.[68] Studies have documented strong correlation between coronary death rates and saturated or trans fat intake as a percentage of calories.[71,72] With the new regulations that require nutrition labeling to include amounts of trans fats, most manufacturers have eliminated these in their products. However, avoidance of hydrogenated vegetable fats (often found in baked goods and convenience foods) is advisable.

Both mono- and polyunsaturated oils increase HDL and decrease LDL cholesterol. The lowest risk of coronary disease was seen with low intake of trans and saturated fats combined with a high proportion of mono- and polyunsaturated oils.[71] Olive oil, canola oil, nuts, and avocados are other good sources of monounsaturated oil. Polyunsaturated oils include corn, safflower, soybean and cottonseed oils.

For women at high risk for heart disease, omega-3 fatty-acid supplements may be added (level B).[68] Omega-3 fatty acids (most commonly found in cold-water fish) prolong bleeding time, increase erythrocyte deformability, and decrease blood viscosity. In the Nurses' Health Study, women with a higher intake of omega-3 fatty acids had a lower risk of coronary disease.[72] Omega-3 fatty acids have been shown to reduce mortality in the first 3 months after a heart attack. The American Heart Association (AHA) recommends fish intake as part of a heart-healthy lifestyle, but gives cautions regarding the use of fish oil supplements because high intakes can cause excessive bleeding.[73]

Fiber

Overall, there is good evidence to support increasing dietary fiber, vegetable, fish, and nut consumption.[74] A pooled analysis of cohort studies concluded that for each 10 gram per day increase in dietary fiber, there was a 14% decrease in coronary events and a 27% reduction in coronary deaths.[9]

Soy protein intake has been consistently found to induce modest reduction of serum cholesterol. The US Food and Drug Administration (FDA) and American Heart Association now agree that 25 grams per day of soy protein, in conjunction with a low fat diet, may reduce the risk of heart disease.

Niacin is available both as a dietary supplement and as a prescription drug. In high doses (1200–3000 mg/day) niacin can raise HDL and lower triglyceride and LDL levels.[75] Hepatotoxicity is a risk, especially with long-acting preparation.

Red yeast rice products contain numerous different HMG-CoA reductase inhibitors.[75] Therefore they can have effectiveness and risks similar to prescription statins. Because they are unregulated and contents are not standardized, these products are best avoided.

Antioxidants (vitamin E, vitamin C, and beta-carotene) in fruits, vegetables, and whole grains are associated with reduced cardiovascular risk (evidence fair). However, supplements of these vitamins have shown no protection for CVD events or mortality and therefore should not be recommended to reduce heart disease risk (evidence strong).[76]

Hypertension

> C. C. is a 51-year-old woman with borderline hypertension. She's been successful in losing a few pounds, and her pressure today is 138/86. She's concerned because the nurse at work told her she needed to cut all salt out of her diet if she wanted to get her pressure down, but the salt-free foods she's tried were awful.

Blood pressure is a highly integrated response to interactions among various anions and cations. In particular, high intake of sodium chloride in conjunction with low dietary potassium, calcium, and/or magnesium increases the risk for hypertension.

Sodium

A reduction in dietary sodium has been shown to lower blood pressure even in those without hypertension.[77] In those with hypertension and/or salt sensitivity (defined as 10% or greater difference in blood pressure on low-sodium versus high-sodium diet) the reduction in blood pressure is even greater.[78] The major predictors of salt sensitivity are body weight, age, blood pressure, kidney function, and race (African-American).

Moderation in salt intake (limiting cured meats, high-salt snacks, and processed foods, for example) is advisable for all, especially those with increasing obesity and hypertension. Current recommendations limit salt intake to no more than 6 grams per day (2400 mg or 100 mmol sodium);[79] its effect is estimated to be 2–8 mmHg.[80] A very low sodium diet is unnecessary for most patients.

Potassium

The higher the sodium intake, the more effect potassium has on lowering blood pressure. A meta-analysis of randomized controlled trials concludes that there is a significant reduction in blood pressure with potassium supplementation.[81] Dietary sources of potassium include milk, fruits, grains and vegetables. The less processed these foods are, the higher the potassium to sodium ratio. For example, potatoes, tomatoes, and milk have high potassium to sodium ratios; potato chips, ketchup, and cheese have high sodium to potassium ratios.

Calcium

A meta-analysis of randomized controlled trials showed that the effect of calcium supplements on blood pressure is small.[82] However, it may act in conjunction with other nutrients to lower blood pressure. An increase in calcium consumption only reduces blood pressure in those with hypertension.

Magnesium

The blood pressure lowering effects of magnesium are small. The Nurses' Health Study showed that women with a magnesium intake >300 mg/day had a 23% reduction of risk for developing hypertension compared to women with a magnesium intake of <200 mg/day.[83] The average dietary intake of magnesium is 300 mg/day.[84]

Alcohol

Alcohol is a significant pressor agent. Heavy drinkers (more than 3 liters of wine per day) have significantly more hypertension than those drinking less than 1 liter of wine per day. Alcohol should be reduced to moderate amounts. Those with resistant or difficult-to-treat hypertension should discontinue alcohol intake. Hypertensive patients with optimal blood pressure control may be allowed light to moderate alcohol consumption. For a woman, this means less than 0.5 oz ethanol (12 oz beer, 5 oz wine, 1 oz 100 proof whiskey) per day, preferably consumed with meals. Decreasing alcohol intake to a moderate level is associated with a reduction of systolic blood pressure of approximately 2–4 mmHg.[85]

Obesity

Increased body weight, particularly abdominal obesity, is a major factor in blood pressure control.

The combined effects of aging and weight gain may affect blood pressure more than either alone. A weight loss of 10 kg has been found to result in a reduction of systolic blood pressure of 5–20 mmHg.[78,86]

Other dietary factors

The DASH Diet (Dietary Approaches to Stop Hypertension) is high in fruits (5 servings per day), vegetables (4 servings per day), low-fat dairy products (2 servings per day), whole grain, poultry, fish, and nuts, with small amounts of red meat. In people with hypertension, the DASH diet has been shown to reduce systolic blood pressure by 11.4 mmHg and diastolic by 5.5 mmHg.[86]

Vitamin C, fish oil, fiber, soy, and the amino acid composition of the diet may affect blood pressure, but not as much as those factors listed above.[87] A diet that is high in fruits, vegetables, and low-fat dairy foods, in conjunction with moderation in sodium intake, is likely to improve blood pressure. These measures, coupled with weight loss and exercise, are the best non-pharmacologic treatments for hypertension.

Cancer

> J. T. is recovering from a mastectomy for breast cancer, and about to undergo a course of chemotherapy. She's always been thin, and is aware that she needs to keep up her intake so she doesn't lose too much weight. The stress has really hurt her appetite, and she's afraid the chemo will make it even more difficult for her to eat.

Malnutrition is the most frequently identified determinant of severity of illness and death among cancer patients.[88] Cancer patients with adequate nutrition have been shown to fare better in general, and specifically have a higher tolerance for side effects related to therapeutic interventions. Many factors determine the severity of side effects, including the type and location of the tumor, and the type, length, and dose of treatment.

Surgery

Pain often leads to anorexia and reduced fluid intake, subsequently causing weakness and fatigue. Nausea, vomiting, and diarrhea further deplete nutritional resources.

Radiation

While all cells exposed to radiation are affected, most normal cells recover. The size of the radiation field, total dose, and number of treatments may adversely affect nutritional status indirectly through loss of appetite, or more directly through damage to the gastrointestinal tract. Side effects typically start during the second or third week of treatment; most end two to three weeks after completion of therapy.

Chemotherapy

Side effects of chemotherapy include loss of appetite, changes in taste and smell, mouth tenderness or sores, nausea, vomiting, changes in bowel habits, fatigue, leukopenia, and weight loss or gain. Many side effects of chemotherapy dissipate quickly. Their frequency and severity depend on initial nutritional status, type and dosage of chemotherapy, and other drugs and treatments given simultaneously.

Maintaining a balanced dietary intake helps replenish nutrients, decreases risk of infection, and accelerates healing and recovery. This will likely improve tolerance to treatment-related side effects. A diet high in protein will facilitate maintenance of weight and strength, tissue regeneration and healing. Small and frequent feedings may be better tolerated than large meals. Multivitamin and mineral supplements can be used in addition to food intake. Adequate fluid intake must also be maintained to avoid dehydration. Adding unsaturated fat to a patient's diet may be appropriate if weight gain is desired. Fats are a concentrated calorie source, and the tastes and textures they add to foods may encourage increased intake.

Dietary interventions may be helpful in the management of side effects of cancer treatment. Because taste alterations are common in patients with cancer, supplements offering a variety of flavors are thought to help taste fatigue.[89] Considerations of the diet for the patient with cancer are included in Table 3.5.

Chronic lung disease

> *S. L. is 58 years old, a smoker since she was 13. She just cut back from two packs a day to one. She's experiencing more frequent acute exacerbations of her chronic bronchitis, and her recovery seems to take longer each time. She is worried that she seems to be losing more and more weight with each bout of bronchitis. She's read that fish oil is supposed to be good for your lungs, and wonders if there's anything she can do with her diet to help.*

One complication of chronic obstructive pulmonary disease (COPD) is malnutrition. Malnutrition, in turn, exacerbates COPD by leading to weakened respiratory muscles and compromised pulmonary function. As a result, COPD patients can become trapped in a cycle in which recurrent pulmonary infections lead to poor intake.

Weight loss in COPD patients has been well documented. Episodic weight loss may result from prolonged or recurrent cytokine production that occurs during infections and exacerbations.[90]

Reversing under-nutrition has proven difficult, and nutritional supplementation programs have received mixed reviews.[91] In one study, short-term nutritional support of COPD patients improved muscle function by 10%–20% without a measurable change in cell mass.[92] Two studies, one a randomized controlled trial, demonstrated creatine supplements combined with rehabilitative exercise resulted in significant weight gain.[93,94,95]

Long-term nutrient supplementation improved nutritional status in some patients. Caloric supplements for at least two weeks resulted in improved pulmonary function, respiratory muscle strength, anthropometric measures, and functional exercise capacity. Studies among hospitalized patients suggest increased caloric input (1.7 times the resting expenditure) should balance the caloric input/output equation.[96]

Recent speculations suggest that foods rich in omega-3 fatty acids (found in fish oils, flax seed oil, green leafy vegetables and olives) may therapeutically benefit COPD patients[97] because the presence of omega-3 fatty acids may displace inflammatory precursors such as arachadonic acid from cell membrane lipids and lower the product of inflammatory eicosanoids.[96] In addition, others reported nutritional support of COPD patients with omega-3 polyunsaturated fatty acids had anti-inflammatory effects and improved exercise tolerance.[98] In one large study, the risk of developing COPD was lower in smokers with a high intake of omega-3 fatty acids.[99] Daily recommended doses are 1800 to 3000 mg/day of combined DHA (docosahexaenoic acid) and EPA (eicosapentaenoic acid).[100]

In summary, encouraging increased caloric intake is important. The intake should be adequate in protein, vitamins, and minerals. Carbohydrate should not be restricted, and supplemental omega-3 fatty acids may be beneficial. A moderate exercise regimen may also be helpful.

Arthritis

N. L. is 55, but she's had problems with pain in her joints since her early 40s. Her biggest problem is her knees. It hurts to walk, so she's decreased her exercise and is gaining weight. Ibuprofen helps the pain, but it's starting to irritate her stomach. The man at the health food store recommended some supplements with glucosamine and chondroitin, and she asks you if it's worth trying.

There are multiple types of arthritis, with differing pathophysiologies. The nutritional issues vary with the type of joint disease.

The most common type of arthritis responsible for symptoms of the large weight-bearing joints is osteoarthritis. The most common cause of this "wear and tear" arthritis is obesity. Patients who are overweight or obese, who complain of pain in the knees and/or hips, should attempt to lose weight. A combination of calorie reduction and a regular pattern of non-impact exercise provides better improvement in function and pain than weight loss or exercise alone.[101]

Gout is a metabolic disease in which acute joint inflammation is caused by uric acid crystals in synovial fluid. Dietary strategies which reduce serum uric acid levels may be useful in decreasing the frequency of recurrences. Urate production for any individual appears to vary directly with body weight; hence, weight loss is recommended. Central obesity has been shown to have a significant effect on gout occurrence independent of BMI.[102] Higher levels of meat, seafood, and alcohol intake are all associated with increased risk of gout.[102,103] Overall purine and protein intake have not shown this association. While limited protein intake was once a standard of therapy for gout, high-protein diets have a uricosuric effect and may actually reduce serum uric acid levels.[103] Consumption of low-fat dairy products, as well as fruits and vegetables, appears protective.[102,103] A limitation of the evidence is that most studies have been performed on men.

Numerous supplements are promoted for help in controlling arthritis pain. Evidence varies as to their safety and efficacy, as does the methodologic quality of reported studies.

Glucosamine appears to be safe and effective, and may stimulate cartilage growth. Taken in doses of 1500 mg/day, it reduces pain and improves function in patients with knee or hip osteoarthritis, and may

Table 3.6 Web sources for good dietary information

A comprehensive discussion of dietary issues of interest to women is beyond the scope of this chapter. Recommended resources for reliable information for patients and providers include the following (URLs valid as of 12/06).

General dietary information American Dietetic Association http://www.eatright.org/

Weight control, diabetes, and other medical disorders

National Institute of Diabetes, Digestive and Kidney Disorders http://www.niddk.nih.gov/health/nutrition.htm

Dietary supplements

National Center for Complementary and Alternative Medicine http://nccam.nih.gov/

Calcium

National Women's Health Information Center http://www.womenshealth.gov/faq/diet.htm

also be helpful in other forms of arthritis (evidence level B).[104] Glucosamine may relieve joint pain from osteoarthritis as well as NSAIDs, with fewer side effects.[104] However, this was not confirmed in a recent randomized clinical trial.[105] Glucosamine is available in several forms; the sulfate is the most studied. Since it is derived from shellfish exoskeletons, there is a theoretic risk of reaction in those with shellfish allergies.[104,106] Concerns about glucosamine increasing insulin resistance are waning,[104] but monitoring of glucose levels in diabetic patients is appropriate.

Chondroitin is often sold in combination with glucosamine, but has not consistently been found to improve symptoms (evidence level B).[107] One recent randomized controlled trial suggests benefit from combined glucosamine and chondroitin for moderate-to-severe osteoarthritis only.[105] Because chondroitin is usually derived from bovine cartilage, there is concern of possible contamination with prions that cause bovine spongiform encephalopathy (BSE, aka mad cow disease).[106] Preliminary research also suggests that chondroitin may stimulate growth in prostate cancer cells.[104] The safer approach is to use glucosamine sulfate in a single ingredient preparation.

S-adenosylmethionine (SAMe) may also be effective in reducing osteoarthritis symptoms, comparably to NSAIDs (evidence level A).[104,106] High cost, low bioavailability, and poor product quality make it impractical for general use at this time.

Avocado/soybean unsaponifiables may reduce pain and slow joint space loss in osteoarthritis (evidence level A). "Unsaponifiable" refers to the residual after hydrolysis of fatty acids in avocado and soybean oil. Use of this supplement appears to be safe for up to two years.[104]

Omega-3 fatty acids reportedly suppress inflammatory cytokines, thereby producing an anti-inflammatory effect which may be helpful in rheumatoid arthritis (evidence level A).[104] Taking fish oil may reduce morning stiffness, but relief may not be noted for up to 12 weeks. Doses over 3 grams per day should be avoided due to antiplatelet effects and risk of bleeding.

Gamma linolenic acid is contained in evening primrose, blackcurrant, and other oils. Some research suggests that these seed oils may be beneficial for rheumatoid arthritis, but study quality is variable (evidence level B).[104] Onset of effect may not be seen for up to 6 months.

Preliminary research has suggested that people with low vitamin D levels have more pain and disability from osteoarthritis than people with sufficient vitamin D, so supplements could be considered for those without sufficient sunlight exposure.[104] Dietary intake high in antioxidants (such as beta-carotene and vitamins C and E) might slow progression of osteoarthritis.[106]

Numerous other dietary supplements have been suggested for arthritis pain, including cat's claw, devil's claw, stinging nettle, phellodendron, ginger, willow bark, turmeric, green tea, quercetin, and resveratrol. There is not yet sufficient evidence to support the use of these (Table 3.6).

References

1. *My Pyramid Background*, http://www.mypyramid.gov, accessed 1/07.

2. American Institute for Cancer Research. *The American Plate*, http://aicr.convio.net/site/PageServer?pagename=pub_nap_index_21, accessed 1/07.

3. Fuchs C. S., Giovannucci E. L., Coldtz G. A. Dietary fiber and the risk of colorectal cancer and adenoma in women. *N Engl J Med* 1999; **340**, 169–176.

4. Trichopoulou A., Orfanos P., Norat T., *et al.* Modified Mediterranean diet and survival: EPIC-elderly prospective cohort study. *Br Med J* 2005; **330**, 991. doi:10.1136/bmj.38415.644155.8F.

5. Dawson-Hughes B. Interaction of dietary calcium and protein in bone health in humans. *J Nutr* 2005; **133**, 852S–854S.

6. Bonjour J.-P. Dietary protein: an essential nutrient for bone health. *J Am Coll Nutr* 2005; **24**, 526S–536S.

7. Wolk A., Manson J. E., Stampfer M. J., *et al.* Long-term intake of dietary fiber and decreased risk of coronary heart disease among women. *J Am Med Assoc* 1999; **281**, 1998–2004.

8. Weickert M. O., Möhlig M., Schöfl C., *et al.* Cereal fiber improves whole-body insulin sensitivity in overweight and obese women. *Diabetes Care* 2006; **29**, 775–780.

9. Pereira M. A., O'Reilly E., Augustsson K., *et al.* Dietary fiber and risk of coronary heart disease: a pooled analysis of cohort studies. *Arch Intern Med* 2004; **164**, 370–376.

10. Van Horn L. Fiber, lipids, and coronary heart disease: a statement for healthcare professionals from the nutrition committee, American Heart Association. *Circulation* 1997; **95**, 2701–2704.

11. McKeown N. M., Meigs J. B., Liu S., Wilson P. W. F., Jacques P. F. Whole-grain intake is favorably associated with metabolic risk factors for type 2 diabetes and cardiovascular disease in the Framingham Offspring Study. *Am J Clin Nutr* 2002; **76**, 390–398.

12. Wylie-Rosett J., Segal-Isaacson C. J., Segal-Isaacson A. Carbohydrates and increases in obesity: does the type of carbohydrate make a difference? *Obes Res* 2004; **12**, 124S–129S.

13. Carleton R. A., Dwyer J., Finberg L., *et al.* Report of the Expert Panel on Population Strategies for Blood Cholesterol Reduction. A statement from the National Cholesterol Education Program, National Heart, Lung, and Blood Institute, National Institutes of Health. *Circulation* 1991; **83**, 2154–2232.

14. American Dietetic Association. *Disorders of Lipid Metabolism Evidence-Based Nutrition Practice Guideline, Executive Summary Recommendations, Evidence Analysis Library*, http://www.adaevidencelibrary.com, accessed 12/06.

15. NIH. *Optimal Calcium Intake*. NIH Consensus Statement Online 1994 June 6–8; **12**(4), 1–31, http://www.ncbi.nlm.nih.gov/books/bv.fcgi?rid=hstat4.chapter.13595.

16. Maserejian N. N., Joshipura K. J., Rosner B. A., Giovannucci E., Zavras A. I. Prospective study of alcohol consumption and risk of oral premalignant lesions in men. *Cancer Epidemiol Biomarkers Prev* 2006; **15**(4), 774–781.

17. Hin-Peng L. Diet and breast cancer: an epidemiologist's perspective. *Crit Rev Oncol Hematol* 1998; **28**(2), 115–119.

18. Engel L. S., Chow W. H., Vaughan T. L., Gammon M. D., Risch H. A., Stanford J. L., Schoenberg J. B., Mayne S. T., Dubrow R., Rotterdam H., West A. B.,

Blaser M., Blot W. J., Gail M. H., Fraumeni J. F. Jr. Population attributable risks of esophageal and gastric cancers. *J Natl Cancer Inst* 2003; **95**(18), 1404–1413.

19. Montalto G., Cervello M., Giannitrapani L., Dantona F., Terranova A., Castagnetta L. A. Epidemiology, risk factors, and natural history of hepatocellular carcinoma. *Ann NY Acad Sci* 2002; **963**, 13–20.

20. Brown L. M., Silverman D. T., Pottern L. M., Schoenberg J. B., Greenberg R. S., Swanson G. M., Liff J. M., Schwartz A. G., Hayes R. B., Blot W. J., *et al.* Adenocarcinoma of the esophagus and esophagogastric junction in white men in the United States: alcohol, tobacco, and socioeconomic factors. *Cancer Causes Control* 1994; **5**(4), 333–340.

21. Gammon M. D., Schoenberg J. B., Ahsan H., Risch H. A., Vaughan T. L., Chow W. H., Rotterdam H., West A. B., Dubrow R., Stanford J. L., Mayne S. T., Farrow D. C., Niwa S., Blot W. J., Fraumeni J. F. Jr. Tobacco, alcohol, and socioeconomic status and adenocarcinomas of the esophagus and gastric cardia. *J Natl Cancer Inst* 1997; **89**(17), 1277–1284.

22. Pischon T., Lahmann P. H., Boeing H., Friedenreich C., Norat T., Tjonneland A., *et al.* Body size and risk of colon and rectal cancer in the European Prospective Investigation Into Cancer and Nutrition (EPIC). *J Natl Cancer Inst* 2006; **98**(13), 920–931.

23. McPherson K., Steel C. M., Dixon J. M., ABC of breast diseases. Breast cancer – epidemiology, risk factors, and genetics. *Br Med J* 2000; **321**(7261), 624–628.

24. Chow W. H., Blot W. J., Vaughan T. L., Risch H. A., Gammon M. D., Stanford J. L. Dubrow R., Schoenberg J. B., Mayne S. T., Farrow D. C., Ahsan H., West A. B., Rotterdam H., Niwa S., Fraumeni J. F. Jr. Body mass index and risk of adenocarcinomas of the esophagus and gastric cardia. *J Natl Cancer Inst* 1998; **90**(2), 150–155.

25. Lagergren J., Bergstrom R., Nyren O. Association between body mass and adenocarcinoma of the esophagus and gastric cardia. *Ann Intern Med* 1999; **130**(11), 883–890.

26. Wu A. H., Wan P., Bernstein L. A multiethnic population-based study of smoking, alcohol and body size and risk of adenocarcinomas of the stomach and esophagus (United States). *Cancer Causes Control* 2001; **12**(8), 721–732.

27. Crew K. D., Neugut A. I. Epidemiology of upper gastrointestinal malignancies. *Semin Oncol* 2004; **31**(4), 450–464.

28. Weiderpass E., Persson I., Adami H. O., Magnusson C., Lindgren A., Baron J. A. Body size in different periods of life, diabetes mellitus, hypertension, and risk of postmenopausal endometrial cancer (Sweden). *Cancer Causes Control* 2000; **11**(2), 185–192.

29. De Luca L. M., Ross S. A. Beta-carotene increases lung cancer incidence in cigarette smokers. *Nutr Rev* 1996; **54**(6), 178–180.

30. Cronin K. A., Krebs-Smith S. M., Feuer E. J., Troiano R. P., Ballard-Barbash R. Evaluating the impact of population changes in diet, physical activity, and weight status on population risk for colon cancer (United States). *Cancer Causes Control* 2001; **12**(4), 305–316.

31. Terry M. B., Gaudet M. M., Gammon M. D. The epidemiology of gastric cancer. *Semin Radiat Oncol* 2002; **12**(2), 111–127.

32. American Cancer Society. *Common Questions about Diet and Cancer*, http://www.cancer.org/docroot/PED/content/PED_3_2X_Common_ Questions_About_ Diet_and_Cancer.asp?sitearea=PED, accessed 12/06.

33. American Cancer Society. *Cancer Prevention and Early Detection – Facts and Figures*, 2005, http://www.cancer.org/downloads/STT/CPED2005v5PWSecured.pdf, accessed 12/06.

34. El-Agamey A., Lowe G. M., McGarvey D. J., Mortensen A., Phillip D. M., Truscott T. G., Young A. J. Carotenoid radical chemistry and antioxidant/pro-oxidant properties. *Arch Biochem Biophys* 2004; **430**(1), 37–48.

35. Wactawski-Wende J., Kotchen J. M., Anderson G. L., *et al.* Calcium plus vitamin D supplementation and the risk of colorectal cancer. *N Engl J Med* 2006; **354**(7), 752–754.

36. Holt P. R., Bresalier R. S, Ma C. K., Liu K. F. *et al.* Calcium plus vitamin D alters preneoplastic features of colorectal adenomas and rectal mucosa. *Cancer* 2006; **106**(2), 287–296.

37. Carroll D. G. Nonhormonal therapies for hot flashes in menopause. *Am Fam Physician* 2006; **73**(3), 457–464.

38. Jellin J. M., Gregory P. J., Batz F., Hitchens K., *et al.*, eds. *Natural medicines in clinical management of menopausal symptoms. Pharmacist's Letter/Prescriber's Letter, Natural Medicines Comprehensive Database.* www.naturaldatabase.com, accessed 11/06.

39. Agency for Healthcare Research and Quality. Management of menopause-related symptoms. *Summary, Evidence Report/Technology Assessment: Number 120.* AHRQ Publication No. 05-E016–1, March 2005. Rockville, MD: AHRQ, 2005, http://www.ahrq.gov/clinic/epcsums/menosum.htm, acessed 11/06.

40. Scott G. N. Soy for preventing aging effects in older women. *Prescribers lett* 2004; **20**, 200914.

41. Tice J. A., Ettinger B., Ensrud K., *et al.* Phytoestrogen supplements for the treatment of hot flashes: the

isoflavone clover extract (ICE) study. *J Am Med Assoc* 2003; **290**(2), 207–214.

42. Dodin S., Lemay A., Jacques H., *et al.* The effects of flaxseed dietary supplement on lipid profile, bone mineral density, and symptoms in menopausal women: a randomized, double-blind, wheat germ placebo-controlled clinical trial. *J Clin Endocrinol Metab* 2005; **90**(3), 1390–1397.

43. North American Menopause Society. *Mother Nature's Treatment for Hot Flashes*, Menopause Flashes 2006, http://www.menopause.org/hotflashes.htm, accessed 1/07.

44. Treatment of menopause-associated vasomotor symptoms: position statement of the North American Menopause Society. *Menopause* 2004; **11**(1), 11–33.

45. Hedley A. A., Ogden C. L., Johnson C. L., Carroll M. D., Curtin L. R., Flegal K. M. Prevalence of overweight and obesity among US children, adolescents, and adults, 1999–2002. *J Am Med Assoc* 2004; **291**, 2847–2850.

46. Ramlo-Halsted B. A., Edelman S. V. The natural history of type 2 diabetes: implications for clinical practice. *Primary Care Clin Office Pract* 1999; **26**, 771–789.

47. McTigue K. M., Hess R., Ziouras J. Obesity in older adults: a systematic review of the evidence for diagnosis and treatment. *Obesity* 2006; **14**, 1485–1497.

48. Lyznicki J. M., Young D. C., Riggs J. A., Davis R. M. Obesity: assessment and management in primary care. *Am Fam Physician* 2001; **65**, 2185–2196.

49. National Heart, Lung, and Blood Institute. *Clinical Guidelines on the Identification, Evaluation, and Treatment of Overweight and Obesity in Adults: The Evidence Report*, NIH Publication no. 98–4083, September 1998, http://www.nhlbi.nih.gov/guidelines/obesity/ob_gdlns.pdf, accessed 1/07.

50. USDA. *The 1987–88 Nationwide Food Consumption Survey (NFCS)*, http://www.ars.usda.gov/Services/docs.htm?docid=7804, accessed 12/06.

51. Cho S., Dietrich M., Brown C. J. P., Clark C. A., Block G. The effect of breakfast type on total daily energy intake and body mass index: results from the Third National Health and Nutrition Examination Survey (NHANES III). *J Am Coll Nutr* 2003; **22**(4), 296–302.

52. Ma Y., Bertone E. R., Stanek E. J., Reed G. W., Hebert J. R., Cohen N. L., Merriam P. A., Ockene I. S. Association between eating patterns and obesity in a free-living US adult population. *Am J Epidemiol* 2003; **158**(1), 85–92.

53. Song W. O., Chun O. K., Obayashi S., Cho S., Chung C. E. Is consumption of breakfast associated with body mass index in US adults? *J Am Diet Assoc* 2005; **105**, 1373–1382.

54. Martin A., Normand S., Sothier M., Peyrat J., Louche-Pelissier C., Laville M. Is advice for breakfast consumption justified? Results from a short-term dietary and metabolic experiment in young healthy men. *Br J Nutr* 2000; **84**, 337–344.

55. Schlundt D. G., Hill J. O., Sbrocco T., Pope-Cordle J., Sharp T. The role of breakfast in the treatment of obesity: a randomized clinical trial. *Am J Clin Nutr* 1992; **55**, 645–651.

56. Wyatt H. R., Grunwald G. K., Mosca C. L., Klem M. L., Wing R. R., Hill J. O. Long-term weight loss and breakfast in subjects in the National Weight Control Registry. *Obesity Res* 2002; **10**(2), 78–82.

57. American Dietetic Association. Eating frequency and patterns, *Evidence Analysis Library*, http://www.adaevidencelibrary.com/, accessed 10/06.

58. LaHaye S. A., Hollett P. M., Vyselaar J. R., Shalchi M., Lahey K. A., Day A. G. Comparison between a low glycemic load diet and a Canada Food Guide diet in cardiac rehabilitation patients in Ontario. *Can J Cardiol* 2005; **21**(6), 489–494.

59. Bouche C., Rizkalla S. W., Luo J., Vidal H., Veronese A., Pacher N., Fouquet C., Lang V., Slama G. Five-week, low-glycemic index diet decreases total fat mass and improves plasma lipid profile in moderately overweight nondiabetic men. *Diabetes Care* 2002; **25**, 822–828.

60. Blanck H. M., Khan L. K., Serdula M. K. Prescription weight loss pill use among Americans: patterns of pill use and lessons learned from the fen-phen market withdrawal. *Prev Med* 2004; **39**, 1243–1248.

61. Kruger J., Galuska D. A., Serdula M. K., *et al.* Attempting to lose weight: specific practices among US adults. *Am J Prev Med* 2004; **26**(5), 402–406.

62. American Dietetic Association. *Evidence Library*, www.adaevidencelibrary.com/, accessed 11/06.

63. American Dietetic Association. Adult weight management, low carbohydrate diets, *Evidence Analysis Library*, http://www.adaevidencelibrary.com/conclusion.cfm?conclusion_statement_id=250234, accessed 12/06.

64. American Dietetic Association. Adult weight management, meal replacement diets, *Evidence Analysis Library*, http://www.adaevidencelibrary.com/conclusion.cfm?conclusion_statement_id=250237, accessed 12/06.

65. Fisher M. The course and outcome of eating disorders in adults and in adolescents: a review. *Adolesc Med State Art Rev* 2003; **14**, 149–158.

66. American Diabetes Association. Position statement: standards of medical care in diabetes – 2006. *Diabetes Care* 2006; **29**, S4–S42.

67. Cryer P. E., Fisher J. N., Shamoon H. Hypoglycemia (technical review). *Diabetes Care* 1994; **17**, 734–755.

68. Mosca L., Appel L. J., *et al.* AHA Scientific Statement. Evidence-based guidelines for cardiovascular disease prevention in women. *Circulation* 2004; **109**, 672–693.

69. Katan M. B., Zock P. L., Mensink R. P. Effects of fats and fatty acids on blood lipids in humans: an overview. *Am J Clin Nutr* 1994; **60**(suppl), 1017S–1022S.

70. Mozaffarian D., Katan M. B., Ascherio A., *et al.* Trans fatty acids and cardiovascular disease. *N Engl J Med* 2006; **354**(15), 1601–1613.

71. Hu F. B., Willett W. C. Optimal diets for prevention of coronary heart disease. *J Am Med Assoc* 2002; **288**, 2569–2578.

72. O'Mara N. B. Fish and fish oil and cardiovascular disease. *Prescriber's Lett* 2002; **9**, 180510.

73. American Heart Association. *Fish and Omega-3 Fatty Acids*, http://www.americanheart.org/presenter.jhtml?identifier=4632, accessed 12/06.

74. Gavagan T. Cardiovascular disease. *Prim Care* 2002; **29**(2), 323–338. http://home.mdconsult.com/das/journal/view/24073294/N/12597644?ja=288950&PAGE=1.html&sid=145542255&source=, accessed 10/06.

75. Jellin J. M., Gregory P. J., Batz F., Hitchens K., *et al.* eds. Natural medicines in clinical management of hyperlipidemia. *Pharmacist's Letter/Prescriber's Letter Natural Medicines Comprehensive Database*. Stockton, CA: Therapeutic Research Faculty, updated 8/16/06. www.naturaldatabase.com, accessed 8/21/06.

76. American Dietetic Association. Disorders of lipid metabolism evidence based nutrition practice guideline, *Evidence Analysis Library*, www.adaevidencelibrary.com.

77. Vollmer W. M., Sacks F. M., Ard J., *et al.* Effects of diet and sodium intake on blood pressure: subgroup analysis of the DASHG-Sodium trial. *Ann Intern Med* 2001; **135**, 1019–1028.

78. Sacks F. M., Svetkey L. P., Vollmer W. M., *et al.* Effects on blood pressure of reduced dietary sodium and the dietary approaches to stop hypertension (DASH) diet. *N Engl J Med* 2001; **344**, 3–10.

79. Keevil J., Stein J. H., McBride P. E. Cardiovascular disease prevention. *Prim Care* 2002; **29**(3). http://home.mdconsult.com/das/journal/view/24073294/N/12597673?ja=295124&PAGE=1.html&sid=145544570 &source=, accessed 11/02.

80. NHLBI JNC-7. http://www.nhlbi.nih.gov/guidelines/hypertension/jncintro.htm, accessed 10/06.

81. Whelton P. K., He J., Cutler J. A., *et al.* Effects of oral potassium on blood pressure. Meta-analysis of randomized controlled clinical trials. *J Am Med Assoc* 1997; **277**, 1624–1632.

82. Van Mierlo L. A. J., Arends L. R., Streppel M. T., *et al.* Blood pressure response to calcium supplementation: a meta-analysis of randomized controlled trials. *J Hum Hypertension* 2006; **20**, 571–580.

83. Song Y., Sesso H. D., Manson J. E. Dietary magnesium intake and risk of incident hypertension among middle-aged and older US women in a 10 year follow-up study. *Am J Cardiol* 2006; **98**(12), 1616–1621.

84. Sacks F. M., Willett W. C., Smith A., Brown L. E., Rosner B., Moore T. J. Effect on blood pressure of potassium, calcium, and magnesium in women with low habitual intake. *Hypertension* 1998; **31**, 131–138.

85. Xin X., He J., Frontini M. F. Effects of alcohol reduction on blood pressure: a meta-analysis of randomized controlled trials. *Hypertension* 2001; **38**, 1112–1117.

86. Appel L. J., Moore T. J., Obarzanek E., *et al.* A clinical trial of the effects of dietary patterns on blood pressure. *N Engl J Med* 1997; **336**, 1117–1124.

87. Whelton P. K., He J., Appel L. J., *et al.* Primary prevention of hypertension: clinical and public health advisory from the national high blood pressure education program. *J Am Med Assoc* 2002; **288**, 1882–1888.

88. Berger A. M., Clark-Snow R. A. Adverse effects of treatment. In Devita V. T., Hellman S., Rosenberg S. A. eds., *Cancer Principles and Practice of Oncology*. Philadelphia, PA: Lippincott-Raven, 1997, p. 2705.

89. Ravasco P. Aspects of taste and compliance in patients with cancer. *Eur J Oncol Nurs* 2005; **9**(Suppl 2), S84–S91.

90. de Godoy I., Donahoe M., Calhoun W. J., *et al.* Elevated TNF production by peripheral blood monocytes of weight losing COPD patients. *Am J Respir Crit Care Med* 1996; **153**, 633–637.

91. Ferreira I. M., Brooks D., Lacasse Y., *et al.* Nutritional support for individuals with COPD: a metaanalysis. *Chest* 2000; **117**, 672–678.

92. Fiaccadori E., Coffrini E., Ronda N., *et al.* A preliminary report on the effects of malnutrition on skeletal muscle composition in chronic obstructive pulmonary disease. In Ferranti R. D., Rampulla C., Fracchia C., Ambrosino N., eds., *Nutrition and Ventilatory Function*, Verona: Bi and GI Publishers, 1992.

93. Fuld J. P., Kilduff L. P., Neder J. A., Pitsiladis Y., Lean M. E., Ward S. A., Cotton M. M. Creatine supplementation during pulmonary rehabilitation in chronic obstructive pulmonary disease. *Thorax* 2005; **60**(7), 531–537.

94. Schols A. M., Soeters P. B., Mostert R., *et al.* Physiologic effects of nutritional support anabolic steroid in patients with obstructive pulmonary disease: a placebo-controlled randomized trial. *Am J Respir Crit Care Med* 1995; **152**, 1268–1274.

95. Griffiths T. L., Proud D. Creatine supplementation as an exercise performance enhancer for patients with COPD? An idea to run with. *Thorax* 2005; **60**(7), 525–526.

96. Berry J. K., Baum C. L. Malnutrition in chronic obstructive pulmonary disease: adding insult to injury. *AACN Clin Issues* 2001; **12**, 210–219.

97. Schwartz J. Role of polyunsaturated fatty acids in lung disease. *Am J Clin Nutr* 2000; **71**(Suppl), 393S–396S.

98. Matsuyama W., Mitsuyama H., Watanabe M., Oonakahara K., Higashimoto I., Osame M., Arimura K. Effects of omega-3 polyunsaturated fatty acids on inflammatory markers in COPD. *Chest* 2005; **128**(6), 3817–3827.

99. Allen J. The therapeutic use of fish oil. *Prescriber's Lett* 1997; **4**, 130624.

100. Smit H. A., Grievink L., Tabak C. Dietary influences on chronic obstructive lung disease and asthma: a review of the epidemiological evidence. *Proc Nutr Soc* 1999; **58**, 309–319.

101. Messier S. P., Loeser R. F., Miller G. D., *et al.* Exercise and dietary weight loss in overweight and obese older adults with knee osteoarthritis: the arthritis, diet, and activity promotion trial. *Arthritis Rheum* 2004; **50**(5), 1501–1510.

102. Lyu L.-C., Hsu C.-Y., Yeh C.-Y., *et al.* A case-control study of the association of diet and obesity with gout in Taiwan. *Am J Clin Nutr* 2003; **78**, 690–701.

103. Choi H. K., Atkinson K., Karlson E. W., *et al.* Purine-rich foods, dairy and protein intake, and the risk of gout in men. *N Engl J Med* 2004; **350**, 1093–1103.

104. Scott G. N. Natural alternatives to rofecoxib (Vioxx). *Pharmacist's Lett/Prescriber's Lett* 2004; **20**(12), 201210.

105. Clegg D. O., Reda D. J., Harris C. L., *et al.* Glucosamine, chondroitin sulfate, and the two in combination for painful knee osteoarthritis. *N Engl J Med* 2006; **354**(8), 795–808.

106. Jellin J. M., Gregory P. J., Batz F., Hitchens K., *et al.* eds. Natural medicines in clinical management of osteoarthritis. *Pharmacist's Letter/Prescriber's Letter Natural Medicines Comprehensive Database.* Stockton, CA: Therapeutic Research Faculty, updated 8/16/06. www.naturaldatabase.com, accessed 8/21/06.

107. FPIN's clinical inquiries: glucosamine and chondroitin for osteoarthritis. *Am Fam Physician* 2006; **73**(7), 1245–1247.

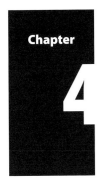

Chapter

4

Physical activity and exercise

Tanya A. Miszko

Introduction

For our ancestors, physical activity was engrained in daily life. In the early 1900s before automobiles were invented and mass-produced, walking was a common mode of transportation. Today, automobiles are used for leisurely one-mile drives to the local video store or half-mile treks to the grocery store. Improved technology has reduced our physical activity level by making life "easier."

This "easier" way of life has led to increases in cardiovascular disease, hypertension, high cholesterol, strokes, heart attacks, osteoporosis, obesity, and diabetes mellitus. Cardiovascular disease is the leading cause of death for women in the United States. The American Heart Association states that one in five women has some form of blood vessel or heart disease, 5.7 million women have physician-diagnosed diabetes mellitus, and almost half (46.8%) of non-Hispanic white women are overweight; 23.2% are obese (www.aha.org). Genetics cannot be ruled out as a contributing factor to these chronic conditions, but it must also not be an excuse.

In addition to increased morbidity, physical inactivity also has a direct effect on the economy, amounting to $76 billion of US health care expenditures.[1] In 2000, obesity related medical costs totaled $117 billion (www.cdc.gov). The yearly cost of medical care for a physically active individual is approximately $330 less than that for an inactive person. Furthermore, if 10% of inactive people became active, $5.6 billion in heart disease costs could be saved (www.cdc.gov). Intuitively, these data would be an incentive for health insurance companies to embrace interventions that focus on the prevention of disease; however, that medical paradigm is not yet emphasized. Because medical costs increase around age 45

to 54 for inactive women, this is a perfect time for women to take charge of their physical, as well as financial, health.[1]

Benefits of exercise

Hattie is a 55-year-old first grade teacher. She has had diet-controlled type II diabetes for 2 years, although her last hemoglobin A1C was 7.8% and her morning fasting blood sugars are running 150 to 180 mg/dL. She weighs 185 lbs. At her regular follow-up, you discuss the effects of exercise and the possibility that it might reduce her sugars and her weight. She shrugs, saying that she is on her feet all day and that should be enough exercise.

A distinction must be made between physical activity and exercise. Physical activity refers to any bodily movement produced by skeletal muscles that results in energy expenditure, such as mowing the lawn, grocery shopping, and doing household chores.[2] Exercise, on the other hand, is physical activity with the purpose of improving some component(s) of fitness (muscle strength and endurance, cardiorespiratory endurance, body composition, and/or flexibility), such as regular participation in an endurance-training or strength-training program at an intensity that will confer physiological and performance benefits.[3]

Exercise and physical activity can improve most aspects of mental and physical health.[4,5,6] The benefits derived, however, are specific to the type of exercise performed (Table 4.1).

Regular physical activity

Moderate levels of physical activity have significant effects on a woman's health. Burning approximately

Handbook of Women's Health, second edition, ed. Jo Ann Rosenfeld. Published by Cambridge University Press.
© Cambridge University Press 2009.

Table 4.1 Benefits of exercise

Resistance training	Endurance training	Yoga	Tai Chi
Increases muscle strength	Increases aerobic capacity	Increases muscular strength and endurance	Reduces fall rate
Increases type II fiber area	Reduces blood pressure	Increases flexibility	Decreases depression
Increases muscle cross-sectional area	Increases bone mineral density	Increases aerobic capacity	Increases positive affect
Increases or preserves bone mineral density	Reduces anxiety (state and trait)		
	Reduces fatigue in cancer patients		

150 kilocalories per day or 1,000 kilocalories per week leads to a reduction in the risk of coronary heart disease by 50% and of hypertension, diabetes, and colon cancer by 30%.[7] After adjusting for covariates such as age, smoking, alcohol use, history of hypertension, and history of high cholesterol, women who are regularly physically active are 50% less likely to develop type II diabetes (relative risk = 0.54) than women who are not regularly active.[8] Vasomotor and psychosomatic symptoms associated with menopause are also reduced with moderate amounts of activity.[5,9] Examples of moderate levels of physical activity are depicted in Table 4.2.

Regular physical activity can also reduce the risk of colon cancer, the third leading cause of cancer incidence and mortality in the United States. The risk of colon cancer is reduced 40% to 50% in highly active people compared to low active individuals.[10] The mechanisms responsible for a reduction in the risk of colon cancer are

- a reduced transit time in the bowel which decreases exposure to carcinogens,
- a reduction in insulin action which decreases colon mucosal cells,
- an increase in prostaglandin F2 α which increases intestinal motility, and
- a reduction in prostaglandin E2 which increases colon cell proliferation.

The evidence for exercise providing a reduction in the risk of breast cancer, however, is equivocal. In a cohort of 37,105 women who exercised regularly, there was lower risk of breast cancer compared to those who did not.[11] The Nurses' Health Study suggests that the risk of breast cancer and mortality from

Table 4.2 Examples of moderate levels of physical activity

LESS VIGOROUS, MORE TIME

Washing a car for 45–60 minutes

Playing volleyball for 45 minutes

Gardening for 30–45 minutes

Wheeling self in wheelchair for 30–40 minutes

Walking 1.75 miles in 35 minutes (20 min/mile pace)

Basketball (shooting baskets) for 30 minutes

Bicycling 5 miles in 30 minutes

Pushing a stroller 1.5 miles in 30 minutes

Raking leaves for 30 minutes

Walking 2 miles in 30 minutes (15 min/mile pace)

Dancing fast (social) for 30 minutes

Water aerobics for 30 minutes

Bicycling 4 miles in 15 minutes

Jumping rope for 15 minutes

Shoveling snow for 15 minutes

Walking stairs for 15 minutes

MORE VIGOROUS, LESS TIME

Source: Adapted from US Department of Health and Human Services. *Physical Activity and Health: A Report of the Surgeon General*, Atlanta, GA: US Department of Health and Human Services, Centers for Disease Control and Prevention, 1996.

breast cancer is reduced in physically active women.[12,13] Decreased body fat and estrogen levels may be responsible for the reduction in breast cancer risk associated with exercise.[14] Although epidemiological evidence supports a positive relationship between physical activity and cancer rates, more research is needed in this area to substantiate the protective effect of exercise against specific cancers.

Small increases in physical activity level and subsequently energy expenditure have a positive effect on psychological outcomes and physiological parameters in most, but especially middle-aged women. Women who increase their level of physical activity by at least 300 kilocalories per week have a smaller reduction in HDL cholesterol with advancing age and are less depressed and stressed than those women who remain at their current activity level.[15] Women who are physically active have higher resting metabolic rates and lower body fat, but similar fat-free mass, body mass index, and body weight compared to their sedentary counterparts.[16] These results suggest that physical activity is a component of a healthy lifestyle.

Resistance training

Although resistance training has been proven to alter positively some modifiable risk factors for disease (obesity, hypertension, low bone mass, etc.), fewer than 20% of the US population between the ages of 18 to 64 years and fewer than 12% of adults over the age of 65 years regularly participate in a resistance-training program.[17] Women who participate in a resistance-training program increase muscle strength and power, alter muscle ultrastructure (type II fiber area), increase or preserve bone mineral density, and improve cardiovascular risk factors for disease.[18,19]

Muscle strength and power are compromised during a woman's middle-aged years because of age-associated changes in the muscle ultrastructure.[20] In a sedentary individual, maximal strength is reduced approximately 7.5% to 8.5% per decade beginning around age 30 and muscle power is reduced approximately 35% per decade.[21] This reduction is relative to the remaining strength and power, so that muscle power in a 50-year-old woman is 35% less than it was when she was 40 years old, but 35% more than she will have when she is 60-years old. Considering that muscle power is lost at a faster rate than muscle strength after age 65 and that muscle power is significantly related to functional performance,[22] having a high strength and power base

before this age could protect against losses later in life, thus serving as a buffer to functional decline.

Regular participation in a resistance-training program has profound effects on muscle ultrastructure. Resistance training attenuates the loss in muscle cross-sectional area, type II fiber area, strength, and bone mineral density commonly associated with aging.[23] Significant increases in maximum torque, electromyography, maximal strength, and type II mean fiber area have been observed in middle-aged women after participating in an explosive-strength training program.

Cross-sectional and longitudinal exercise data support the efficacy of resistance training as an effective modality for the prevention and treatment of osteoporosis. A recent meta-analysis demonstrated that resistance training can increase or preserve bone mineral density in premenopausal and postmenopausal women.[24] With the cessation of exercise, bone mineral density will return to pre-exercise levels at a rate similar to age-matched controls. Thus, the continued participation in a resistance-training program is essential for bone health.

Endurance training

> Sarah is a 42-year-old bank teller with no known cardiac risk factors who was found to have a fasting total cholesterol level of 299 mg/dL with an LDL of 179 mg/dl at a recent screening. After 3 months of vigorous change of diet to a low-fat diet, she returns for a fasting lipid profile. Total cholesterol has only decreased to 245 mg/dL with an LDL of 145. She asks what else she can do without starting on pharmacotherapy.
>
> You suggest walking three times a week for 30 minutes each day as a form of exercise. She agrees; six months later, she has lost 4.5 kg, and her total cholesterol level is 195 mg/dl, with an LDL of 120 mg/dL.

Endurance training can reduce some of the risk factors associated with cardiovascular disease such as hypertension, high cholesterol, and inactivity. As little as two to three days per week are required to gain health benefits from a moderate-intensity (50% maximum oxygen consumption) endurance training program. These health benefits include a reduction in blood pressure, total cholesterol, body mass index, and an increase in HDL cholesterol.[25,26] Brisk walking for three or more hours per week can reduce the risk of cardiac events in middle-aged women (relative risk = 0.65).[27] Becoming physically active also reduces the risk of cardiac events; exercise is preventive medicine.

Despite the age-associated reduction in aerobic capacity, endurance training can have a positive effect on the cardiovascular system. On average, maximal aerobic capacity declines at a rate of approximately 7.5% to 9% per decade after age 25.[28] Although endurance athletes have a greater absolute rate of decline in aerobic capacity than sedentary women, their relative (ml/kg·min^{-1}) rate of decline in aerobic capacity is smaller.[29] Older endurance trained women have higher aerobic capacities throughout life, thus serving as a physiological reserve against functional decline.

In addition to improvements in the cardiovascular system, endurance exercise also improves a woman's psychological outlook and the skeletal system. Women who exercise regularly are less neurotic, have greater self-esteem, and are more satisfied with life compared to their sedentary counterparts.[30] Weight bearing activities such as walking increase or preserve bone mineral density by approximately 5%.[31] However, as with resistance training, the positive effects of exercise are negated when exercise is discontinued or reduced (fewer than 3 days per week). Regular exercise clearly has a significant impact on the human body.

Non-traditional exercise

Non-traditional styles of exercise, such as Yoga and Tai Chi, have also demonstrated positive improvements in health.[32] Yoga involves various standing, seated, and supine postures and breathing and relaxation techniques designed to enhance functioning of the various physiological systems by supporting a natural posture. Tai Chi incorporates slow body movements (forms) that concentrate on balance and body weight transfers. Young and old men and women have performed yoga and Tai Chi for centuries in Eastern countries. Both have been purported to focus concentration and relax the body.

Yoga practice has been shown to improve muscular strength, endurance, flexibility, gait parameters, and aerobic capacity.[6] Evidence suggests that yoga practice reduces sympathetic activity, improves aerobic capacity, reduces perceived exertion after maximal exercise, and reduces heart rate and left ventricular end diastolic volume at rest. From a functional perspective, people who practice yoga demonstrate improved gait parameters, reduced pain and symptoms associated with knee osteoarthritis, and

reduced disability, which collectively or independently has the potential to reduce the risk of falls.[33] When compared to standard care for chronic low back pain, yoga is more effective at reducing pain, use of medications, and improving physical function.[34] Additionally, yoga practice may retard the progression and increase the regression of atherosclerosis in patients with coronary artery disease. Thus, research demonstrates yoga's efficacy to improve health.

Tai Chi practice improves mood states, physical function, and hemodynamic parameters.[35] A reduction in anger, total mood disturbance, tension, confusion, and depression and an increase in self-efficacy are evident after regular Tai Chi practice.[35] Improvements in self-reported physical function and a reduction in falls is also reported.[36] Patients suffering from acute myocardial infarction can reduce blood pressure after practicing Tai Chi.[37] Tai Chi is an effective modality for improving several aspects of health.

Empirical evidence has demonstrated the positive benefits of exercise, such as improved strength, reduced anxiety, improved blood lipid profile, and decreased risk of cardiovascular disease. The modality required to obtain these benefits can vary from a structured exercise program (resistance training and walking/running) and non-traditional programs (yoga and Tai Chi) to daily physical activity (mowing the lawn and climbing stairs).

Exercise prescription for healthy populations

The type of exercise performed depends on the desired goal. If a woman wants to build muscular strength, then resistance training is appropriate. Endurance training (walking, running, cycling, swimming) is required if a woman wants to improve her cardiovascular health and endurance. Yoga and Tai Chi are therapeutic alternatives to the rigors of strength and endurance training that can reduce stress, increase strength and flexibility, and improve cardiovascular parameters. A certified yoga or Tai Chi instructor should be consulted for more information on the styles of each.

Resistance training

Resistance training is the mode of exercise performed to stimulate the neuromuscular system. Variations of the number of sets, repetitions, rest period, and

Table 4.3 Resistance training exercises

Muscle group	Exercise
Quadriceps and hamstrings	Squat*
	Lunge*
	Leg press*
	Leg curl
	Step-up*
Pectoralis major and minor	Bench press (barbell or dumbbell)*
	Push-up*
	Fly
Lumbar extensors, latissimus dorsi, rhomboids	Lat pull-down*
	Row (seated or dumbbell)*
	Trunk extension
	Side lateral raise
Deltoids	Rear deltoid raise
	Military press (with dumbbells)*
Triceps and biceps	Triceps extension (cable, single arm or double arm)
	Biceps curl (dumbbell or barbell)

Note: *Multi-joint exercises

weight lifted determines the outcome of the training program. Programs designed to increase strength are typically performed at a high intensity (80% of the one-repetition maximum, 1RM) with long rest periods (2 to 3 minutes) and low to moderate volume (2 to 3 sets of 8 to 10 repetitions), whereas programs designed to promote muscle hypertrophy are performed at a moderate to high intensity (60% to 80% 1RM) with shorter rest periods (30 to 60 seconds) and higher volume (3 to 4 sets of 10 to 12 repetitions).[38] A 5% increase in resistance is suggested when 12 to 15 repetitions can be performed.

In a generally healthy population, resistance training can be performed with exercise machines or with free weights. Examples of resistance training exercises are provided in Table 4.3. Multi-joint, multi-planar exercises commonly associated with free weights may be more functional because their motor patterns mimic motor patterns of daily tasks.[39]

Machines offer more safety for beginners and isolate muscle groups more so than free weights; however, free weights require an individual to use accessory/stabilizer muscles as they would naturally do in daily life and improve strength more than training on machines.[40] Free weights also concurrently train balance, strength, and coordination – similar to the demands of daily activities. Household items (rice bags, jugs of water, soup cans, etc.) and elastic resistance bands can also be used for resistance instead of metal weights or a cable system. For an individual with no resistance training experience, machines should be used initially to increase strength so that a progression to free weights can be safely made.

The design of the program is somewhat more of an art than a strict, regimented science. Science provides the basis for sound training principles, but creativity is needed to continually manipulate the training volume, exercise selection, and order of exercise. The exercise prescription can be written for specific combinations of muscle groups (back and hamstrings, chest and arms, etc.), agonist versus antagonist (leg extension versus leg curl, chest press versus seated row), and upper versus lower body (legs on Monday then chest, back, and shoulders on Tuesday, etc.) muscle groups.

Regardless of the design of the program, specific guidelines should be followed. Within each session, individuals should perform large muscle groups (prime movers) before smaller muscle groups (secondary movers) to avoid fatigue of the larger muscles. However, smaller stabilizing muscles (rotator cuff, hip adductor/abductor, neck muscles, etc.) should not be neglected. If left untrained, these smaller stabilizing muscles are at risk of injury. The Valsalva maneuver, holding the breath during exertion, should never be performed. To avoid a reduction in venous return to the heart and a significant increase in blood pressure, individuals should exhale on exertion. As always, medical clearance should be sought prior to beginning an exercise program if an individual has a condition that may be made worse by exercise.

Endurance training

The cardiovascular system is most effectively improved by endurance training. Endurance training involves rhythmic movements of large muscle groups. For example, running/walking, bicycling, swimming,

47

and dancing are effective and common modes of endurance exercise. However, a combination of modalities within an exercise session might provide extra motivation and reduce boredom.

The exercise prescription for endurance training offers variety, similar to resistance training. The American College of Sports Medicine recommends 20 to 60 minutes a day, 3 to 5 days per week at an intensity equal to 60% to 90% of age-predicted maximum heart rate ($HR_{max} = 220 -$ age).[41] Intensity and duration are inversely related, so that a reduction in intensity requires an increase in duration. Any of these variables can be manipulated within and between exercise sessions. For example, in a three day a week exercise program, day 1 is 40 minutes of treadmill walking at 65% HR_{max}, day 2 is 10 minutes of bicycling at 70% HR_{max}, 10 minutes of intervals at 90% HR_{max}, then 5 minutes at 60% HR_{max}, and day 3 is 20 minutes of swimming at 80% HR_{max}. All three variations can provide health and fitness benefits.

To maximize benefits and reduce the risk of injury, specific guidelines should be followed. Because large muscle groups utilize more oxygen and generate more adenosine triphosphate (ATP) than smaller muscle groups, they should be incorporated into every exercise routine. Thus, more calories are expended when training larger muscle groups.

Manipulating certain extraneous factors reduces the risk of injury while exercising outdoors. Because the ambient temperature is hottest at mid-day, outdoor exercises should be performed in the morning or evening when the temperature is cooler. Loose fitting, light-colored clothing is appropriate for warmer climates in order to circulate air and facilitate evaporative cooling.[42] In cooler temperatures, however, layers of dark-colored clothing should be worn to trap heat or to be removed as the body temperature rises.[43] The inner layer of clothing should be made from a wicking material that carries moisture away from the body. Proper footwear with a supportive arch and adequate cushioning is also necessary. These guidelines can help improve performance while reducing the risk of injury.

Exercise prescription for special populations

The athletic woman

Exercise prescriptions for a female athlete are specific to the demands of her sport. Differences in energy system requirements dictate the intensity and design of the program. Training of an anaerobic athlete (sprinter, swimmer, etc.) requires high intensity, short duration activities, whereas an aerobic athlete (runner, triathlete, road cyclist, etc.) requires low to moderate intensity for longer durations. Periodized endurance- and strength-training programs alter the training variables (speed, intensity, volume, etc.) to maximize performance. The metabolic demand of the sport should match the metabolic demand of the training sessions. Thus, these programs are sport specific and require assistance from a professional in the field such as a Certified Strength and Conditioning Specialist or an Exercise Physiologist.

The career woman

Women with busy daily schedules can still find time to exercise and take care of their health by manipulating their daily routine. The American College of Sports Medicine has recently stated that 30 minutes of continuous exercise is not necessary to elicit health benefits, rather 30 minutes of total accumulated time is required (a minimum of 10-minute bouts).[44] The time commitment is less restrictive, which allows a woman to plan exercise sessions around her work and family schedule. For example, a 10-minute walk in the morning before work, 10-minute stair climbing during work, and a 10-minute bike ride or walk after dinner would satisfy the recommendation for 30 minutes per day. The intensity should be in the range of 65% to 90% of age-predicted HR_{max} and the exercise should be performed most days of the week.

With respect to strength training, the career woman should focus on multi-joint functional exercises. Utilizing large muscle groups in a whole-body training program increases the metabolic demands of each training session, which elicits a greater caloric expenditure per exercise session. Because leisure time is a limited resource, maximizing the amount of calories burned per workout is highly beneficial and effective.

Middle ages

During a woman's middle-aged years, many physiological changes occur, some of which are modifiable. Regular physical activity can reduce the risk of premature death from coronary artery disease, colon cancer, hypertension, and diabetes mellitus.[3] However, more than 60% of adult Americans are not regularly physically active, 50% of adolescents aged 12–21 years do not participate in vigorous activities, 25% of adult Americans are not active at all, and women continue to be less active than men, regardless of age.[3] The World Health Organization states that "age 50 marks a point in middle age at which the benefits of regular physical activity can be most relevant in avoiding, minimizing, and/or reversing many of the physical, psychological, and social hazards which often accompany advancing age."[45] Middle age is an opportune time for the middle-aged woman to make lifestyle changes and take charge of her life.

While much research is published about the effects of exercise in older (>60 years) and younger (18 to 25 years) women, less is available for middle-aged women (45 to 60 years). This may be due partially to the plethora of physiological changes that are occurring during these years, especially the changes in the hormonal milieu. To capture the exercise needs of women of all ages, exercise prescription guidelines for older and younger women, as well as certain medical conditions/diseases pertaining to aging women and the application of exercise as a primary or secondary preventative tool will be briefly discussed. Regular physical activity and exercise can improve all aspects of health, spirit, mind, and body.

Older women

With an increase in age there are certain physiological changes occurring that impact the ability of an older adult to complete daily tasks. Thus, exercise prescriptions for older adults aim to improve physical function by impacting the most influential variables, such as muscle strength, muscle power, and aerobic capacity. Various exercise programs for older adults have demonstrated efficacy to improve muscle strength, bone mineral density, aerobic capacity, and physical function, and to reduce falls. Recent research has questioned whether power training (fast speed of concentric movement) improves physical function more so than does strength training (slow speed of concentric movement). While power training has been proven to be more effective than strength training for improving certain functional tasks[46] and bone mineral density,[47] strength training repeatedly demonstrates increases in muscle strength, cross-sectional area, improved functional task performance, and preservation of bone mineral density.[48] Based on available evidence, the following regimen can be

prescribed for older adults: strength or power training 2 days/week, 50–85% 1RM, 3 sets of 10–15 repetitions; endurance training 4–5 days/week, 60–70% HR_{max}, 30 minutes/day; flexibility training daily, holding each stretch for 30 seconds.

Adolescents

With an alarming increase in the incidence of obesity, diabetes, and the metabolic syndrome among adolescents in America, the need for regular physical activity and exercise is overwhelming.[49] Diet and exercise can reduce variables of the metabolic syndrome in youth to a level that "declassifies" them as having the metabolic syndrome, meanwhile improving lipid profiles, insulin sensitivity, and reducing blood pressure and body weight.[50,51] Awareness that low body satisfaction in adolescents is associated with health-compromising behaviors (i.e. dieting, unhealthy weight control measures, smoking) suggests that exercise strategies be designed to encourage a healthy body weight and image.[51] Establishing a healthy mind, body, and spirit in adolescence sets the stage for a future of better health and less morbidity.

Strength training should be a component of any exercise program for any woman, regardless of age. A whole-body, multi-joint strength program performed 2 to 3 days per week could include exercises such as a lunge, squat, medicine ball swing, standing dumbbell row, and stability ball dumbbell chest press. (Refer to the list of resources at the end of the chapter for more information.) These exercises can be performed in the home with little equipment needed and can be adapted to fit any schedule and available space.

Disease considerations

The most common causes of morbidity and mortality in the United States are associated with modifiable risk factors, such as obesity, sedentary lifestyle, smoking, and poor diet (www.cdc.gov). Exercise is important as a preventative measure as well as a treatment option for certain diseases, combined with a healthy balanced diet, relaxation practice, and continued supervision/treatment from a physician. Exercise prescriptions can be modified for those persons who have a diagnosed disease. Exercise guidelines are given in Table 4.4 for select diseases.

In November 2000, the Centers for Disease Control and Prevention released a report on the health and economic burden of chronic disease.[52] Seventy

49

Table 4.4 Exercise guidelines for select diseased populations

Disease	Fitness parameter	Mode	Frequency	Intensity	Duration
Arthritis	Aerobic capacity	Non-weight bearing activities, low-impact activities (swimming, cycling)	3–5 days/ week	60–80% peak heart rate**	5–10 minutes to begin then progress to 30–45 minutes
	Muscle strength	Circuit strength training	2–3 days/ week	1–2 sets of 3–12 repetitions (start at 3 and progress to 12)	
	Flexibility	ROM exercises	Every day	Slight discomfort, no pain; never bounce	Hold each position for approximately 30 seconds
Diabetes	Aerobic capacity	Walking, cycling	4–7 days/ week	50–90% peak heart rate**	20–60 minutes/ session
	Muscle strength	Free weights, machines	2–3 days/ week	1–2 sets of 8–10 repetitions	
Osteoporosis	Aerobic capacity	Weight bearing activities (walking, stair climbing)	3–5 days/ week	40–70% peak heart rate**	20–30 minutes/ session
	Muscle strength	Free weights, machines	2 days/ week	2–3 sets of 8 repetitions	
	Flexibility	ROM exercises, stretching	5–7 days/ week	Slight discomfort, no pain; never bounce	Hold each stretched position for approximately 30 seconds
Myocardial infarction	Aerobic capacity	Large muscle activities	3–4 days/ week	40–85% heart rate reserve*	20–40 minutes/ session 5–10 minutes of warm-up and cool-down
	Muscle strength	Circuit training	2–3 days/ week	1–3 sets of 10–15 repetitions	
Valvular heart disease	Aerobic capacity	Large muscle activities	3–7 days/ week	60–85% peak heart rate** (resting heart rate + 30 beats after surgery)	20–60 minutes/ session
	Muscle strength	Machines	2–3 days/ week		
Cancer[†]	Aerobic capacity	Large muscle groups (walking, cycling)	3–5 days/ week	50–75% heart rate reserve	20–30 minutes/ session, continuous

Source: Modified from ACSM's *Exercise Management for Persons with Chronic Diseases and Disabilities*. Champaign, IL: Human Kinetics, 1997.
Notes: [†]From Courneya K. S., Mackey J. R., Jones L. W. Coping with cancer. Can exercise help? *Phys Sports Med* 2000; **28**(5), 49–73.
*Heart rate reserve = [(% intensity)(220 − age − heart rate at rest)] + heart rate at rest.
**Peak heart rate = maximal heart rate obtained during an exercise test.

percent of Americans who die, die of a chronic disease. For women age 35 to 64 years old, cardiovascular disease and lung and breast cancer are the three leading causes of death. One sixth of the American population has arthritis, the primary disabling disorder. Fifty percent of individuals with osteoporosis cannot walk unassisted and 25% require long-term care. Clearly, there is a need for exercise intervention to help mitigate the effects of aging, prevent chronic disease, and enhance quality of life.

Summary

Because of the multitude of physiological changes that start occurring during early middle age, these years are a welcomed opportunity for a woman to directly impact her current and future health. Exercise and physical activity can forestall the age-associated changes (reduced muscle strength, power, aerobic capacity, and bone mineral density) that can lead to dependence and disability. As a minimum, women (and all adults) should be active for at least 30 minutes on most, if not all, days of the week to gain health benefits. To improve certain aspects of fitness (muscular strength, cardiovascular endurance, flexibility, aerobic capacity, body composition), however, a more vigorous exercise regimen would have to be adhered to.

Regular physical activity and exercise result in positive improvements in health and fitness. Moderate amounts of physical activity can reduce the risk of certain types of cancer, heart disease, diabetes, and obesity. Resistance training can preserve or increase bone mineral density, increase muscle fiber area, strength, and power. Endurance training can reduce resting heart rate, improve blood lipid profiles, decrease blood pressure, and increase aerobic capacity. Tai Chi and yoga complement these programs by reducing stress, increasing flexibility, reducing falls, and increasing strength. The available evidence strongly suggests that physical activity and exercise have a positive effect on morbidity and mortality, thus attenuating functional decline and increasing quality of life which could lead to a more able old age. Never let age itself be a deterrent to exercise; the human body is capable of adapting at any age.

Further resources

Books
Chu D. *Explosive Power and Strength*, Champaign, IL: Human Kinetics, 1996.

Coulter H. D., McCall T. *Anatomy of Hatha Yoga: A Manual for Students, Teachers, and Practitioners*, Indianapolis, IN: Body and Breath, 2001, ISBN 0980800601.

Goldenberg L., Twist P. *Strength Ball Training*, Champaign, IL: Human Kinetics, 2002.

Videos
Santana J. C. Functional Training. (Perform Better, 1–888–556–7464)

Santana J. C. The Essence of Stability Ball Training. (Perform Better, 1–888–556–7464)

Johnson M. Tai Chi for Seniors: Self Healing Through Movement. (1–800–497–4244 or http://www.taichiforseniorsvideo.com)

Johnson J. A. Power Tai Chi: Total Body Workout, 1999. (http://www.amazon.com)

On-line yoga classes available at http://www.yoga4realpeople.com.

References

1. Pratt M., Macera C. A., Wang G. Higher direct medical costs associated with physical inactivity. *Phys Sports Med* 2000; **28**(10), 63–70.

2. American College of Sports Medicine. *Guidelines for Exercise Testing and Prescription*. Philadelphia, PA: Lea & Febiger, 1991.

3. US Department of Health and Human Services. *Physical Activity and Health: A Report of the Surgeon General*. Atlanta, GA: US Department of Health and Human Services, Centers for Disease Control and Prevention, National Center for Chronic Disease Prevention and Health Promotion, 1996.

4. Hakkinen K., Kraemer W. J., Newton R. U., Alen M. Changes in electromyographic activity, muscle fibre and force production characteristics during heavy resistance/power training in middle-aged and older men and women. *Acta Physiol Scand* 2001; **171**, 51–62.

5. Slaven L., Lee C. Mood and symptom reporting among middle-aged women: the relationship between menopausal status, hormonal replacement therapy, and exercise participation. *Health Psych* 1997; **16**(3), 203–208.

6. Tran M. D., Holly R. G., Lasbrook J., Amsterdam E. A. Effects of hatha yoga practice on health-related aspects of physical fitness. *Prev Cardiol* 2001; **4**(4), 165–170.

7. Warburton D. E. R., Nicol C. W., Bredin S. S. D. Health benefits of physical activity: the evidence. *Can Med Assoc J* 2006; **174**(6), 801–809.

8. Hu F. B., Sigal R. J., Rich-Edwards J. W., *et al*. Walking compared with vigorous physical activity and risk of

type 2 diabetes in women: a prospective study. *J Am Med Assoc* 1999; **282**(15), 1433–1439.

9. Ueda M., Tokunaga M. Effects of exercise experienced in the life stages on climacteric symptoms for females. *J Physiol Anthropol* 2000; **19**(4), 181–189.

10. Colditz G. A., Cannuscio C. C., Frazier A. L. Physical activity and reduced risk of colon cancer: implications for prevention. *Cancer Causes Control* 1997; **8**, 649–667.

11. Moore D. B., Folsom A. R., Mink P. J., *et al.* Physical activity and incidence of postmenopausal breast cancer. *Epidemiology* 2000; **11**, 292–296.

12. Holmes M. D., Chen W. Y., Feskarich D., Kroenke C. H., Colditz G. A. Physical activity and survival after breast cancer diagnosis. *J Am Med Assoc* 2005; **293**(20), 2479–2486.

13. Rockhill B., Willett W. C., Hunter D. J., Manson J. E., Hankinson S. E., Colditz G. A. A prospective study of recreational physical activity and breast cancer risk. *Arch Intern Med* 1999; **159**(19), 2290–2296.

14. Singh M. A. F. Exercise comes of age: rationale and recommendations for a geriatric exercise prescription. *J Gerontol Med Sci* 2002; **57A**(5), M262–M282.

15. Owens J. F., Matthews K. A., Wing R. R., Kuller L. H. Can physical activity mitigate the effects of aging in middle-aged women? *Circulation* 1992; **85**, 1265–1270.

16. Gilliat-Wimberly M., Manore M. M., Woolf K., Swan P. D., Carroll S. S. Effects of habitual physical activity on the resting metabolic rates and body compositions of women aged 35 to 50 years. *J Am Diet Assoc* 2001; **101**, 1181–1188.

17. Trends in strength training – United States, 1998–2004. *MMWR Morb Mortal Wkly Rep* 2006; **55**(28), 769–772.

18. Nelson M. E., Fiatarone M. A., Morganti C. M., Trice I., Greenberg R. A., Evans W. J. Effects of high-intensity strength training on multiple risk factors for osteoporotic fractures. *J Am Med Assoc* 1994; **272**, 1909–1914.

19. Hakkinen K., Kallinen M., Izquierdo M., Jokelainen K., Lassila H., Malkia E., Kraemer W. J., Newton R. U., Alen M. Changes in agonist-antagonist EMG, muscle CSA, and force during strength training in middle-aged and older people. *J Appl Physiol* 1998; **84**(4), 1341–1349.

20. Larsson L., Grimby G., Karlsson J. Muscle strength and speed of movement in relation to age and muscle morphology. *J Appl Physiol* 1979; **46**(3), 451–456.

21. Skelton D. A., Greig C. A., Davies J. M., Young A. Strength, power and related functional ability of healthy people aged 65–89 years. *Age Ageing* 1994; **23**, 371–377.

22. Bassey E. J., Fiatarone M. A., O'Neill E. F., Kelly M., Evans W. J., and Lipsitz L. A. Leg extensor power and functional performance in very old men and women. *Clin Sci* 1992; **82**, 321–327.

23. Hagberg J. M., Zmuda J. M., McCole S. D., Rodgers K. S., Ferrell R. E., Wilund K. R., Moore G. E. Moderate physical activity is associated with higher bone mineral density in postmenopausal women. *J Am Geriatr Soc* 2001; **49**, 1411–1417.

24. Kelley G. A., Kelley K. S., Tran Z. V. Resistance training and bone mineral density in women. *Am J Phys Med Rehabil* 2001; **80**, 65–77.

25. Okazaki T., Himeno E., Nanri H., Ikeda M. Effects of a community-based lifestyle-modification program on cardiovascular risk factors in middle-aged women. *Hypertens Res* 2001; **24**(6), 647–653.

26. O'Hara R. B., Baer J. T. Effect of a culturally based walking program on blood pressure response in African-American women. *Med Sci Sports Exerc* 2000; **32**(5), S313.

27. McCartney N., Hicks A. L., Martin J., Webber C. E. Long term resistance training in the elderly: effects on dynamic strength, exercise capacity, muscle, and bone. *J Gerontol Med Sci* 1995; **50A**, B97–B104.

28. Tanaka H., DeSouza C. A., Jones P. P., *et al.* Greater rate of decline in maximal aerobic capacity with age in physically active vs. sedentary healthy women. *J Appl Physiol* 1997; **83**(6), 1947–1953.

29. Eskurza I., Donato A. J., Moreau K. L., Seals D. R., Tanaka H. Changes in maximal aerobic capacity with age in endurance-trained women: 7-yr follow-up. *J Appl Physiol* 2002; **92**(6), 2303–2308.

30. Brown D. R., Wang Y., Ward A., *et al.* Chronic psychological effects of exercise and exercise plus cognitive strategies. *Med Sci Sports Exerc* 1995; **27**(5), 765–775.

31. Dalsky G. P., Stocke K. S., Ehsani A. A., *et al.* Weight-bearing exercise training and lumbar bone mineral content in postmenopausal women. *Ann Intern Med* 1988; **108**, 824–828.

32. Li F., Harmer P., McAuley E., Duncan T. E., *et al.* An evaluation of the effects of Tai Chi exercise on physical function among older persons: a randomized controlled trial. *Ann Behav Med* 2001; **23**(2), 139–146.

33. Kolasinski S. L., Garfinkel M., Tsai A. G., *et al.* Iyengar yoga for treating symptoms of osteoarthritis of the knees: a pilot study. *J Alt Compl Med* 2005; **11**(4), 689–693.

34. Sherman K. J., Cherkin D. C., Erro J., Miglioretti D. L., Deyo R. A. Comparing yoga, exercise, and a self-care book for chronic low back pain. *Ann Intern Med* 2005; **143**, 849–856.

35. Green J. S., Stanforth P. R., Gagnon J., *et al.* Menopause, estrogen, and training effects on exercise hemodynamics: the HERITAGE study. *Med Sci Sports Exerc* 2002; **34**(1), 74–82.

36. Li F., Harmer P., McAuley E., Fisher K. J., Duncan T. E., Duncan S. C. Tai Chi, self-efficacy, and physical function in the elderly. *Prev Sci* 2001; **2**(4), 229–239.

37. Channer K. S., Barrow D., Osborne M., Ives G. Changes in haemodynamic parameters following Tai Chi Chuan and aerobic exercise in patients recovering from acute MI. *Postgraduate Med J* 1996; **72**, 349–351.

38. Pollock M. L., Franklin B. A., Balady G. J., *et al.* Resistance exercise in individuals with and without cardiovascular disease. Benefits, raltionale, safety, and prescription: an advisory from the Committee on Exercise, Rehabilitation, and Prevention, Council on Clinical Cardiology, American Heart Association. *Circulation* 2000; **101**, 828–833.

39. Rutherford O. M., Greig C. A., Sargeant A. J., Jones D. A. Strength training and power output: transference effects in the human quadriceps muscle. *J Sports Sci* 1986; **4**(2), 101–107.

40. Santana J. C. Machines versus free weights. *Strength Conditioning J* 2001; **23**(5), 67.

41. American College of Sports Medicine. The recommended quantity and quality of exercise for developing and maintaining cardiorespiratory and muscular fitness in healthy adults. *Med Sci Sports Exerc* 1990; **22**, 265–274.

42. Gisolfi C. V. *Preparing Your Athletes for Competition in Hot Weather*, GSSI: Coaches' Corner, 1996.

43. Pate R. R. *Tips on Exercising in the Cold*, GSSI: Coaches' Corner, 1996.

44. Pollock M. L., Gaesser G. A., Butcher J. D., *et al.* The recommended quantity and quality of exercise for maintaining cardiorespiratory and muscular fitness, and flexibility in healthy adults. *Med Sci Sports Exerc* 1998; **30**(6), 975–991.

45. Chodzko-Zajko W. J. The World Health Organization issues guidelines for promoting physical activity among older persons. *J Aging Phys Act* 1997; **5**(1), 1–8.

46. Miszko T. A., Cress M. E., Slade J. M., *et al.* Effect of strength and power training on physical function in community-dwelling older adults. *J Gerontol Med Sci* 2003; **58A**(2), 171–175.

47. Stengel S. V., Kemmler W., Pintag R., *et al.* Power training is more effective than strength training for maintaining bone mineral density in postmenopausal women. *J Appl Physiol* 2006; **99**, 181–188.

48. Englund U., Littbrand H., Sondell A., Pettersson U., Bucht G. A 1-year combined weight-bearing training program is beneficial for bone mineral density and neuromuscular function in older women. *Osteoporosis Int* 2005; **16**, 1117–1123.

49. James P. T., Rigby N., Leach R. The obesity epidemic, metabolic syndrome, and future prevention strategies. *Eur J Cardiovasc Prev Rehabil* 2004; **11**, 3–8.

50. Sideraviciute S., Gailiuniene A., Visagurskiene K., Vizbaraite D. The effect of long-term swimming program on body composition, aerobic capacity and blood lipids in 14–19-year aged healthy girls and girls with type 1 diabetes mellitus. *Medicina (Kaunas)* 2006; **42**(8), 661–666.

51. Neumark-Sztainer D., Paxton S. J., Hannan P. J., Haines J., Story M. Does body satisfaction matter? Five-year longitudinal associations between body satisfaction and health behaviors in adolescent females and males. *J Adolescent Health* 2006; **39**, 244–251.

52. Centers for Disease Control and Prevention. *Unrealized Prevention Opportunities: Reducing the Health and Economic Burden of Chronic Disease.* Atlanta, GA: Centers for Disease Control and Prevention, US Department of Health and Human Services, 2000.

Chapter

5

Psychosocial health of well women through the life-cycle

Cathleen Morrow

Introduction

Primary care providers are uniquely positioned to assess the psychosocial health of women. While most individuals who seek care are "patients," – those who require or request care for specific problems – women are frequently seen when they are well. Whether for Pap smears, prenatal care, or general physical exams, primary practitioners will more likely encounter healthy women throughout their lives. Psychosocial health is the substrate from which a woman adapts to the complex world that comprises her life. As such, whether seen in illness or in health, the provider always has an abiding interest in the psychosocial state in which the individual presents herself.

Definitions and background

1. "Psychosocial" refers generally to the psychological status of an individual within the context of their social environment.
2. "Well woman" refers both to the absence of disease and the experience of health. This implies a broad definition of health to include cognitive, emotional, physical, psychological, spiritual, and environmental factors.
3. Assessment of and screening for psychosocial health is deeply connected to the quality of the provider–patient relationship. The life and clinical experience of the provider has a profound impact on decisions about the value, methodology, and approach toward assessment of psychosocial health. Some providers feel this is not an essential role for the clinician, and others see the relationship as a potentially powerful tool toward understanding the individual, enhancing a

relationship with them and potentially favorably influencing the patients future health.

> The provider–patient relationship is a potentially powerful tool for understanding an individual, enhancing the relationship and potentially favorably influencing future health.

4. There is, inherent in relational work, the potential for affecting a provider's own satisfaction with the daily work of supplying medical care to diverse peoples. It can be delightfully refreshing to provide medical care for a "well" person even if there is considerable variation in what the parameters of that care might include.
5. Each provider brings to the exam room a set of knowledge, beliefs, and experiences rooted in their own upbringing, family system, and education and training experiences. Depending on the era of the provider's training, his/her own knowledge base about the normal psychological development of women (and men) will vary widely.
6. Many physicians, nurse practitioners and physician assistants have had little to no training or educational background in healthy women's psychological development. Their approach and understanding to psychosocial issues might then be limited to their own family's system and their clinical experience. Other providers may have had extensive training in traditional psychology that, historically, has viewed women's psychological development as deviant from that of men.
7. In the last two decades, feminist thinkers have advanced alternative theories about women's psychological development that have influenced the thinking and approach of mental health and

Handbook of Women's Health, second edition, ed. Jo Ann Rosenfeld. Published by Cambridge University Press.
© Cambridge University Press 2009.

primary care providers. For some practitioners exposure to the "biopsychosocial model" came during their clinical training and is rooted in family systems theory and thinking. The practitioner's knowledge base, wherever rooted, significantly affects his/her ability to attend to psychosocial issues in a woman's life. All practitioners should be fully aware of the strengths and limitations of their own experience in this regard.

Theories of early psychological development

1. Theoretical constructs of psychological development have been rooted for much of the twentieth century in theories based on observations and studies of men. Theories designed to describe normal psychological development of men, thus, resulted in description of women's development as aberrant or arrested.[1]

> Theories designed to describe normal psycho-logical development of men, thus, resulted in description of women's development as aberrant or arrested.

2. While extensively debated over the decades, the works of Freud and Erickson remain, to this day, the underlying sets of assumptions about the earliest psychological development of infants and young children. These principles emphasize separation, autonomy and independence of the infant from the (mother) caretaker with evolution toward emphasis on generativity, the development of rules and universal principles. Pediatric and family medicine texts continue to offer these understandings as norms for early childhood development.[2]

3. Accepting that these constructs may be relevant for male infants and children, they leave behind female infants and children as problems that need explaining. As such, these theories often concluded that females were wanting, less evolved, and less capable of achieving the highest levels of development.[1]

4. In the 1970s, women psychologists and psychotherapists began to critique and expand upon ideas of early female psychological development. Rather than an approach that tended to see what it was not relative to male development, these theorists began to describe how the experience of attachment, separation, growth and individuation might be different for women. These ideas assumed femaleness as uniquely itself, rather than as "other." Further, the truth that caretakers of infants and children were overwhelmingly female was bound to be relevant. Might not, these theorists argued, the experience of attachment and separation differ for male and female infants, particularly in light of the powerful gender identification that highlights caretakers and the cultures from which they come? These questions ultimately led to a theory of development that has relationship at its core.

> The experience of attachment, separation, growth and individuation might be different for women. Attachment is the norm.

5. This relational approach to developmental theory holds that being-in-relation is the core experience for female infants and children. In other words, attachment is the norm, particularly in light of the gendered caretaker (mother) from whom separation is not required. Given the sameness, or identification with, the mother caretaker, the process is more likely to be of relationship to rather than separation from.

6. By this formulation, ideas of empathy, relationship, connectedness and mutuality come to the forefront of the development process and remain there throughout a woman's life,[3] in contrast to ideas of separation, autonomy and independence. Thus, "relationship is seen as the basic goal of development: i.e. the deepening capacity for relationship and relational competence . . . other aspects of self (e.g. creativity, autonomy, assertion) develop within this primary context . . . There is no inherent need to disconnect or to sacrifice relationship for self development" (page 53).[3]

7. In adolescence, therefore, relational theory would describe a transformation in the pattern of the parent–child bond rather than a break in the bond. Adolescent identity formation is realized in individuated relationships in which differences are freely expressed within a basic context of connectedness."[4]

8. Female adolescents traverse the complex terrain of individuation within the context of relatedness. They must forge new identities while remaining rooted in the mutuality of their families. The emphasis on friendships during this time does not necessarily imply a separation from the family of origin, but rather a new context in which to be individuated and broaden the range of their relationships.[5] These are formidable challenges and important times for psychosocial assessment and care.

Women's psychological development

Relational theory sees women in a context broader than that assigned by their reproductive abilities or gender driven caretaking roles. If development is understood as unfolding from infancy onward via one's affiliations, there will be a much broader context from within which to understand women as they are self defined rather than as role or gender defined. Being "self defined" means recognizing that women are both self defined and in relationship to others, whatever the context of that "other" might be.

Relational theory, therefore, would suggest that autonomy means being in relation and caring, but not to caring which is dependent or oppressive.[2] Candib asks us to consider what is requisite to create a working model of adult development for clinical practice (Table 5.1).[2]

> Relational theory suggests that autonomy means being in relation and caring, but not to caring which is dependent or oppressive.

Racism must be taken into consideration in looking at the experience of women of color in relational theory. Moreover, such a model must consider development within the context of relationships rather than separate from them, and it must view critically the idea that development consists in striving toward the goal of male-defined autonomy.[2]

This discussion of relational theory attempts, with broad brush strokes, to describe a methodology for thinking about psychosocial issues in women's lives. It is, for purposes of this chapter, a brief overview. The interested reader is strongly encouraged to understand more deeply by reading any of the references cited, but particularly relevant to the practicing

Table 5.1 Requirements of a relational theory of women's development

Incorporate a historical and social context

Be applicable to women without limiting their development to their biology

Consider the centrality of work as well as family to women's lives

Be broad enough to consider women who make a variety of choices – single, without children, with children, working, in-career, non-career, lesbian, transgendered, heterosexual

clinician is the excellent discussion found in *Medicine and the Family* by Dr Lucy Candib.[2]

Principles of psychosocial care for women

The busy provider, hustling through a day packed with sick patients and interspersed with physicals on well children and adults, has her doubts about all this. For many, taking care of ill people and performing well care with the requisite attention to preventive counseling and screening, and doing this well, is more than a day's work. Nonetheless, it is also true that when practitioners enter the exam room and ask "how are you?" they begin the process of providing good psychosocial care.

The principles of good psychosocial care are both simple and complex. A caring, attentive ear that remains alert to the woman's own understanding of her life in relation to self, to others, and to the systems and institutions that comprise her life is a beginning. Fueled by genuine interest and curiosity, good psychosocial care has, at its heart, a deep and abiding respect for women and their enormous strengths and vulnerabilities. It is dependent upon relationship; that exists and is developing each moment of an encounter. For most providers, this is knowledge acquired over time, both in the general sense and in the specific.

> The broader culture has not inculcated providers with a sense of deep respect for women.

The broader culture has not inculcated providers with a sense of deep respect for women. Many come to the practice of medicine with biases and stereotypes about the roles and capabilities of women. Even if providers are raised in families with positive messages about women, popular culture has muddled that message to some extent.

Good psychosocial care of women respects relationships as fundamental and is capable of viewing the world through relational lenses. It avoids judgment and labeling and is willing to accept a world view different from one's own. It demands some fearlessness about feeling and asks for, at times, reconsideration of the more traditional medical rules about boundaries. It may, at times, call for emotional investment on a provider's part and remains open to that possibility. Nonetheless, thoughtful psychosocial care fully respects appropriate boundaries.

Good psychosocial care is sensitive to the dilemmas faced by women in the culture and does not trivialize them. Respect for the burdens placed by assumptions and prescribed roles that have oppressed women is critical.

Good psychosocial care does not fail to acknowledge these hard realities and appreciate the power of them, and it does not shirk from addressing them. It respects the enormous diversity of women's lives and does not make assumptions of normalcy. It remains sensitive to the dilemmas faced by women within the medical culture and seeks to improve upon them.

If the relational model is used to consider health care, the major risk factors threatening psychosocial health become more apparent. Those events and influences that lead to major disconnection will be the most likely to disturb the well-being of an individual woman. The potential dislocations that occur as a result of social change, coupled with the significant mobility of the culture provide enormous opportunity and potential for major disconnection.

Disconnections such as death (particularly of a child), job loss, divorce, partnership dissolutions, domestic violence, trauma, or illness may seriously threaten a woman's sense of her self and her world. Women remain particularly at risk for economic dislocation, whether by earning less then men for equivalent work, or through divorce, partnership dissolution, or spousal death. Psychological and biological health are all at substantial risk during such times when a woman's sense of control over her environment and life is seriously threatened. Her ability to process, grieve, and ultimately grow through such events is predicated upon her own internal and external support systems that may facilitate, or may threaten, her survival.

Table 5.2 Seven features of the resilient individual

Insight
Independence
Relationships
Creativity
Humor
Morality
Initiative

Source: Taken from Wolin S., Wolin S. *The Resilient Self*, New York: Villard Press, 1993.

The potential dislocations that occur as a result of social change, coupled with the significant mobility of the culture provide enormous opportunity and potential for major disconnection. Women remain particularly at risk for economic dislocation, whether by earning less then men for equivalent work, or through divorce, partnership dissolution, or spousal death.

A helpful model for considering the coping styles of women facing major disconnections is that of resiliency, the ability to rebound from adversity. Wolin and Wolin have described seven features of the resilient individual from their work with survivors of troubled families (Table 5.2).[6] These features will cluster in varied fashion depending on the personality and circumstances of the loss or disconnection faced, and a given woman may utilize one or several of these qualities in coping. For the provider, assessment of the ability and diversity of such strategies may highlight risks and illuminate strengths, while suggesting other potential strategies for improved coping.

Knowledge of the individual, her experience with previous coping strategies that were successful or not, and awareness of the presence or absence of support may all serve to help the provider care for and work with an ill woman. A past experience of acceptance by a provider is very powerful. Knowledge that she will be accepted for her coping strategy and heard empathically rather than lectured to about what she "should" do is powerful.

Well-meaning friends and cultural mores often dictate to women how they should cope or grieve. Mores about acceptable grief, whether temporal or topical, often tyrannize women. A climate of acceptance, a sense that she is right to do it her way, in her own time is very powerful. Avoiding a tendency to immediately medicate signs and symptoms of psychological distress may also be valuable and appropriate. Many women will benefit from a steadying hand from their provider rather than a prescription.

> Avoiding a tendency to immediately medicate signs and symptoms of psychological distress may also be valuable and appropriate. Yet, the provider need also exercise caution about minimizing and downplaying distress.

Yet, the provider should exercise caution about minimizing and downplaying distress. Supporting women through periods of reactive depression, overwhelming grief, and intense feeling without judging or pathologizing can be among the most important and powerful clinical interventions practitioners will ever perform.

Nonetheless, there are circumstances when prescriptions, active interventions, and referrals are absolutely necessary. The clinical judgment of the provider must always be alert for the signs and symptoms of major depression, suicidality, and life threatening behaviors. In fact, an environment of trust and relationship improves the likelihood that dangerous disconnections will be more readily identified by the provider and interventions more readily accepted.

Many women have had their feelings and concerns minimized in the medical setting. Some arrive to these environments primed to be ignored or to have their feelings discounted. Lesbian women and women of color have often been the victims of insensitive and irrelevant care. **Women are much more likely than men to have had their behavior and symptoms labeled**. Providers who are inclined toward curiosity rather than judgment, understanding instead of diagnosis, and mutuality rather than strict doctor–patient roles may find they are more successful at providing good psychosocial care.

Psychosocial health through the life-cycle – adolescents

Providing humane, thoughtful psychosocial care to young women during the period of enormous transition and growth that marks adolescence is exciting and often very challenging for the provider. The stakes may be high and there is significant content in screening, assessment, and risk factor identification that need to be covered. Often adolescents do not really want to talk, and there are medical aspects of a visit with which to contend.

The 1990s brought an explosion of work, both scholarly and popular, about the risks and transitions for adolescent girls in western culture. Galvanizing public attention to the issue, the American Association of University Women Study of 1990 looked at 3,000 young girls and boys age 9 to 15. The results clearly identified the costs and risks of coming of age in America within a patriarchal cultural and educational system. The study found that the passage to adolescence was particularly treacherous for girls, marked by decreased confidence, decreasing abilities in math and science, and an increasingly critical attitude toward their own body.[5]

> Passage to adolescence was particularly treacherous for girls, marked by decreased confidence, decreasing abilities in math and science, and an increasingly critical attitude toward their own body.

More recent studies of academic success show that girls achieve substantially higher than boys in reading literacy (in the developed world) while continuing to lag in mathematics and science achievement. However, those differences are narrower than in past decades.[7]

Relationally speaking, girls begin to lose their voice. The pressures and messages about being female in a western culture sufficiently quieted the strong and confident younger girls as they learned to be nice, get along, and accommodate others. "At the crossroads of adolescence, the girls in the study describe a relational impasse that is familiar to many women: a paradoxical or dizzying sense of having to give up relationship for the sake of 'relationships'" (page 216).[5]

Thoughtful psychosocial care can be provided by attending to this fact. By caring about and creating relationship with adolescent girls, providers come to know them and identify those risks that arise from this dissociation from self. The clinician can seek to identify relationships that may be sources either of strength and support, or discord and vulnerability.

Table 5.3 presents one series of inquiries that may be used as screening questions regarding relationship. A question might lead to a series of others that illuminate a conflict or highlight a strength. Keeping an

Table 5.3 Psychosocial relational adolescent screening

A. Tell me about your important relationships. Who matters in your life right now? Mom? Dad? Friends? Siblings? Pets?

B. How do you feel about your body now? Do you like it? Why or why not? Sports, exercise, diet, etc.

C. How do you feel about school? Work, if any? Other? e.g. church, volunteering?

D. What are your recreations? Hobbies? Drugs? Alcohol?

E. Have there been any big losses in your life since I saw you last? Conflicts? Problems or obstacles that you felt like you couldn't solve?

F. How about successes? Accomplishments?

G. Tell me about your dreams? Goals? Aspirations?

ear attuned to a sense of disconnection, whether from parents, friends, school, or others can provide the tip-off to other questions to pursue in more depth. Listening carefully to an adolescent's version of their relationship to others helps to avoid the land mines of assumptions, whether about sexuality, values, or "normalcy."

Adolescent girls value relationship. They describe most anxiety about abandonment and they may be most at risk when they abandon themselves,[1] by dissociating from their own confident younger girl voices in order to accommodate to the pressures and expectations of the culture around them.

Studies that have attempted to isolate correlates of psychosocial health through these turbulent years have identified active participation in all girl sports teams as a positive factor.[8] Sports involvement helps not only with body image issues as girls come to view their bodies as competent and strong, but ongoing support of other girls in relationship to themselves can help in weathering the doubt and self-negation so ubiquitous during this time.

> Sports involvement helps with body image issues as girls come to view their bodies as competent and strong, and by providing the ongoing support of other girls.

A study of resilient adolescent teens who became mothers identified relationships, insight, and initiative as the positive correlates of coping well with this major transition.

An additional strategy might be called responsibility/rebellion. This may be a quality particularly valuable for adolescents. Some young women who were determined to prove that they would not fail or do poorly as all the surrounding systems predicted, thrived.[9]

Given the value placed on relationship, the primary care provider should appreciate the relationship with an adolescent over time and not despair of the limited "progress" that seems to be made in any given individual visit. Many a provider has been suprised and pleased to learn how strongly the young girl identifies them as "my doctor."

Creating the environment of trust necessary for a productive care relationship with an adolescent if the provider also cares for the extended family, is challenging. Issues of confidentiality need to be addressed directly and adhered to faithfully for the provider to sustain credibility with the adolescent. Identification as "my doctor" will be facilitated by seeing the adolescent alone.

> The primary care provider should appreciate the relationship with an adolescent over time and not despair of the limited "progress" that seems to be made in any given individual visit.

Adult women

As women emerge from adolescence into adulthood, issues of relationship persist, but the complexities of attaining a livelihood, sustaining oneself, and possible partnering come more directly to the fore.

Many young adult women will be continuing to traverse tasks of adolescence, while many others will have long since been pushed prematurely into assuming sets of responsibilities normally thought of as adult. The developmental tasks faced in adulthood are numerous (Table 5.4). These broadly apply to most women in a western culture but will be affected powerfully by ethnicity, culture and circumstance.

Few women, if any, follow a smooth developmental trajectory. Economic forces will shape this trajectory tremendously and poverty is consistently identified as a major source of psychosocial stress.

Sexual orientation may have significant influence on the accessibility of social supports upon which one might depend. Changing social mores may affect how openly a woman remains single, is lesbian, adopts

Table 5.4 Developmental tasks facing adult women

1. Solidifying a self identity independent of one's family of origin yet remaining in relation to them.

2. Creating independence as a single person or in a relationship.

3. Participating in many and varied adult relationships at home and work. Possible partnering/marriage.

4. Supporting self and potentially others.

5. Considering becoming, or choosing not to become, a parent.

6. If raising children, establishing and maintaining a secure environment in which to raise them.

7. Continued extended family involvement, establishing newly configured adult relationships with parents.

8. Finding balance between work, family, and social responsibilities.

9. Balancing own personal, emotional, psychological, spiritual, and health needs.

Table 5.5 Psychosocial relational adult screening

1. Who do you care for at this time? Children? Partner? Siblings? Parents? Extended family?

2. How do you care for yourself? Who helps care for you? Where do you go for help when you need it?

3. Tell me about work (in or out of home). Does it nourish/stress you? Is the balance right?

4. Are there other environments besides home/work that matter to you? Church? School? Volunteer work?

5. Tell me about your successes and accomplishments.

6. How about losses? Conflicts that were difficult to resolve or remain a source of a lot of distress?

7. Do you feel as though your life is under your control?

children of color, and lives her life. Job and legal changes may allow closeted women to live more openly than previously, or the reverse may occur.

Threats of violence, harassment, and intimidation are daily facts of life for millions of women. Constructing a model for "normalcy" in women's lives is not reasonable. There are simply as many variations as there are women. Table 5.5 presents some suggestions for psychosocial screening questions that may facilitate a deeper discussion of these issues.

> Constructing a model for "normalcy" in women's lives is not reasonable.

Research that explores psychosocial correlates of health has highlighted attributes that may be relevant for the provider. One large study examined psychosocial factors and their relationship to coronary heart disease in 750 women between the age 45 and 64. Women who developed angina and coronary heart disease were 2–3 times more likely to score higher on scales measuring type A behavior (emotional lability, ambitiousness, and "non-easygoing"), suppressed hostility and anger, tension and anxiety.[10] A follow-up study examining this same group 20 years later revealed similar findings but added low educational level, lack of vacations, and perceived financial status among employed women as risk factors.[11] Measurable associations exist between divorce, lower socioeconomic class, lower educational attainment, and limited social supports, on the one hand, and cardiovascular disease, cardiac arrhythmias, sleep disturbance, depression, and anxiety, on the other.[12,13]

Conversely, overall health has been shown to have strong correlations with role satisfaction (particularly work related),[14] higher socioeconomic class, caring for a family, strong social supports, high self esteem, and larger social networks.[15,16,17]

Clear differences exist in mortality between lowest and highest income women and educational attainment level. Many argue that the higher rates of morbidity and mortality found in low income groups are solely explained by differences in health related behaviors such as alcohol and tobacco consumption. While no doubt a factor, other studies refute these as the major etiology and find that education level, social stresses, and social roles at work and home are independent risk factors.[18,19]

Women are the caretakers in the culture; this role can be a source of great satisfaction, identity and fulfillment, but can also be the source of enormous stress and frustration.

How caretaking affects women will be highly dependent on a host of associated factors: support systems, relief from the role, degree of caretaking, presence of more than one generation requiring caretaking, and the nature of the caretaking relationships, among many others.

The full time working woman (some 65% of women) who is responsible not only for young children but also aging parents or relatives is at high risk of being overwhelmed by these responsibilities.

Relationships with those being cared for may be warm and loving or may be fraught with anger, unresolved issues, and confusion.

The provider should be aware of the caretaking responsibilities of their patients and how these will affect psychosocial and overall health. Providers can serve not only as a source of this needed caretaking but also assist women in realistic assessment of the demands upon them, and assist with finding alternatives where needed.

Older women

Although poverty is an enormous issue in the psychosocial life of any woman, this issue becomes more important in elderly women. Women older than the age 65 constitute the fastest growing segment of the population and comprise the significant majority of that total population.

By the year 2012, people age 65 and older will comprise 14% of the total population, twice the number in 1956.[20] Moreover, women comprise an even higher percentage of the elderly poor (72%), and twice as many African-American women live in poverty as Caucasian. Elderly women are half as likely as men to have pensions and four times more likely to become indigent and require Medicaid for nursing home or other care.[21]

As women age, life-cycle tasks evolve significantly. There is enormous diversity of life experience, health status, economic conditions and overall social supports each individual woman experiences. Many providers will first come to know women during this time as the frequency of visits tends to increase with the development of health problems. Eighty percent of elderly women older than age 65 have at least one chronic health condition. Concerns about health may well dominate over psychosocial concerns as well as substantially impact quality of life.

> Eighty per cent of elderly women older than age 65 have at least one chronic health condition.

Attention to psychosocial health may reap significant benefits. The aging woman may have more time for reflection, more knowledge about herself and life, and be less driven by sociocultural norms of success and achievement. This age has the potential to be a time of enormous satisfaction. A lifetime of caretaking for others may be turned, finally, toward the self. Women may need permission to do so, and may benefit from support and encouragement to see the value in evolving roles.

It can also be deeply unsettling to no longer be needed in familiar roles. What is perceived as a time of freedom and independence to some can be a source of depression and loss for others.

Major financial changes, whether caused by retirement, death of a supporting partner, or divorce can dramatically alter the course of an older woman's life. Statistically, a woman in America who reaches age 65 can expect to live another 19 years, a lengthy period of time to finance and survive.

Several psychosocial challenges are likely to present themselves as women age. Loss of partners, loved ones, spouses, and siblings may place a woman at risk of isolation, living alone, and marked diminution of social supports.

Women who have enjoyed lifelong independence may find themselves facing gradual dependence secondary to physical decline. Our profoundly mobile society may mean that children, grandchildren, and other potential sources of support may be substantial distances from each other. Retirement from work may be associated with pleasure and joy in newfound freedom or may result in a loss of sense of identity, value and importance.

In this culture, aging women are not usually revered and beloved for their wisdom and past work, though surely, such family systems exist as places of support for some. An individual's ethnicity will influence, to some extent, how older women are valued within a family and community. Western culture, and thus providers, tend to focus on loss in the elderly rather than gain.

As chronic medical conditions mount, numbers of prescriptions increase, and visits to the office become regular, the provider and the individual can both lose sight of the health that does remain. Gains of this time in a woman's life should be celebrated. A new grandchild, volunteer work that is meaningful, travel, pleasure in time spent with loved ones all contribute to the health of an aging individual. These should be acknowledged and celebrated in the course of the care as surely as the blood pressure should be monitored.

Isolation is one of the greatest psychosocial risk factors, and can lead to, or be a symptom of, depression. Recognition by the provider that an aging individual is becoming isolated can be an important step in preventive care.

> Isolation is one of the greatest psychosocial risk factors, and can lead to, or be a symptom of, depression.

End of life issues are challenging for all providers, and perhaps even more so for patients with whom practitioners have developed strong relationships. Yet the fruits of long relationship can be realized powerfully in such times. All wish for a peaceful death. If the provider genuinely knows the patient, then s/he genuinely knows their wishes.

Inevitably, except for sudden unexpected deaths, the process of physical decline, diagnosis, work up, and treatment often moves women away from the primary care arena into specialty and intensive care settings. Primary providers can lose touch with their patients, yet this is a time when their continued presence can be quite valuable. Occasionally, the provider will be the only individual who has had direct and clear conversation about a woman's wishes toward the end of life. A provider's responsibility clearly extends through the end of life in such cases.

Confusion and conflict within families, particularly gatherings of those from distances, may demand the distinct voice of the provider who has had these important conversations. It is a component of good psychosocial care to assist the extended family in such times, and honors a provider's relationship with the individual. Countless patients have experienced a sense of abandonment by providers as the time for medical intervention passes and the time arrives for allowing the inevitable to occur. "A peaceful death can only be possible if it is understood that the power of death in the end triumphs over human science and artifice, and that only a stepping aside to allow it to happen can be faithful to the force of nature and the respect owed to patients."[22] Practitioners must remain present in order to see these relationships through, to facilitate that stepping aside if need be, and to continue the process of providing good psychosocial care to those left behind.

Conclusions

Providing excellent psychosocial care to women throughout the life-cycle is one of the most complex and rewarding tasks a primary provider will undertake. The attention, time, and focus by the provider to the broad spectrum of emotional, developmental, economic, cultural, and social issues that will impact one's health will be time well spent. Women, by virtue of their unique caretaking, childrearing, and employment responsibilities, have special concerns that require care and attention. Respect and appreciation for the value of psychosocial care will not only lead to better care of patients, but better satisfaction by providers.

This chapter has focused on the psychosocial health care of women and suggested shifts in the paradigm of the approach in order to meet the needs of women that may be unique to them. However, many feel that the precepts and principles of relational thinking are relevant to both genders and support an overall approach that is more sensitive to the needs and realities of all. Viewing one's patients, regardless of gender, through a relational lens offers the possibility of humanism as a guiding ideal for medicine. Perhaps, as practitioners care for the caretakers in our culture, this ideal might be better realized throughout medicine.

References

1. Gilligan C. In *A Different Voice: Psychological Theory and Women's Development*. Cambridge, MA: Harvard University Press, 1952, pp. 5–12.

2. Candib L. *Medicine and the Family*. New York: Basic Books, 1995, pp. 4–13.

3. Surrey J. L. The self-in-relation: a theory of women's development. In Jordan J. V., Kaplan A. G., Miller J. B., Stiver I. P., eds., *Women's Growth in Connection: Writings from the Stone Center*, New York: Guilford Press, 1991, pp. 51–66.

4. Grotevant H. D., Cooper C. R. Individuation in family relationships: a perspective on individual differences in the development of identity and role-taking skill in adolescence. *Hum Dev* 1956; **29**, 93–94.

5. Brown L. M., Gilligan C. *Meeting at the Crossroads: Women's Psychological and Girls Development*. Cambridge, MA: Harvard University Press, 1992, pp. 216–220.

6. Wolin S., Wolin S. *The Resilient Self*, New York: Villard Press, 1993.

7. Halpern D. F. *Girls and Academic Success: Changing Patterns of Academic Achievement. Handbook of Girls'*

and Women's Psychological Development, Oxford: Oxford University Press, 2006, pp. 272–274.

8. Pipher M. *Reviving Ophelia*, New York: Ballantine Books, 1995, pp. 266–267.

9. Carey G., Ratcliff D., Lyle R. Resilient adolescent mothers: ethnographic interviews. *Families Systems Health* 1995; **16**(4), 347–364.

10. Haynes S. G., Feileib M., Kannel W. B. The relationship of psychosocial factors to coronary heart disease in the Framingham Study. *Am J Epidemiol* 1950; **III**(1), 37–55.

11. Eaker E. D., Pinsky J., Castelli W. P. Myocardial infarction and coronary death among women: psychosocial predictors from a 20 year follow-up of women in the Framingham Study. *Am J Epidemiol* 1992; **135**, 554–564.

12. Horsten M., Erickson M., Perski A., Wamala S. P. Psychosocial factors and heart rate variability in healthy women. *Psychosomatic Med* 1999; **61**(1), 49–57.

13. Owens J. F., Mathews K. A. Sleep disturbances in healthy middle aged women. *Maturitas* 1995; **30**(1), 41–50.

14. Rosenfeld J. A. Maternal work outside the home and its effect on women and their family. *J Am Med Women Assoc* 1992; **47**, 47–53.

15. Thomas S. P. Psychosocial correlates of women's health in middle adulthood. *Issues Mental Health Nurs* 1995; **16**(4), 255–314.

16. Denton M., Walters V. Gender differences in structural and behavioral determinants of health: an analysis of the social production of health. *Soc Sci Med* 1999; **45**(9), 1221–1235.

17. McQuaide S. Women at midlife. *Social Work* 1995; **43**(1), 21–31.

18. Lantz P. M., House J. S., Lepkowski J. M., Williams D. R., Mero R. P., Chen J. Socioeconomic factors, health behaviors, and mortality: results from a nationally representative prospective study of US adults. *J Am Med Assoc* 1995; **279**(21), 1703–1705.

19. Gottlieb N. H., Green L. W. Life events, social network, life-style, and health: an analysis of the 1979 National Survey of Personal Health Practices and Consequences. *Health Educ Q* 1954; **11**(1), 91–105.

20. Butler R. N., Oberlink M., Schechter M. *The Elderly in Society: An International Perspective. Brocklehurst's Textbook of Geriatric Medicine and Gerontology*, 5th edition, New York: Churchill Livingstone, 1995, p. 1445.

21. Goldstein M. Z. Gender issues in geriatric psychiatry. In Sadock B. J., Sadock V. A., eds., *Kaplan and Sadock's Comprehensive Text book of Psychiatry*, 7th edition, Lippincott, Williams & Wilkins, 1999, p. 3174.

22. Callahan D. The value of achieving a peaceful death. In Cassel C. K., *et al.*, eds., *Geriatric Medicine*, New York: Springer Verlag, 1997, pp. 1035–1104.

6

Sexuality through the life-cycle

Jo Ann Rosenfeld

Introduction

1. Sexuality is a significant aspect of all individuals' lives. Physicians and health care professionals who provide continuing care to individuals and families have an opportunity and responsibility to provide appropriate counseling, anticipatory guidance and education. Many women consider their physicians as experts in the area of human sexuality.

2. Sexual issues are frequently ignored in practice. Sexuality provides individuals a way to express their feelings, demonstrate caring and communicate and develop intimacy with another person. Sexual expression becomes a source of pleasure and fulfillment. For couples, it is a powerful form of conversation.

3. Many medical, psychological, and developmental concerns impact sexual behavior. These include psychosocial development, contraception, STDs, and the impact of various illnesses such as depression, substance abuse, physical disability, heart disease and diabetes on sexuality. If not discussed, this may be ignored.

4. When talking with the woman about sexual histories and concerns, consider the age, culture and religious background of the individual. For some this may be embarrassing or inappropriate, whereas many women will seize the opportunity with welcome relief.

Sexuality and adolescence
Initiation of sexual intimacy

1. Adolescence is a time of great physiological, emotional and psychological change. It is a time of exploration, emancipation, and a search for self-identity. Sexual intimacy is one aspect of accomplishing this transition.

2. Many women, especially teenagers, define themselves by their relationships to others. Having sexual relations may cement these relationships.

3. In the USA, more than three-quarters of boys and two-thirds of girls have had sexual intercourse by their senior year of high school. Nearly half of all 15–19 year olds have had sex at least once.[1] By age 19, 70% of teenagers have had sex.

4. US teenagers are waiting longer on average to have sex than they did previously. Three-quarters of girls state that they started sex in the context of a relationship with a "steady" boyfriend.[1]

5. The onset of sexual intimacy varies among adolescents. Peer pressure, feelings of love and attraction, curiosity, and wanting to be "grown up," are all among the reasons cited by teenagers for initiating sexual experimentation.[2] Family factors such as divorce or single-parent homes and abuse also influence the initiation of sexual activity.[3] Environmental and behavioral factors such as drug and alcohol use, delinquency, poor self-esteem, and decline in school grades have also been linked to premature sexual experimentation among adolescents.[4]

6. Physicians should be sensitive to the issue of emerging and possible confusing sexuality in gay and lesbian adolescents. As many as 10% of all adolescents have concerns about sexual identity issues.[5]

7. In some teenage girls, sexuality is related to poor self-esteem. Reminding them that they have a right to refuse, to enjoy, and to request is important.

Handbook of Women's Health, second edition, ed. Jo Ann Rosenfeld. Published by Cambridge University Press. © Cambridge University Press 2009.

STDs and pregnancy

1. Relatively few adolescents admit to planning sexual encounters. However, more sexually experienced teenagers are using contraceptives and most of these are using condoms, especially at first intercourse.
2. Lack of comfort with their bodies, poor self-image, and embarrassment may interfere with a teen's willingness to consider contraception.
3. Teens may be reluctant to discuss these issues with their physicians. Establishment and assurances of confidentiality and its limits will help create an atmosphere of trust.
4. Adolescents, especially those who begin their sexual activity at a younger age, are more likely to have multiple sexual partners over time, exhibiting a type of serial monogamy, which also places them at a higher risk for STDs or pregnancy.
5. Adolescents need reassurance of their normality and the normality of their concerns, reaffirmation of the need for contraception and prevention of STDs, and confirmation for their right to enjoyment and lack of pain and ability to refuse.
6. Exploring the teen's understanding of sexuality, including dreams, fantasies, homosexual thought, masturbation, hormonal and body changes, reproduction, contraception and prevention of STDs is important.

Pregnancy

1. Pregnancy creates many physical and psychological changes in the woman's and couple's relationship. The woman may have body image changes, physical discomfort, and fears for the safety of the pregnancy.
2. Sexual desire decreases during the first trimester, increases during the second trimester, and decreases again in the final trimester. Some studies have linked advanced pregnancy to decreased sexual desire and satisfaction.
3. For couples who want to continue sexual intimacy throughout pregnancy, the physician may recommend positional changes that are more comfortable for the woman and can accommodate the enlarging fetus. Use of pillows under the woman's head and back or reclining to decrease the shortness of breath that comes with lying flat will help the sexual relationship. Alternative positions, such as side to side or the woman on top, may be preferable. Sex without penetration may be more comfortable.
4. Unless the woman is at high risk for or develops premature labor, there is no medical reason, except discomfort, to stop having sexual relations during pregnancy.

Postpartum

1. Following delivery, women gradually return to former levels of sexual desire and interest, although physiological factors such as vaginal bleeding or dyspareunia may contribute to decreased sexual interest during the postpartum period.
2. Fatigue, lack of sleep, psychological concerns, role overloads, and stress may also have a negative impact upon the resumption of sexual activity in the new mother.
3. The husband's fear of injuring his partner may impact the couple's resumption of sexual activity. The family physician can offer guidance as to ways to cope with the numerous adjustments a couple experience when they become parents.

Medical problems and sexuality
Cancer

1. The diagnosis of cancer has a profound effect upon the woman, her partner and her family. Loss, fear, anxiety, anger, and depression are common responses to the diagnosis. Loss may be related to expectations of fertility, of experiences as becoming less whole, less feminine, and more vulnerable to the exigencies of life. Fears associated with the treatment, pain, loss of control, change in perceived desirability, and death are frequent responses. Those cancers that affect sexual organs are traumatic for the patient and her partner. Since cancer provokes crises in a woman's life, exploring the nature and quality of significant relationships is essential.
2. Partners of cancer patients also experience reactions to the illness that may include fear of loss and hurting the patient, irrational fears of contamination or contracting the disease, or a decreased sense of her desirability. Communication between partners is crucial.

The physician can facilitate communication, provide information about the treatment and outcomes, and explore the patient's understanding of what cancer means to them.

3. Pain, or the anticipation of experiencing pain, may have a negative effect on the woman's interest in sexual intimacy. Premature resumption of sexual activity before the woman is ready physically, psychologically, and emotionally may occur in order to relieve anxiety about her partner's perceived sexual needs and a need to affirm her desirability as a woman.

Gynecological cancers

1. While the sexual consequences of gynecological cancers vary according to the treatment needed, dyspareunia is more common among women who have radiation than surgical interventions.[6]
2. Vaginal dilators may be used for women experiencing dyspareunia following radiation treatment or surgical interventions. Use of the dilator two or three times a week may reduce anxiety about pain and enable the woman to resume sexual activity more comfortably and experience penetration without pain.[7]
3. Different positions may be used so that the couple can find the better ones for themselves.

Breast cancer

1. A diagnosis of breast cancer brings numerous psychological, emotional, relational, and sexual ramifications for the woman, her partner and her family. Cultural and personal views of the breast as a symbol of femininity and attractiveness and conversely as a source of life and nutrition, play a role in how the woman and her partner respond to the diagnosis.
2. Assessing the woman's self concept, her body image, expectations of fertility, and her sense of femininity when discussing treatment options are important. Women also fear the response of their partners to potentially disfiguring surgeries. Involving the partner in the treatment is important. The adjustment process can be improved by encouraging the partner to view the surgical site early, discussing issues of revulsion or avoidance (of the breast and the partner) and addressing concerns about sexual activity causing pain.

3. Sexual dysfunction occurs frequently among breast cancer patients. However, the source of the dysfunction has not been linked solely to the diagnosis and treatment of breast cancer. The sequelae of treatments, premature menopause, depression, the impact of medication and chemotherapy and preexisting sexual problems may all contribute to dysfunction in breast cancer patients.
4. A relationship exists between menstrual status and sexual functioning in the woman who has breast cancer. Chemotherapy induced menopause causes vaginal dryness, and other hormonal changes exacerbate sexual problems.[8] Women who have had chemotherapy and younger women who have had premature menopause are more likely to have problems with sexual function.
5. Women who have undergone reconstructive surgery following mastectomy often complain of loss of sensation and pain in the breast.[9] Direct stimulation of the breast is no longer as pleasurable and may affect the quality of the sexual interactions between the woman and her partner. Women who have had total mastectomies and reconstructive surgery are more likely to experience significant sexual problems than those who have undergone lumpectomies.

Disability

1. Studies have addressed the sexual needs of spinal-cord injuries, little research has assessed the sexual health needs of persons born with physical and intellectual disabilities. Societal attitudes toward sexual expression among people with intellectual disabilities have not been favorable. Families, fearing exploitation and abuse, may shield their impaired children from obtaining any sexual knowledge or keep them from participating in appropriate sex education programs.
2. Clearly, an assessment of the intellectual capabilities of the individual is needed to determine the person's ability to consent to sexual overtures. Similar problems may arise among individuals with congenital physical disabilities. In both cases, the physician must address the concerns of the parents, provide education, anticipatory guidance to the child or young adult, and encourage responsible sexual behavior.

3. Appropriate confidentiality is important also. Treading the difficult line between giving the non-independent woman appropriate confidential information and consultation and helping her work within her family system may be challenging. Understanding guardianship and family relations will help.

Chronic illness

Many individuals begin to experience the onset of chronic illnesses during the fifth and sixth decades of life. Diseases such as cardiac and circulatory problems, diabetes, arthritis, osteoporosis, chronic obstructive pulmonary disease, hypertension, neurological disorders, and depression, among others, have a profound impact on sexual functioning (Table 6.1).

1. **Heart disease**

    The effects of cardiac illness on men have been well researched. Few studies have addressed the specific issues of women following a cardiac event and their unique counseling needs. Women may receive less counseling, including referral to cardiac rehabilitation, than men do. Resumption of sexual activity following a cardiac event may elicit fear and anxiety. Women may choose to avoid returning to their previous level of sexual activity fearing a reinfarct or death. Symptoms such as chest discomfort, shortness of breath, and excessive sweating are deterrents to the resumption of sexual activity in women.

    a. Women can resume sex when climbing two flights of stairs no longer causes anxiety or chest pain. Education regarding the impact of the sexual response cycle on cardiac function is essential.

    b. Explaining the number of metabolic equivalents (METs) used during sex as compared with common daily activities can help to reduce anxiety. Patients must understand the need to avoid heavy eating and drinking prior to sex to reduce the potential stress on the heart. Patients should be advised to discontinue sexual activity if they become short of breath, experience chest pain, or become too anxious, and to notify their physician of their symptoms as soon as possible. Reassurance and education can help to reduce anxiety among women with cardiac disease.

Table 6.1 Effects of medical disease on sexuality in women

Disease	Effects
Gynecological cancers	Fertility concerns, fear of partner rejection, pain, dyspareunia
Breast cancer	Altered self-image and fears of loss of sexuality
Chemotherapy, menopause	Vaginal dryness
Heart disease	Fear of restarting sexual intercourse, chest pain
Hypertension	Sexual dysfunction caused by medications
Diabetes	Orgasmic difficulty
Renal failure	Anhedonia, decreased lubrication, anorgasmia, hypoactive sexual desire disorders
Spinal cord injuries	Loss of self-esteem, body image problems, social role problems, penetration difficulties, dyspareunia
Decreased mobility	Decreased ability to participate
Multiple sclerosis	Decreased libido, delayed and decreased lubrication, decreased orgasmic capacity
Arthritis	Reduced mobility, detrimental effect on sexual function
Scleroderma	Vaginal dryness, dyspareunia, decreased orgasmic function

2. **Hypertension**

    Hypertension medications may affect the sexual response cycle negatively (Table 6.2).

3. **Diabetes**

    a. While impaired or decreased sexual functioning is a complication of diabetes in men, the sexual impact of diabetes on women is not well defined. Early studies found that women with diabetes often suffer significant orgasmic difficulty.[10] Few more recent studies have investigated this information. Results of subsequent research have been inconclusive or contradictory.

    b. Sexual dysfunction has been reported in 42% of women with type 2 diabetes and in 18–27% of women with type 1 diabetes.[11] Women with

Table 6.2 Some medications that affect sexual functioning in women

Medication	Effect
Amphetamines	Decreased orgasm
Antipsychotics	Decreased desire, hypoactive sex drive
Antihypertensives	
ACEIs	Decreased arousal
Beta-blockers	Decreased arousal, desire
CNS active drugs	Decreased arousal, anorgasmia
Thiazides	Decreased arousal, desire
Antihistamines	Decreased desire and arousal
Danazol	Increased or decreased desire
Narcotics	Decreased desire, arousal, orgasm
Sedatives	Decreased desire, arousal, orgasm
Benzodiazepines	Anorgasmia
Antidepressants	Decreased desire, arousal, orgasm; delayed orgasm
Alcohol	Decreased arousal, orgasm

Note: Data from Crenshaw T. L., Goldberg J. P., eds. *Sexual Pharmacology: Drugs that Affect Sexual Function*, New York: W. W. Norton, 1996.

more diabetic complications are more likely to have sexual dysfunction.

c. Neuropathies alone have not been found to contribute to sexual dysfunction in women diabetics.

d. Many psychosocial problems that are associated with diabetes can impact sexual functioning.

e. Renal failure has been linked to several types of sexual dysfunction in women. Anhedonia, decreased vaginal lubrication, and anorgasmia have been associated with women on dialysis.[12] Women with chronic renal failure often have a hypoactive sexual desire disorder. The source of this dysfunction may be multifactorial, including chronic disease, medications, and psychosocial issues.

4. **Spinal-cord injuries**

a. Spinal-cord injuries result in multiple types of losses for the patient and her partner.

Self-esteem, perceptions of body image, social roles, and feelings of dependence are all affected. The degree of impairment dictates the effect on sexual function. For example, muscle spasticity may make penetration difficult.

b. Therefore, an assessment of the patient's sensory capacity and mobility are important in offering anticipatory guidance. Recommendations may include encouraging the patient to improve self-esteem and self-image and to make advanced preparations for sexual intimacy. The woman should tend to bowel and bladder care before initiating sex to avoid any accidents that would have psychological consequences.

c. The timing of the sexual activity may be important to avoid fatigue or spastic responses.[13] Sensate focus exercises may be helpful to the patient and her partner. Experimenting with different positions may also be helpful.

5. **Decreased mobility problems**

a. Diseases that result in decreased mobility or flexibility, such as multiple sclerosis, arthritis, or connective tissue disorders, often lead to sexual inactivity. Joint stiffness, decreased flexibility, muscle spasms and increased tone, pain and other symptoms affect a woman's ability to engage in sexual intimacy.

b. Multiple sclerosis has been associated with decreased libido, delayed and decreased lubrication, decreased orgasmic capacity, and anorgasmia in many women. Fatigue, spasticity, contractures, loss of manual dexterity and incontinence may contribute to sexual problems.[14]

c. The use of assistive devices, muscle relaxants, and vibrators may help to alleviate the distress and disability caused by contractures, muscle weakness, and spasms.

d. Bowel and bladder training programs may be recommended when incontinence is a problem.

e. For some patients, the use of corticosteroids has produced improvement in sexual functioning.

f. For women with arthritis, timing of sexual activity to coincide with optimal physical

69

mobility and pain relief may help. Specific suggestions, such as positional changes (side-by-side, woman on top, use of chairs, or use of hot tubs) can aid the arthritic woman maintain her sexual activity.

6. **Scleroderma**

   a. Scleroderma can have negative effects on sexual functioning. Women with scleroderma and Sjogren's syndrome have high rates of sexual dysfunction.

   b. Common problems include vaginal dryness, dyspareunia, and decreased orgasmia. Other changes such as joint pain, contractures, and muscle weakness may interfere with a woman's sexuality.

Facilitation

1. Physicians can best assist their patient to maintain healthy sexual functioning by taking a sexual history and exploring a patient's sexual concerns, fears, and expectations.

2. Physicians may suggest positional changes, environmental changes (placement of pillows, use of hot tubs or waterbeds) and alternative activities to penetrational intercourse such as hugging, caressing, cuddling, and mutual masturbation.

3. Both the patient and her partner must be willing to consider suggestions regarding alternative positions and practices.

4. Good communication between the partners is essential. The partners should be encouraged to discuss their concerns and reservations.

5. Referrals to certified sex therapists and to chronic disease support groups or on-line support groups or chat rooms may be helpful.

Aging
Midlife

1. Women in midlife, age 40 to 65, can use guidance regarding the impact of chronic illness, hormonal changes, and medications on sexual functioning. Women at this age may be experiencing changes in family structure and the psychosocial adjustments these demand. The variety of needs is amazing. Midlife women may be trying to become pregnant, be menopausal, be widowed, or caring for young children or grandchildren.

2. Women may express fears about the effect of time and hormones on their self-image and desirability. Information about physiological changes that do occur and exploration of the woman's beliefs about sexuality at this age are essential.

3. Most physiological changes associated with aging affect the sexual response cycle of the older woman. Estrogen-deficient vaginitis, insertional dyspareunia, and reduced lubrication are common complaints associated with menopause. The use of artificial lubricants can reduce the symptoms and pain.

4. As women age, the excitement phase of the sexual cycle can occur more slowly. For many menopausal women, it may take 5 minutes rather than 10 to 15 seconds in the excitement phase to achieve lubrication. More and more direct genital stimulation may be needed during the arousal or excitement phase.

5. The plateau phase may also become longer. The orgasmic phase may become shorter and orgasms may be painful. Contraction may be spasmodic rather than rhythmic. Nonetheless, women retain the potential to return to the excitement phase and to experience multiple orgasms.

Interest

1. Most studies of middle-aged and older women demonstrate that interest in sexual intimacy continues into advanced old age. Prevalence varies by area, country and population surveyed. From 30% of community dwelling US women older than age 65 to 95% of community dwelling Danish women the same age have stated that they have regular intercourse. According to a length study conducted by the Consumers' Union, most women over age 65 engaged in sexual activity at least once a week.[15] Older women report less sexual activity than men the same age, correlating with the availability of a socially sanctioned partner.[16]

2. The most important correlation between continued sexual activity in older women is availability of a healthy partner. Women often marry older men, who may develop chronic illnesses, disability, or die before women. Women who are widowed, divorced or single are less likely to continue their sexual activity. Various studies

have noted a sharp decrease in sexual interest and activity among women in their late 60s. For many women, this may be a source of considerable frustration. Societal expectations and misconceptions about the physiological effects of aging on sexuality contribute to this distress. Aging signs may result in feelings of decreased sexual attractiveness.

3. For women without a partner, masturbation may be an option.

4. However, sensitive inquiry about sexual beliefs, practices, and concerns will be needed before any recommendations can be made. Providing education will enable the woman to make informed decisions.

5. Many social issues may contribute to a lack of sexual interest or responsiveness, such as monotony, preoccupation with career and finances, physical and mental fatigue, overindulgence in food and drink, and fear of failure in sexual performances. Excessive life stressors, socioeconomic issues, patterns of disinterest in sexual activity as a young adult also may decrease middle age sexual intimacy.

6. Arthritis and stiffness can make sex difficult. Asking the partners to come into the office in comfortable clothes or sweatsuits is a method of helping them to try different and more comfortable positions. Taking an acetaminophen or NSAID before sex may help stiffness.

7. Refraining from alcohol and heavy meals before sex is helpful.

8. Reviewing drugs used by either partner may allow the substitution of one that affects sexual functioning.

9. Lubrication with exogenous creams may help.

The elderly
Dementia

1. Dementia presents special difficulties for the older woman and her partner. Common sexual consequences of dementia include anhedonia, depression, impotence, incontinence, and anorgasmia. During the early and middle stages of disease, however, sexual intimacy remains a viable option for couples.

2. Some individuals feel better withdrawing from their partners prematurely because of guilty feeling about continuing sex in light of the cognitive impairment. Role changes, distaste for sexual intimacy because of poor hygiene, or as a means of coping with the increasing demands of caregiving are also reasons for stopping sexual relationships.

3. Desexualization of the demented spouse often helps the caregiver meet the personal and intimate demands of caregiving.

4. As individuals develop dementia, touch may no longer be perceived as pleasurable or soothing. Physical touch and intimacy may result in increasing agitation or anxiety.

5. Individuals who have a minimental status examination score of less than 15 are unlikely to understand the nature of sexual activity and, therefore, may be unable to give consent.

6. While overt and inappropriate sexual behavior of demented patients is not common, caregivers may be at risk for sexual abuse by their demented spouses, or vice versa. Family physicians need to explore this issue gently with the caregiver. Such circumstances may result in the filing of elder abuse charges.

Sexual relationships in long-term facilities

1. Older women residing in assisted living and extended care facilities often lose their privacy and suffer a loss of sexual freedom.

2. Sexual intimacy between married or unmarried and consenting individuals may present difficulties for facility staff who are concerned about safety and legal issues. Family members may also object to the expression of intimacy between their aging relative and others in the facility. The family physician can serve an important role in addressing the concerns of the family and the older patient.

3. Practitioners can advocate for their patients in allowing privacy and conjugal visits, or permission medically stable individuals to participate in home visits.

Common sexual dysfunctions
Decreased sexual desire

1. According to the DSM-IV, 4th edition, hypoactive sexual desire (HSD) disorders are characterized

by persistent or recurrent absence of sexual fantasies and desires, not associated with other medical conditions.

2. This common disorder has a prevalence from 1–30% in women. The etiology is multifactorial, including physical, psychological and social causes.

3. A variety of treatments have been recommended for individuals with HSD. These range from the more insight-oriented approaches to cognitive-behavioral ones. Most treatments use sensate focus techniques. These exercises are designed to increase sexual communication between partners and to identify impediments to sexual arousal and enjoyment.

Sexual arousal disorders

1. Sexual arousal involves both physiological and psychological factors.

2. Physiologically, vaginal lubrication occurs during the excitement phase of the sexual response cycle.

3. Prevalence of this disorder varies by population studied. Women with cancer have high rates of arousal disorders, as do those who have a history of sexual abuse or trauma.

4. Treatment approaches frequently include sensate focus techniques and training in masturbation. Other therapists recommend assertiveness training for women who have been non-initiators of sexual intimacy.

Orgasmic disorders

1. A variety of factors – inability to relax, inconvenient timing of sexual activity, lack of communication, limited sexual knowledge, fatigue, body image distortions, absence of sufficient foreplay, and lack of sexual interest – have been associated with orgasmic problems in women.

2. At the same time, many women have been socialized to view sex as a duty, not as an act to be enjoyed or considered pleasurable. Sexual scripts, such as the good girl image, may contribute to orgasmic difficulties.

3. Primary care physicians can assist their patients by education and referral to appropriate therapists.

4. Treatment usually includes assessment of body image and introduction to masturbation. Self-help books can be adjunct to treatment.

Conclusions

Sexuality is a natural part of human existence, yet there is considerable variability in the ways in which individuals express themselves sexually. Normative changes occur in the sexual life of the individual. The onset of illness or chronic disease may have a significant impact on how and when a woman engages in sexual activity.

References

1. Abma J. C., *et al.* Teenagers in the United States: sexual activity, contraceptive use, and childbearing, 2002. *Vital Health Stat* 2004, Series **23**, No. 24.

2. Alexander E., Hickner B. First coitus for adolescents. Understanding why and when. *J Am Board Fam Pract* 1997; **10**, 96–103.

3. Goodson P., Evans A., Ednundson E. Female adolescents and the onset of sexual intercourse: a theory-based review of research from 1984 to 1994. *J Adolesc Health* 1997; **21**, 147–156.

4. Orr D. P., Beiter M., Ingersoll G. Premature sexual activity as an indicator of psychosocial risk. *Pediatrics* 1991; **87**, 141–147.

5. Braverman P. K., Strassburger V. C. Adolescent sexual activity. *Clin Pediatr* 1993; **56**, 658–668.

6. Shover L. H. *Sexuality and Cancer: For the Woman with Cancer and her Partner*, New York: American Cancer Society, 1990.

7. Auchinloss S. S. After treatment: psychosocial issues in gynecologic cancer survivorship. *Cancer* 1995; **76**, 2117–2124.

8. Ganz P. A., Rowland J. H., Desmond K. A., Meyerwitz B. E., Wyatt G. E. Life after breast cancer: understanding women's health related quality of life and sexual functioning. *J Clin Oncol* 1998; **16**, 501–514.

9. Wilmott M. C., Ross J. A. Women's perception: breast cancer treatment and sexuality. *Cancer Pract* 1997; **5**, 353–359.

10. Kolodny R. C. Sexual dysfunction in diabetic females. *Diabetes* 1971; **20**, 557–559.

11. Enzlin P., Mathieu C., Van den Bruel A., Bosteels J., Vanderschueren D., Demyttenaere K. Sexual dysfunction in women with type 1 diabetes: a controlled study. *Diabetes Care* 2002; **25**, 672–677.

12. Kaiser F. E. Sexuality in the elderly *Geriatr Urol* 1996; **1**, 99–109.

13. Berard E. I. The sexuality of spinal cord injured women. *Paraplegia* 1989; **27**, 99–112.

14. Demirkiran M., Sarica Y., Uguz S., Yerdelen D., Aslan K. Multiple sclerosis patients with and without sexual dysfunction: are there any differences? *Mult Scler* 2006; **12**(2), 209–214.

15. Brecher E. M., ed. *Love Sex and Aging: A Consumers' Union Report*, Boston, MA: Little, Brown and Co. 1984.

16. Mooradian A. D., Brieff V. Sexuality in older women. *Arch Intern Med* 1990; **150**, 1033–1036.

Contraception

Kathryn Andolsek

Contraception is an inherent part of good health care for women. Fertility is not a disease, and therefore contraception is not a purely medical concern but an area for collaborative care in which the woman and clinician, as well as frequently her partner(s), exchange knowledge, values and options in planning and/or preventing her pregnancies.

Introduction

The "modern" birth control era began in the USA in 1912 with Margaret Sanger's efforts. These were perhaps initiated by her own mother's experience of 18 pregnancies and 11 live births. Table 7.1 provides a historical timeline of contraception in the USA.[1]

The proportion of reproductive age women using contraception and the percentage of women using contraception at "first intercourse" continues to increase. Also, the percentage of sexually active women not using contraception has declined among most major US ethnic groups including African-Americans, Hispanics, and whites.

Despite these successes, 49% of the over six million pregnancies in the USA each year are "unintended." Five percent of US women of reproductive age report an unintended pregnancy yearly: nearly half (48%) end in abortion. Unintended pregnancy rates are substantially higher among younger women (aged 18–24), unmarried, low-income, those who did not complete high school and minority women. While the unintended pregnancy rate rose among women without a high school diploma, it fell among college graduates between 1994 and 2001.[2,3,4]

Women who do not use contraception and have unintended pregnancies are equally as likely to have a therapeutic abortion as to continue the pregnancy and have a live birth. Therefore, effective contraception for more women would most likely reduce the number of abortions.[5]

Family size continues to decline, thereby increasing the number of years that contraception is necessary for each woman. The average American family had 7.0 children in 1800, 3.5 children in 1900 and 2.0 children in 1972. The average woman will need to practice contraception for more than 20 years, if she wishes only two children. Most women will use several different contraceptive methods to meet this need.[3]

Clinicians should consider making every visit with a reproductive aged woman a "contraceptive" visit. They should assess the woman's need for contraception, satisfaction with her current method(s) and desire for change(s). Counseling about unintended pregnancy is graded as a Level III recommendation by the Institute for Clinical Systems Improvement (ICSI), indicating that there is "... insufficient evidence to prove their effectiveness and/or ... important harms ... insufficient evidence does not mean the service is not effective, but rather that the current literature is not sufficient to say whether or not the service is effective." It should be noted that this is the same designation ICSI gives advanced directive counseling, clinical breast exam screening, nutrition and physical activity counseling, skin cancer screening, PSA screening and digital rectal exam of the prostate,[6] Which are customarily accepted as part of routine health care. Many facets of effective counseling and the systems issues beyond individual clinician efforts which are necessary to enhance efficacy are considered in the white paper, "Patient Centered Contraceptive Services: Closing the Counseling Gap."[7]

Women and their partner(s) must consider many factors when selecting a contraceptive method

Handbook of Women's Health, second edition, ed. Jo Ann Rosenfeld. Published by Cambridge University Press.
© Cambridge University Press 2009.

Table 7.1 Timeline for US contraception

Year	Event
1873	US federal law made it illegal to send any "obscene, lewd, and/or lascivious" materials through the mail, including contraceptive devices and information
1914	Margaret Sanger arrested for distributing birth control information
1916	First birth control clinic, Brooklyn, NY, closed after 7 days; Sanger imprisoned
1925	First manufacture in USA of diaphragms
1928	Timing of ovulation established
1937	American Medical Association endorses birth control
1937	North Carolina is first state to include birth control in a public health program
1960	First birth control pill approved by FDA
1960	Intrauterine device approved by FDA
1965	Supreme Court (Griswold vs. Connecticut) declares state laws prohibiting contraceptive use by married couples unconstitutional
1972	Medicaid funding for family planning services authorized and contraception "allowed" to be used by unmarried couples
1973	Supreme Court legalizes abortion (Roe vs. Wade)
1990	Norplant approved by FDA
1992	Depo Provera approved by FDA
1993	Female condom approved by FDA
1997	Emergency use of OCPs approved by FDA
2004	Subcutaneous DMPA 104 mg approved by FDA
2005	Today® sponge returns to market
2006	Plan B emergency contraceptive approved as OTC by FDA for women over age 18
2006	Implanon™ FDA approved

Note: Modifed from Milestones in family planning: United States 1900–1997. *MMWR Morb Mortal Wkly Rep* 1999; **48**, 773–780.

Table 7.2 Factors important in the selection of a contraceptive method

Efficacy

Safety

Cost

Accessibility

Acceptability to partners

Degree of involvement from both members of the couple

Ease of use

Reversibility

Tolerability of side effects

Presence of non-contraceptive benefits

Mechanism of action

Ambivalence

Note: Data from *Contraception in the United States: Current Use and Continuing Challenges,* The Alan Guttmacher Institute © May 2004, http://www.guttmacher.org/presentations/contraception-us.ppt#2.

contraceptive method to the individual or couple will influence the success or failure of the method. Ethnicity and socioeconomic status may also influence contraceptive failure and success.[8]

Contraceptive method effectiveness in terms of "failure rate" is reported in terms of "perfect" and/or "typical" use. The difference between perfect use and typical use is highest (about 7% to 15% variation) for those methods that must be used at each time of sexual intercourse. Table 7.3 lists the failure rates for the currently available contraceptive methods.

Contraceptives are, in general, considered as safe, and typically result in less morbidity and mortality than does pregnancy for women younger than age 45 years.[9] However, some hormonal contraceptives may be riskier than a pregnancy for women older than age 45 years who smoke cigarettes: there are "safer" contraceptive choices for them.

Women with chronic conditions such as diabetes mellitus, heart disease, hypertension, and collagen vascular diseases may have higher morbidity and mortality from some contraceptive methods than do women without these conditions. However, these conditions frequently increase a woman's risk from pregnancy and pregnancy-related complications. Therefore the "risk" of the contraceptive method

(Table 7.2). There is no one "perfect" contraceptive method for a couple at one point in time or throughout their reproductive lives. The decision is reached through compromise among various factors. Most couples desire a highly efficacious, reliable, safe, accessible and inexpensive method. The "fit" of the

Table 7.3 Percentage of US women experiencing contraceptive failure during first 12 months of use

Method	% Failure	
	Typical use	Perfect use
None	85	85
Cervical cap: parous women	32	26
Spermicide	29	15
Withdrawal	27	4
Periodic abstinence		
Calendar method	25	9
Ovulation method	25	3
Symptothermal method	25	2
Postovulation method	25	1
Female condom	21	5
Cervical cap: nulliparous women	16	9
Diaphragm	16	6
Spermicide-containing sponge	13–16	9–11
Male condom	15	2
OCPs	8	0.3
Progestin-only OCPs, POPs	3	0.3
Contraceptive patch	1–2	0.3
Vaginal ring	1–2	0.3
Combination hormonal injection	<1	<1
Copper-containing IUD	0.8	0.6
Female sterilization	0.5	0.5
Male sterilization	0.15	0.1
Levonorgestrel intrauterine system	0.2	0.1

Note: Data from Herndon E. J., Zieman M. New contraceptive options. *Am Fam Physician* 2004; **69**, 853–860.

must be individualized against the risk of pregnancy for each individual.[10]

Access to the desired contraceptive method is an important ingredient in its success. Some methods are available "over the counter" while others require a clinician visit. Partners must find the method "acceptable" and commit to the necessary level of involvement required for its success. For example, condoms require participation of both partners, injectable progesterone or Implanon™ does not.

The ease of use is important for many women. For some, a one-time decision, such as an intrauterine device, is easier than a method that requires a "decision" and a "behavior" with each act of intercourse, such as with the diaphragm. Some women will find a "permanent" method desirable. Others prefer methods with more immediate reversibility.[11]

Virtually all methods have side effects. The perceived benefits of the method must outweigh the adverse effects. Some of these effects are medically significant, if infrequent, such as uterine perforation associated with intrauterine device (IUD) insertion. Others are "nuisance," such as perceived weight gain from injectable progesterone. Clinicians, however, should not disregard "nuisance" symptoms as "less significant" because they may indeed be highly significant to the woman and impact the adherence necessary for the success of the regimen.[12]

Some side effects constitute desirable benefits. Many barrier methods combine protection from sexually transmitted infections and diseases with their contraceptive effect. The incidence of some cancers may be reduced with use of some methods. Dysmenorrhea, iron-deficiency anemia, and acne can be decreased in users of oral contraceptives.[13]

Some individuals are concerned with the method's mechanism of action, especially methods that may work by affecting "postfertilization" mechanisms. This may be extremely important to individuals with ethical or religious views that would preclude any interference of embryonic development once fertilization of the egg by the sperm had occurred.[14]

Table 7.4 lists the contraceptive choices of women in 2002. Nine percent of users utilize a combination of more than one method. Some do this to "improve" the success of contraception. Others desire enhanced efficacy with additional benefits. The most common combination of contraceptives is the condom and the pill.[15]

Even if the clinician does not actively choose to incorporate contraceptive planning into a routine visit, knowledge of contraceptive status is critical even for the "non-contraception" office visit. For example, prescribing isotretinoin (Accutane) for a sexually active woman with acne vulgaris should only occur if she is known to consistently use a reliable method of contraception.[15] Non ace inhibitor antihypertensives

Table 7.4 2002 contraceptive choices for US women

Method	% contraceptive users
OCPs	30.6
Female sterilization	27.0
Condom	18.0
Male sterilization	9.2
Combination hormonal injection	5.3
Withdrawal	4.0
IUD	2.0
Periodic abstinence, calendar	1.2
Implant or patch	1.2
Other methods	0.9
Periodic abstinence, natural family planning	0.4
Diaphragm	0.3

Note: IUD, intrauterine device. Data from Mosher W. D., Martinez G. M., Chandra A., *et al. Use of Contraception and Use of Family Planning Services in the United States: 1982–2002, Advance Data, 2004.* Number 350.

may be a better choice for a woman with high blood pressure who may become pregnant.

Finally, even if the patient is not interested in contraception, discussing the nature and frequency of sexual activity with patients provides an opportunity to assess the risk of common sexually transmitted infections. If the woman is "at risk," counseling can include safe sex practices such as abstinence. Barrier methods, such as the male and female condoms, may be recommended as a strategy to decrease risk while providing some contraceptive benefit. Screening for cervical dysplasia and sexually transmitted infections such as gonorrhea, chlamydia, syphilis, hepatitis B and HIV may be recommended. Primary prevention against hepatitis B and HPV can be offered through vaccination. If, on the other hand, the woman is interested in becoming pregnant, she may benefit from preconception assessment and counseling, such as folic acid supplementation.

Office visits can also provide an opportunity to discuss the availability of emergency contraception or "EC" (see below) because even the woman who uses contraception may experience method "failure." EC is now available without prescription for US women over 18 years of age. Younger women may choose to keep a prescription for EC "on hand" in much the same way as women with infrequent asthma may opt to have a rescue inhaler available.

Emergency contraception (EC)

EC is birth control used to prevent pregnancy after known or suspected failure of contraception or unprotected intercourse, including sexual assault. A national survey of women in the USA reported that even though two-thirds of women were aware of EC, only 6% reported ever having used it.[16]

EC in the USA continues to provoke controversy because of ethical perspectives on prevention and termination of pregnancy, and concerns about the impact of over-the-counter availability.[17] Even so, in August 2006, the FDA approved the sale of progestin-only EC without a prescription to women and men 18 years of age and older. Some clinicians may still use estrogen/progestin containing oral contraceptives as EC because of their availability.

EC hinders or delays ovulation, prevents fertilization, and may affect implantation. It does not interrupt or disrupt an already established pregnancy. On average, eight of 70 women will become pregnant from a single act of unprotected intercourse. Progestin containing EC results in 1 pregnancy per 70 women, (about 89% effective) depending upon its timing in relation to unprotected intercourse.[18] If 70 women used combination estrogen/progestin as EC, two would become pregnant; if 700 women had an IUD placed followed unprotected intercourse, only one would become pregnant.

The World Health Organization regards the only contraindication to either combination estrogen/progestin EC or the progestin-only EC is a known pregnancy, primarily because the treatment will not work in already pregnant patients.

There have been sporadic case reports of ectopic pregnancies following EC. Patients with a history of salpingitis or ectopic pregnancy should be counseled regarding the potentially increased risk of an ectopic pregnancy regardless of EC use or non-use. Progestin-only EC does not increase the risk of ectopic pregnancy; there is no evidence demonstrating EC is teratogenic.

For individuals with chronic health conditions in which estrogen containing OCs are contraindicated, combination EC may still be offered because the duration of use is extremely short. However, progestin-only regimens may be prefered for those with with known hypercoagulable states, such as a history of blood clots or hereditary hypercoagulopathies or thrombophilias.

Because pregnancy may itself increase the risk of adverse outcomes in women with these health conditions, contraceptive benefit and availability of ECs may outweigh any risks.

Concurrent use of certain medications such as some antiepileptic drugs, St John's wort, medications to treat human immunodeficiency virus, the antibiotic rifampin, and the antifungal griseofulvin may reduce the efficacy of OCs and, thus, potentially combination EC, but not affect efficacy of the progestin-only EC.

Currently available methods of EC are listed in Table 7.5, and include oral hormones similar to those available in many OCPs , the progestin-only EC, and the copper T intrauterine device.[19]

Doses and medication

Some clinicians still informally prescribe combinations of available birth control pills "off label" particularly if women have a medication already on hand. In 1997, the US Food and Drug Administration (FDA) recognized that seven OCPs available at that time could be safely and effectively used as EC.[20] These included the medications listed in Table 7.5. The drawback is that they require taking a relatively large number of tablets at one time.

Only Plan B is currently marketed specifically for EC in the USA. Although it can be started within 120 hours of unprotected intercourse, it is most successful if used immediately. There have been virtually no contraindications. Emergency oral contraception is of such short duration and utilizes such a low hormonal dose that it is not thought to pose a risk for women at risk of stroke, deep vein thrombosis, or cardiovascular disease, even those who are not usually considered candidates for combination oral contraceptives. For almost all of these women, their risk from an unintended pregnancy is far greater than their risk from the medication. Plan B, the progestin-only OCPs, or the IUD is recommended for women who absolutely must avoid estrogen completely. Some changes in the following menstrual cycle (amount, duration, timing) can be anticipated in about 7% of women.

Preven, an EC previously available in the USA consisted of four tablets, each composed of 0.25 mg of levonorgestrel and 0.05 mg of ethinylestradiol. It is no longer marketed in the USA. Its dose is mimicked by many of the OCPS listed in Table 7.5.

Plan B, which became available in 1999, consists of two tablets of levonorgestrel, 0.75 mg. According to the product labeling, one tablet is taken initially and the second tablet is taken in 12 hours; both tablets should be taken within 72 hours of unprotected intercourse. While research data indicate both tablets may be taken initially at one time within 120 hours of unprotected intercourse with no change in efficacy,[21] it is more successful when initiated closer in time to the episode of unprotected intercourse. Neither a pelvic examination nor a pregnancy test is necessary before use. The mechanism of action appears to influence fertilization.

Another form of emergency contraception is the copper IUD; since an actual visit to a clinician is required for placement it is not as "convenient" as oral methods. Its "window" of efficacy is longer as it can be inserted within five days of unprotected intercourse. Copper IUDs are over 99% efficacious and have the additional advantage of providing continuing contraception for the woman who desires it.

Mifepristone (RU 486) is approved by the FDA for medical pregnancy termination, but not EC. It has been used at a lower dose as EC in China. It prevents 85% of the pregnancies expected to occur without treatment and can be given up to 120 hours after unprotected intercourse. The only side effect is delayed onset of the next menses. Dosages of 600 mg, 50 mg and 7 mg have been similarly efficacious. The smallest dose is associated with the lowest incidence of side effects.[11,22]

Providers may consider counseling women about EC and encouraging them to have a method "on hand." Women who do not use regular contraception, women who have a history of a past unintended pregnancy, and those who use contraceptive methods with a high rate of method failure may find EC particularly beneficial.

Women who use EC should be given additional opportunities to consider whether a more permanent or better method of contraception is warranted.

An excellent resource is the Emergency Contraception website accessible at http://ec.princeton.edu/questions/index.html which has information for a lay audience and health professionals. It also lists options for access by zip code.

Table 7.5 Medications used as emergency contraception; adapted from http://ec.princeton.edu/questions/dose.html#dose

EC method	First dose	Second dose	Ethinyl estradiol per dose (μg)	Levonorgestrel per dose (mg)	Comments
Prevens					No longer marketed in the USA
Plan B	2 white pills	None; although the label for Plan B says to take one pill within 72 hours after unprotected intercourse, and another pill 12 hours later, recent research has found that both Plan B pills can be taken at the same time.	0	1.5	Prescription not necessary if >18 years of age; the purchaser must be >18 years of age (not necessarily the intended "user"). See FDA Q and A at http://www.fda.gov/cder/drug/infopage/planB/planBQandA20060824.htm
Alesse,	5 pink pills	5 pink pills	70	0.5	
Aviane	5 orange pills	5 orange pills	70	0.5	
Levlen	4 light orange pills	4 light orange pills	120	0.6	
Levlite	5 pink pills	5 pink pills	70	0.5	
Lo Ovral	4 white pills	4 white pills	120	0.6	
Nordette	4 light orange pills	4 light orange pills	120	0.6	
Ovral	2 white pills	2 white pills	70	0.5	
Preven					
Seasonale	4 pink pills	4 pink pills	120	0.6	
Seasonique	4 light blue green pills	4 light blue green pills	120	0.6	
TriLevlen, Triphasil	4 yellow pills	4 yellow pills	120	0.5	
Copper IUD					Inserted within 5 days of intercourse; most effective of all listed; can continue contraceptive effect for up to 7 years

Abstinence

Abstinence is the only 70 percent effective contraceptive, if used 70 percent of the time; in reality, it may be difficult to practice. Patients may benefit from practical suggestions about how to implement abstinence in situations in which they feel pressured. This includes using "role play" and practicing actual word choices and responses in certain predictable situations.

Once adolescents have had a sexual experience, they may be even more open to reconsidering "abstinence" and should be encouraged to consider abstinence as a potential choice. The American Academy of Pediatrics recently updated its positions on adolescents and contraceptive counseling, commenting that

> Most successful prevention programs include multiple and varied approaches to the problem, including both abstinence promotion and contraception information and availability, sexuality education, school-completion strategies and job training; current research indicates that encouraging abstinence and urging better use of contraception are compatible goals … sexuality education that discusses contraception does not increase sexual activity, and programs that emphasize abstinence as the safest and best approach, while also teaching about contraceptives for sexually active youth, do not increase sexual activity and improve teens' knowledge about access to reproductive health.[23]

Fertility awareness

Fertility awareness methods identify the relatively few "fertile days" of each menstrual cycle: the couple then avoids genital sexual contact during those days. The number of fertile days can range from 7 to 15 days each cycle. Many couples prefer these methods because no hormones, chemicals or appliances interfere with their sexual activity. There are several methods typically classified as "fertility awareness." Their efficacy varies.

"Calendar" rhythm, a method that predicts the fertile days by "extrapolating" from the length of the previous menstrual cycles, is historically unreliable.

The symptothermal methods of natural family planning incorporate predictable physiological changes that coincide with ovulation or the immediate period prior to ovulation. "Thermal" refers to the characteristic temperature elevation associated with progesterone levels.

Just prior to ovulation, a woman's temperature declines approximately 0.1 to 0.2 °C from her usual baseline and then rises 0.5 to 0.6 °C and remains elevated for 12 to 15 days until the onset of menstruation. These changes are best assessed by a woman taking her "basal body temperature," or the temperature each morning at the same time daily before rising, eating, drinking, or smoking.

Unfortunately other conditions may affect temperature, including febrile illness and alcohol consumption. Women can also use non-prescription kits that measure the presence in urine of leutenizing hormone. However, these kits are expensive to use in this manner. "Sympto" includes the predictable

physiological changes associated with ovulation such as Mittelschmerz pain (mid cycle ovulatory pain), moliminal symptoms (breast tenderness) and changes in cervical consistency. For many couples, the most consistent "symptom" is the predictable change in cervical mucus that correlates with various portions of the menstrual cycle. Classes taught by experienced health educators or couple-to-couple instruction help couples to reliably recognize and interpret mucus changes and establish the days that require "abstinence." The couple who wishes to identify the time of peak fertility can also use these methods.

Lactational amenorrhea is another fertility awareness method described in greater detail under the section "Special populations." Its efficacy was assessed in a recent Cochrane Review.[24]

The Cochrane collaborative identified three trials, one from Colombia and two from California. Because of significant methdologic weaknesses including issues in recruitment, high drop-out rates, and poor research methods they were unable to compare how well fertility awareness-based methods work.[20]

Coitus interruptus/withdrawal

Coitus interruptus (CI)/withdrawal is the withdrawal of the penis from the vagina prior to ejaculation. Failures most commonly occur with lack of clear communication and because sperm are present in the pre-ejaculatory seminal fluids released before withdrawal. Although the failure rate is high, it is better than "no method." Couples who plan to use this method may benefit from knowledge regarding EC.

Spermicides/spermicide-containing sponge

Methods

Spermicides are chemicals that are "toxic" to sperm.[25] They either kill or inactivate sperm, without harming either partner. Most contain nonoxynol-9 or octoxynol-9 as the active ingredient. They can be used by themselves or in combination with condoms, diaphragms, or cervical caps.

STI prevention

Spermicides may reduce the risk of acquiring some sexually transmitted infections but, unfortunately, not

HIV. In fact, some experts suggest that the risk of HIV transmission may increase because of associated local irritation of genital tissue. A recent report from South Africa found that women who used vaginal gel with condoms became infected with HIV at an approximately 50% higher rate than women who used a placebo gel.[26]

Spermicides are available as gels, creams, jellies, foam, film, and suppositories. Creams may contain a higher concentration of the active ingredient. No clinical trials have compared the contraceptive efficacy of one product to another and choice is usually dependent on partners' preferences. Suppositories and tablets dissolve in less than 30 minutes and are generally effective for less than 1 hour. Either partner may develop a hypersensitivity to these products. Spermicides containing at least 70 mg nonoxynol-9 per dose proved more effective than those containing less. There were no statistical differences in pregnancy rates comparing the gel, film and suppository at doses of at least 70 mg; pregnancy was more likely at the lowest does. There were no differences in patient acceptability among the five formulations tested.[27]

Sponge

The Today® Sponge provides a physical barrier that contains spermicide and provides protection for 24 continuous hours. Made of polyurethane, sponges should be moistened with at least two tablespoons of water prior to insertion. They should be left in place at least 6 hours following the last act of intercourse and not worn for more than 30 continuous hours. It is more effective in nulliparous than in parous women. See http://www.todaysponge.com/index.html for marketing information.

Condoms
STI prevention

Certain types of condoms provide some protection against sexually transmitted infections, in addition to contraception. All condom materials do not provide the same protection. Animal-based condoms do not protect against HIV. However, latex products offer good if not perfect protection against HIV. To a lesser extent they reduce the risk of gonorrhea, syphilis, chlamydia, chancroid, trichomoniasis, HPV, herpes, and pelvic inflammatory disease.

Table 7.6 Compounds that impair latex integrity

Butoconazole, ticonazole, miconazole, clindamyin 2% vaginal cream
Conjugated estrogens (cream), estradiol (cream)
Baby oil, mineral oil, massage oil, suntan oil and lotions
Cold creams, hand and body lotion, petroleum jelly
Butter, cocoa butter, shortening, vegetable or cooking oils whipped cream
Rubbing alcohol, petroleum jelly, aldara cream

Table 7.7 Lubricants compatible with condoms: safe lubricants

Egg white, saliva, water
Glycerin, aloe
Nonoxynol-9, Gynol II
KY jelly, Astro Glide, Gynol II, Prepair, Ramses personal lubricant, Probe, Aqualube, Cornhuskers lotion, deluge, ForPlay, silicone lubricant, I-D (Cream, Glide, Juicy Lube, Millennium, Pleasure)

Cervical cancer effect

Condoms decrease the risk of cervical cancer by as much as 50%, probably because of their impact on sexually transmitted infections such as HPV.

Efficacy

The addition of spermicidal products increases their efficacy. Products that impair latex integrity should be avoided, see Table 7.6. Non-latex condoms, generally polyurethane, became available in 1995. They may provide less contraceptive efficacy, primarily due to increased breakage, but are acceptable alternatives for those with allergies, sensitivities or preferences that might prevent the use of latex condoms.[28]

Lubricants that are compatible with condoms are listed in Table 7.7.

Female condoms were FDA approved in 1993. The most common has two flexible rings on each end of a polyurethane sheath. One ring inserts into the vagina similarly to a diaphragm; the other end remains on the vulva. Female condoms should be removed immediately following intercourse and before standing. In laboratory studies, HIV transmission has been prevented but there are no clinical studies available. One study in Africa has suggested that use of female condoms, in addition to male condoms, by women with husbands with AIDS may further reduce the transmission rate.[29] Latex sensitivity is not an issue, because they are not made of latex. Therefore, oil-based products can be used. Compared with male condoms, the female condom breaks less frequently, slips more and is not as effective in pregnancy prevention. Experience improved results for both.[30]

Clinicians should strongly consider discussing the availability of EC with condom users because condoms can break (1/70), slip (5/70), leak (3.5 to 7/70), and be used inconsistently. Some couples also report less sexual sensitivity and latex-sensitive individuals cannot use latex condoms.

Diaphragm

Method

Most diaphragms are composed of soft latex. They are available in sizes from 50 to 70 mm in 2.5 mm and 5.0 mm increments. Diaphragms must be properly fitted, and several varieties are available.

Use

They are placed anteriorly just under the symphysis pubis and the posterior fornix, acting as a physical barrier to sperm. Spermicidal cream or gel is applied to the rim. The diaphragm is inserted up to two hours before intercourse. If intercourse is repeated, additional spermicide is inserted without removal of the diaphragm; it should be left in place for a minimum of 6 to 8 hours following intercourse. Diaphragms are less effective with increased episodes of intercourse. As with condoms, products that affect latex integrity should be avoided (Table 7.6). Soap and water can be used in cleansing. The woman should be instructed about correct insertion, placement, and removal. Diaphragms should not be used during menses or any vaginal bleeding because toxic shock syndrome can occur if they are left in place for more than 24 hours.

The risk of urinary tract infections is increased two-fold in women who use diaphragms. If they occur, a smaller diaphragm or one with a different rim can be substituted.

Diaphragms are more effective than the sponge or the cap for parous women. They should be refitted yearly and after pregnancy, miscarriage, abortion, pelvic surgery, or weight change of more than 4.5 kg (7 lbs).

Cervical caps

FemCap™ is essentially a smaller diaphragm made of silicone rubber which fits snugly over the cervix, providing continuous contraceptive protection for 48 hours. It comes in three sizes, small for the nulliparous woman, medium for a woman with a pregnancy of more than two weeks, a prior abortion or cesarean section and large, for women with a prior vaginal birth. The second generation FemCap™ approved by the FDA in 2003 is the only product which should be used. The addition of spermicides improve efficacy. The FemCap™ should be inserted into the vagina with the long brim entering first and the dome-side down, pushed towards the rectum and then up and onto the cervix. The patient should check to ensure the cervix is completely covered. The FemCap™ must stay in place 6 hours after last intercourse and not longer than 48 hours. It is made from silicone.

Women should be instructed to watch the instructional video very carefully before using the FemCap™, a back-up contraceptive method should be used during the learning phase and the FemCap™ should be inserted before any sexual arousal. EC should be employed if the FemCap™ was not used or used incorrectly. See http://www.femcap.com/selection.htm for more details on use.

The Prentif cavity rim cervical cap is no longer available in the USA.

Lea's Shield® is a silicone cup with an air valve and a loop. There is only one size and no fitting is required. The device should be slid into the vagina with the valve facing down and the thickest end inserted first. It must be left in the vagina for at least 8 hours after the last act of intercourse but not more than 48 hours and not during menstruation or any vaginal bleeding. A clinician instructional video is available at http://www.leasshield.com/clinicians.htm.

Oral contraceptive pills (OCPs)

OCPs are hormonal methods of birth control. There are two general varieties: combination oral contraceptive pills (COCs) consist of estrogen (usually 20–50 µg ethinylestradiol) and progesterone (e.g. levonorgestrel, norethindrone, desogestrel, norgestimate); the progestin-only pills (POPs) contain only progesterone. By comparison, the estrogen dose in COCs available 30 years ago was at a dose of 50 to 80 µg and even higher.

COCs are further classified as monophasic (fixed dose of estrogen and fixed dose of progestin), biphasic (fixed dose of estrogen with two different progesterone doses), or triphasic (fixed concentration of estrogen and three increasing concentrations of progesterone). One COC varies the dose of estrogen throughout the cycle with a single fixed dose of progesterone. There are no documented clinically significant differences among these combination pills.

POPs or "mini pills" contain one of two different kinds of progesterone. They are used by fewer than 1% of OCP users and are less effective than COCs. Their efficacy is very sensitive to the timing of the doses and ideally they should be taken at the same time of day each day. A back-up contraceptive should be instituted if the dose is delayed by more than 3 hours. Menses may be irregular or absent.

Newer COCs have been developed that offer additional options in dosing. "Very low dose estrogen" pills contain less than 20 μg. Although very low dose estrogen pills minimize the risk of venous thromboembolism compared with older estrogen doses greater than 50 μg, they have not been proven to be safer than OCPs with an intermediate estrogen dose of 30 to 50 μg. They are associated with more breakthrough bleeding, which may be problematic for patients.

Most COCs combine 21 days of "active pill" with 7 days of placebo during which withdrawal bleeding occurs.

More recent COCs have been introduced that reduce or even eliminate the 7 day placebo interval. Two 28 day products, Yaz® (3 mg of drospirenone and 20 mcg ethinyl estradiol) and Loestein®24 FE (1 mg norethindrone acetate and 20 mcg ethinyl estradiol) provide active hormone for 24 instead of 21 days followed by four (not seven) inert pills.

There are also currently extended pill regimens, which reduce the number of withdrawal bleeding episodes per year. Seasonale® (levonorgestrel 150 μg/ethinyl estradiol 30 μg), has 84 days of active pills, followed by 7 inert pills for a hormone-free week. Seasonique™ (84 tablets of 150 μg levonorgestre/estradiol 30 μg and 7 tablets containing 10 μg ethinyl estradiol) completely eliminates the hormone free interval by using seven days of low-dose estrogen (10 μg ethinyl estradiol) during what otherwise would be the pill-free interval. Breakthrough bleeding and spotting are more common but decline with time. The total dose of estrogen for women with these products

Table 7.8 Conditions that appear to be decreased in incidence or severity by oral contraceptives

Ectopic pregnancy

Premenstrual syndrome, menstrual flow, dysmenorrhea

Endometriosis, endometrial cancer

Ovarian cysts, ovarian cancer

Uterine fibroids

Benign breast disease

Toxic shock syndrome

Risk of hospitalization

Rheumatoid arthritis

Osteoporosis

Acne

Hirsutism

is greater than for the traditional 28 day pills, but the clinical significance of this is unknown.[31]

OCPs using new progestins, such as norgestimate and desogestrel, are referred to as third-generation progestins. They are associated with fewer androgenic side effects such as acne and hair loss, they do not affect weight or blood pressure, and are associated with negligible changes in blood glucose, plasma insulin or lipids. A few years ago some studies linked them to an increased risk of thromboembolism; however, the evidence is inconclusive.

OCPs offer many non-contraceptive benefits.[10] The newer progestin-containing OCPs increase high density lipoprotein cholesterol (HDL-C). Perimenopausal users of OCPs with 50 μg of estrogen demonstrate increased bone density and may reduce their risk of hip fracture by 44%. Triphasic OCPs combining norgestimate are as efficacious as topical tretinoin, benzoyl peroxide, and topical or systemic antibiotics for the treatment of moderate acne vulgaris. Table 7.8 lists other conditions ameliorated or lessened by the use of oral contraceptives.

OCPs protect against certain reproductive cancers of the endometrium and ovary. The risk of ovarian cancer is decreased by 40% among OCP users; this benefit persists for up to 20 years following discontinuation of the pill. Women who use OCPs for ten or more years reduce the risk of ovarian cancer by 80%. BRCA-positive women experience similar reductions in risk. The risk of endometrial cancer is decreased by

40% in women who use OCPs for at least two years, and 60% if OCPs are used for at least four years.

The link between OCP use and breast cancer is less conclusive. A 1996 collaborative analysis of over 53,000 women with breast cancer enrolled in 53 studies from 25 countries concluded that "ever users" of OCPs had a 1.07 relative risk of breast cancer unrelated to dose or duration of use. However, OCP users had a lower risk of metastatic disease ($R = 0.88$ compared with non-users).[32]

For most women, pregnancy and/or abortion are associated with a greater risk of mortality and morbidity than oral contraceptives. In attempting to assist the individual woman and her clinician in decision-making, the World Health Organization has replaced a single list of "contraindications" with four categories of increasing "precautions" for women considering OCPs.[33] Category 1 consists of conditions for which no restrictions to pill use are necessary. Category 2 contains medical conditions for which the advantages of OCPs outweigh known risks. Category 3 includes conditions for which the clinician should exercise caution but not necessarily refrain from prescribing. Only category 4 conditions are felt to be so significantly linked to OCP use that WHO recommends patients with these conditions should refrain from using OCPs (Table 7.9).

Thromboembolism, found in category 4, is believed to be related less to the dose of hormone than to the duration of use; there is a decreased risk over time.[34]

Some medical conditions may worsen with the use of OCPs. If this occurs, an oral contraceptive with a lower estrogen dose or progestin-only oral contraceptive can be substituted. Women with well-controlled diabetes mellitus, hypertension, and hypertriglyceridemia (triglycerides <750 mg/dL) should be followed closely but most will do well on OCPs. OCPs are generally contraindicated in women over 35 years of age who smoke cigarettes. Newer OCPs with low doses of estrogen or progestin-only pills are associated with less risk of heart disease. Women who have migraines may have risks associated with OCPs. If a woman's migraines are controlled, she may try a lower dose estrogen COC or POP. If headaches worsen, OCPs should be discontinued and another method used.

Side effects

Most women will experience breakthrough bleeding (BTB) within the first three months of OCP use. If pregnancy has been excluded, BTB is not necessarily a reason to change pills. Breakthrough bleeding is more common with POPs. It may be managed with NSAIDs, a change to COCs, a second- or third-generation COC, or 7–13 days of oral estrogen although there are no randomized trials which support the efficacy of any of these regimens over another.

If the patient develops hair thinning or acne, a product containing a low androgenic progestin such as desogestrel or norgestimate can be considered. Most women using OCPs will have a blood pressure rise of less than 5 mmHg, which generally resolves within three months of discontinuing the pill. Mood changes and fatigue are usually related to the progestin component. A change to a different progestin or a decrease in dose may ameliorate symptoms.[35] Some women prefer amenorrhea to continued end-of-cycle bleeding. This will usually be accomplished by continuing directly with the active pills from the next pack once a pack is completed, and neither "stopping the pills for seven pill free days," nor using the "placebo" pills. Women with uncomfortable premenstrual symptoms that occur during the pill free or placebo days may benefit from continuing directly with the first active pill from the next pill pack.

Missing pills

If a woman misses one pill she should take two pills the next day and continue with the rest of the pack as usual. If she misses two pills in the first two weeks of the cycle, she should take two pills each day for two days and then complete the pack as usual using a back-up method of contraception. If she misses two pills in the third week or misses additional pills, the pack should be discarded and a new pack used. She should use a back-up method of contraception for at least seven days.[36]

Teratogenic effects

Teratogenic effects have probably been overstated in the past. If a woman inadvertently becomes pregnant while using OCPs, the pills should be discontinued but therapeutic abortion is not necessary.

Vacations and subsequent fertility

Pill free periods are unnecessary. When she wishes to conceive, the woman needs only to discontinue the pill. Over 50% of women will become pregnant in three months and 80% in one year. Folic acid supplementation is a desirable preconception addition

Table 7.9 WHO Precaution categories for OCP use

Category 1 (no restrictions)	Category 2 (advantages outweigh risks)	Category 3 (exercise caution)	Category 4 (refrain from use)
Postpartum ≥21 days; Postabortion, abortion performed in 1st or 2nd trimester		Postpartum <21 days	Pregnancy
		Lactation (6 weeks to 6 months)	Lactation (<6 weeks postpartum)
Irregular vaginal bleeding patterns without anemia; Past history of PID; Current or recent history of PID		Undiagnosed vaginal or uterine bleeding	
Vaginitis without purulent cervicitis; Cervical ectropion; Uterine fibroids	Cervical cancer		
Current or recent history of STD; Increased risk of STD; HIV-positive or at high risk for HIV infection			
Benign breast disease; Family history of breast, endometrial, or ovarian cancer	Undiagnosed breast mass	History of breast cancer, but no recurrence in past 5 years	Breast cancer
Varicose veins	Family history of premature myocardial infarction; BP 140/70 to 159/79 mmHg		Venous thromboembolism; Cerebrovascular or coronary artery disease; Structural heart disease; Hypertension (BP >160/70 mmHg)
Mild headaches	Severe headaches after initiation of OCPs		Headaches with focal neurological symptoms
History of gestational diabetes	Diabetes mellitus		Diabetes with complications
Viral hepatitis carrier	Family history of lipid disorders	Gallbladder disease	Liver disease
Thyroid conditions			
	Sickle-cell disease or sickle-cell hemoglobin C disease		
Obesity			
	Age >50 years	Age >35 years and smoke <20 cigarettes per day	Age >35 and smoke ≥20 cigarettes per day
	Major surgery without prolonged immobilization		Major surgery with prolonged immobilization
	Conditions predisposing to medication non-compliance	Interacting drugs	
Past ectopic pregnancy			

Notes: PID, pelvic inflammatory disease; OCPs, oral contraceptive pills; BP, blood pressure.

because OCPs may deplete folic acid stores. The woman does not need to wait three months after discontinuing the pill before conception.

Medications

OCPs may affect, or be affected by, the concurrent use of other medications, especially seizure medication and some antibiotics.

Pathophysiology

Although the primary mechanism of OCPs is to inhibit ovulation, secondary mechanisms also occur, especially with the low dose pills, progestin-only pills, and inconsistent use of OCPs. These include "post-fertilization" effects. Larimore and Stanford suggest that the evidence is compelling enough that patients should be fully informed about the mechanisms of action so that individuals with reservations involving postfertilization mechanisms have the opportunity to make a truly informed decision.[37]

Starting OCPs

A complete physical examination, Pap smear and pelvic examination do not need to be performed prior to initiating OCPs.

A quick-start method has been described, and has the advantage of simplicity.

Contraceptive patch

The combination contraceptive patch (OrthoEvra®) was introduced in 2002 and offers ease of use with weekly replacement. It combines continuous systemic doses of norelgestromin and ethinyl estradiol. The patch is applied weekly three of four weeks; the fourth week no patch needs to be applied. Risks, benefits and potential drug interactions in general are similar to those for oral contraceptives. The patch is associated with 60% higher total exposure to ethinyl estradiol than with the 35 µg pill, but peak estrogen levels are lower. The significance of these data is currently unknown. With typical use, its efficacy is reported to be greater than that of an oral contraceptive and it is easily reversible.[38] In November 2005 the FDA added information to the OrthoEvra label about the increased exposure to estrogen in women who use the patch compared with oral contraceptives containing norgestimate and 35 µg ethinyl estradiol. In September 2006 the FDA announced an update to the OrthoEvra product label stating that users may

be at increased risk of thromboembolism (VTE) when compared with OCP users and advising that women with concerns or risk factors to talk with their health care provider about using OrthoEvra versus other contraceptive options. The FDA warning was based on analysis of two studies. One study found the risk of VTE doubled, another found no increased risk in users of the patch. Women immobilized due to surgery or injury should discontinue the patch because of the associated risks for venous thrombo-embolic events.[39,40]

The patch may be less effective in women weighing more than 198 pounds. One study reported less bleeding in women who applied the patch for more weeks before the patch-free week.[41]

Injectable progestin

Approximately 1% of US women elect to use injectable depot medroxyprogesterone acetate (DMPA). Intramuscular DMPA (150 mg) provides effective contraception for 12 weeks. A new, lower DMPA formulation at a 30% decreased dose (104 mg) administered subcutaneously is currently available. It has been demonstrated to be equally efficacious as the higher does. Although as yet no controlled trial has compared it directly to the 150 mg dose, anecdotally the side effects are similar.[42]

There is an increased risk of pregnancy if the injection is delayed to 14 weeks and if given beyond 12 weeks. In these cases, a back-up contraceptive should be used for two to four weeks.

The lower dose, subcutaneous 104 mg medroxyprogesterone acetate injectable, FDA approved in 2004, is available as prefilled syringes that can be administerd into the thigh or abdomen every 12–14 weeks. It can be given by the clinician or the woman herself, much as individuals give themselves insulin. The dose does not need to be adjusted based on body weight.

Fertility usually returns in four to nine months, but may take as long as 18 months. Duration of use is not related to the length of time before fertility returns. This is particularly effective if temporary excellent contraception is required as during the use of isotretinoin or other medicines, or while waiting for confirmation of vasectomy success.

Side effects

Menstrual disturbances are common. Bleeding can be treated with NSAIDs, combined combination oral contraceptives, or 7 to 13 days of oral estrogen. Amenorrhea is common; over half of women develop amenorrhea within the first year, and three-quarters after the second year. Weight gain has been an issue for many women. The average weight gain is 2 kg (5 lbs) during the first year of use and 5+ kg (11+ lbs) during the second year. Overweight and obese women have lower efficacy rates. Other side effects include bloating, decreased libido, dizziness, mood changes, acne, palpitations, depression, breast tenderness, and headache. Total cholesterol and LDL may increase while HDL decreases.

Bone recovery

Bone mineral density may be reduced in women younger than age 20 years. Duration of use also plays a role, and women who use this method for more than five years are at particular risk. In 2004, the FDA added a "black box" warning to the labeling indicating that women who use Depo-Provera contraceptive injection may lose significant bone mineral density; bone loss is greater with increasing duration of use and may not be completely reversible. It is unknown whether use of Depo-Provera contraceptive injection during adolescence will reduce peak bone mass and increase the risk for osteoporotic fracture in later life. Depo-Provera contraceptive injection should be used as a long-term birth control method (e.g. longer than two years) if other methods are "inadequate."

There is a relatively high rate of discontinuation from this method, perhaps because it is associated with irregular bleeding, weight gain, and increased headaches.

Alternatives

The availability of alternative contraceptive strategies should be discussed at each visit. Adolescents, in particular, may simply not return for a subsequent injection and yet fail to substitute an effective contraceptive.

Subdermal implants

The Norplant system was a six-rod progestin implant that was implanted in the skin of the arm and released 50 to 80 µg levonorgesterel the first year and 30 and 35 µg per year for each of the following four years. In 2000, the manufacturer issued an advisory that the contraceptive efficacy of certain lots of the implants could not be guaranteed, and it was withdrawn.

Implanon™ was approved in 2006. It is a single rod progestin subdermal implant that is about the size of a match stick. It continually releases a steady dose of progestin (etonogestrel) for up to three years. Its effect is quickly reversible. A woman's fertility returns within 24–72 hours of removal. Its primary mechanism of action is to inhibit ovulation although it also increases the viscosity of cervical mucus. It can be used for lactating women after the fourth postpartum week.[43]

It is placed in the groove between the biceps and triceps muscles and can only be inserted and removed by clinicians who complete a formal training program.

Efficacy

Six pregnancies have been reported in 20,648 cycles.

Side effects

Side effects include irregular menses and headache. Bleeding irregularities usually decrease over the first six to twelve months and after that time most women experience amenorrhea. At the end of the first year the mean cumulative weight gain was 2.8 pounds and by the end of the second year 3.7 pounds. Less common side effects are acne, change in appetite, change in libido, ovarian cysts, discoloration or scarring of the skin over the implant, dizziness, hair loss, headache, nausea, nervousness, pain at the insertion site or sore breasts.

Contraindications

Contraindications include active liver disease, active thrombophlebitis, known or suspected breast cancer, undiagnosed abnormal gynecological bleeding, pregnancy, or hypersensitivity to the drug.

Some medications may make Implanon™ less effective. These include barbiturates, griseofulvin, rifampin, phenylbutazone, phenytoin, carbamazepine, felbamate, oxcarbazepine, topiramate, and modafinil as well as possibly herbal remedies such as St. John's Wort.

Interested clinicians should register at the website http://www.implanon-usa.com/hcp/index.asp?C=571 37391742296759259&OrgDom=www.implanonusa.com or http://www.implanon-usa.com/hcp/index.asp?svar qvp2=0 for information on training.

Intrauterine devices (IUDs)

IUDs are the most cost-effective efficacious methods of contraception if used for at least two years.[44] IUDs are the most widely used reversible contraceptive worldwide used by 12% of women. However, in the USA, fewer than 2% of women use IUDs, even though user satisfaction is greater than with any other contraceptive method.

The two IUDs currently available in the USA, the copper-releasing ParaGard T 380A intrauterine contraceptive and levonorgestrel-releasing intrauterine system (IUS), are both T-shaped and have monofilament tails. They can be inserted at any time of the menstrual cycle. The copper variety may be used as an "emergency contraceptive method" if inserted within five days of unprotected intercourse. If used postpartum, it should be inserted within 7 minutes of delivery of the placenta or at 6–8 weeks.

The copper IUD is effective for seven years. Its failure rate is 0.7% in the first year of use. The copper IUD impairs sperm motility and viability, disrupts oocyte division and the formation of fertilizable ova. Changes also occur in the endometrium that could interfere with the implantation of a fertilized ovum. Its primary disadvantage is an average 55% increase in monthly blood loss and dysmenorrhea.[45]

Both IUDs have efficacy rates comparable to sterilization. The levonorgestrel-releasing IUD is the most effective of the currently available IUDs. Its first-year failure rate is 0.1%. Progesterone-releasing IUDs thicken cervical mucus, impeding the movement of sperm. They inhibit sperm capacitation, survival and motility, suppress ovulation (in some women), thin and suppress the endometrium, and stimulate an inflammatory reaction that may impede sperm function and prevent implantation. It may affect tubal mobility and implantation. In addition to contraception, it can be used to treat menorrhagia, dysmenorrhea, and endometriosis. It can also be used for supplemental progesterone in women who take estrogen for hormone replacement therapy (HRT).

Side effects

While IUDs do not increase the risk of pelvic inflammatory disease (PID), this can occur within the first 20 days following insertion. The incidence of PID decreases from 7/700 within the first 20 days to 1/700 after 21 days. IUD users may acquire PID, either during the insertion process and/or from sexual activity. To decrease this risk, IUDs are generally not indicated if either the woman or her partner have multiple sexual partners and are therefore more likely to develop sexually related PID. The routine use of

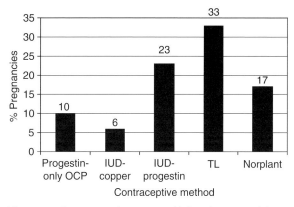

Figure 7.1 Percentage of pregnancies likely to be ectopic if the woman becomes pregnant while using a contraceptive method. OCP, oral contraceptive pill; IUD, intrauterine device; TL, tubal ligation.

antibiotics administered orally one hour before insertion is not recommended.[46,47] Even though antibiotic prophylaxis against subacute bacterial endocarditis is appropriate for women with valvular heart disease, prophylactic antibiotics are unnecessary for women with mitral valve prolapse. Actinomyces-like organisms are common in the genital tract. Symptomatic IUD users with positive actinomyces findings on a Pap smear should be treated with appropriate antibiotics and their IUD removed. Asymptomatic IUD users do not require IUD removal or antibiotic therapy.

Complications also include uterine perforation and expulsion. Uterine perforation during insertion is rare. The expulsion rate is 2–7% within the first year. There is a higher risk of expulsion in nulliparous women and in women with severe dysmenorrhea or excessive blood flow. If a woman experiences expulsion, she has a 30% risk of having a second IUD expelled.

Contrary to a widespread misperception, copper IUDs actually reduce the risk of ectopic pregnancy. In fact, the rate of ectopic pregnancy is 90% lower than in women who use no form of birth control. If a woman becomes pregnant while using the IUD, there is a 5% risk of an ectopic pregnancy.

Any woman who conceives while using any method of contraception should be assumed to have an ectopic pregnancy until proven otherwise. A woman who conceives using the subdermal implant has a 17% chance of an ectopic pregnancy. A woman using a progestin-only OCP and who conceives has a 7% chance of an ectopic pregnancy, and a woman with tubal sterilization who conceives has a 33% chance (Figure 7.1).[48]

Table 7.10 Contraindications to use of intrauterine devices (IUDs)

Pregnancy	Wilson's disease (Copper IUD)
Active PID only (acceptable IUD indications now include women with a history of PID without active PID)	Current PID
Known pelvic tuberculosis	Women with copper allergy (Copper IUD)
Uterine or cervical malignancy	Undiagnosed abnormal uterine bleeding
Known anomalies or fibroids that distort the uterine cavity in a way that is incompatible with IUD insertion	Immediately after puerperal sepsis or septic abortion

Note: PID, pelvic inflammatory disease.

An IUD user who has an intrauterine pregnancy has a 50% risk of a spontaneous abortion. This risk can be reduced by the early removal of the IUD, if necessary under ultrasound guidance.

Contraindications

Nulliparity is not a contraindication to IUD use, although any potential IUD user should be counseled about the potential risk of PID and subsequent sterility. Parous women are not reported to have demonstrable changes in future fertility compared to users of other contraceptive methods; there are conflicting data in nulliparous women.[49] Contraindications to IUD use are listed in Table 7.10.

The levonorgestrel-releasing IUD can be used to treat menorrhagia and anemia and as an alternative to hysterectomy in women with bleeding.[50]

Follow-up

Patients who do not practice safe sex are probably not good candidates for IUDs. If PID develops, the infection should be treated and the IUD should be removed if symptoms fail to improve within 72 hours after treatment begins. If a sexually transmitted infection (STI) is diagnosed, the infection should be treated but IUD removal is not necessary. If the patient cannot feel the IUD string and it cannot be visualized, pregnancy should be excluded. The

clinician can probe for string presence in the cervical canal or a pelvic ultrasound can be used to evaluate whether the IUD is still present and within the uterine cavity.

Vaginal ring[51]

Introduced in the USA in 2001, the vaginal contraceptive ring (NuvaRing®) is a flexible single-size (approximately 2 inches in diameter) ring that releases 5 μg of ethinyl estradiol and 120 μg of etonogestrel daily.

It is worn continuously for three weeks, and then removed for one week. The ring can also be removed for up to three hours at a time if desired. The majority of women in a clinical study considered insertion and removal of the vaginal ring to be easy. The failure rate from the study was 0.65%.

Sterilization
Female sterilization

Female sterilization has the advantage of being a single decision which is best thought of as a "permanent decision." The most common procedures are tubal ligation and Essure® tubal occlusion. In terms of the tubal ligation method, anesthesia, sepsis and hemorrhage can cause mortality, but at a very low rate of 1 to 2 per 70,000. The Essure® tubal occlusion procedure was approved in 2002 and involves placing titanium-dacron coils (micro inserts) into the Fallopian tubes during hysteroscopy. This method involves no surgery and no general anesthesia. Over the course of 3 months, the micro inserts cause tissue to form and block the Fallopian tubes (http://www.essuremd.com/).

As many as 6 to 22% of women report subsequent "regret" about their sterilization decision, although only 1% elect to reverse the procedure.[52,53] The likelihood of regret is increased in women who have been provided with inadequate counseling, women younger than age 30 years, women who have had postpartum procedures, and women who have experienced a change in their marital status or relationships.

Sterilization should be considered a permanent non-reversible option. Although it may be technically possible to reverse some sterilization methods, it is expensive, requires major surgery, and medical insurance does not typically reimburse this expense; success is not guaranteed. The success rate for a subsequent pregnancy is 43 to 86% and assisted reproductive technologies are frequently required.

Women seeking this method should be counseled about the availability of other methods, such as OCPs, injectables and IUDs that are effective if used consistently, and more easily reversible.

The failure rate for tubal ligation though low, is greater than was once appreciated.[54] An average of 18.5 out of 700 women will become pregnant within the seven-year period following sterilization. One-third of the pregnancies that occur are ectopic. The highest risk of pregnancy is among young women sterilized with bipolar coagulation (54.3/700) or by clip occlusion (52.1/700).

Postpartum tubal ligations are less effective than ligations performed at other "interval" periods. The clinician should have a low index of suspicion in ordering a pregnancy test in the evaluation of an individual with relevant symptoms or signs. A pregnant patient with a previous tubal ligation should be assumed to have an ectopic pregnancy unless proven otherwise.

Complications

Mortality: 1 to 2 deaths/70,000 women compared to a maternal mortality rate of 12.1/70,000 live births.

Morbidity

Excessive bleeding or hemorrhage, infection, anesthesia-related complications, trauma to abdominal organs, future risk of ectopic pregnancy complications. Sterilization does not cause of lack of libido, loss of femininity, or weight gain.

Three primary methods are used: tubal ligation, mechanical occlusion of the Fallopian tubes, and electrocoagulation (the most common and simplest to perform).

Mechanical occlusion techniques include clips, rings, or microinserts. Microinserts are relatively new, approved by the FDA in 2002 and inserted transcervically by hysteroscopic visualization. Patients must undergo a hysterosalpingogram three months after surgery and use back-up contraception until occlusion has been confirmed.[55]

Partner/spousal permission is not required but discussing the decision with the partner may improve the quality of the decision making. Federally funded sterilizations may not be performed on anyone under 21 years of age or incapable of informed consent. There is a 30-day waiting period which extends from the signing of the consent form to the time the procedure is performed.

Male sterilization

Male sterilization is the most cost-effective contraceptive method, with a failure rate of 0.1 to 4%. Compared with tubal ligation, it is less expensive, results in fewer complications and surgical risks, necessitates a briefer recovery time with less time away from work, and poses no long-term health risk.

One-half to two-thirds of men will develop sperm antibodies, but their significance is at the present time, unknown.

Reversibility though theoretically possible is difficult and entails additional expense and risk. Male sterilization therefore should be assumed to be a permanent method. Success of reversal is related to the length of time from the original procedure. The overall success rate is 16 to 79%.

Special populations[10,56]
Adolescents[57,58]
Abstinence[59]

Increased abstinence accounted for one-quarter of the drop in the US teen pregnancy rate observed between 1988 and 1995. This decline was caused by lower pregnancy rates among sexually experienced women aged 15–19 years, and not because of a rise in abortions. Abstinence, if a method chosen by the adolescent, should be actively supported and accompanied by specific peer negotiating strategies. Abstinence programs may help adolescents to postpone first intercourse. It may also be a valid method for teens who have been sexually active in the past, but now choose to defer further activity; it can be combined with other methods.

EC

Counseling regarding the availability of EC may provide a back-up method should abstinence not always succeed.

Hormonal therapy

OCPs are excellent choices because teens may benefit from non-contraceptive effects such as more regular periods, less dysmenorrhea, and improved acne. The contraceptive patch and Implanon may also be well tolerated. IUDs are generally avoided though data on future fertility in nulliparous women are conflicting. Injectable DMPA may adversely affect bone density and if weight gain occurs this symptom may be less well tolerated among adolescents. If used by adolescents it should be confined to less than two years unless there is convincing evidence that no other method is acceptable.

Condoms should be encouraged to enhance whatever contraception the woman chooses as they provides additional contraceptive benefit and some protection from STIs.

Information on EC should be offered and a prescription provided if a "back-up" method is desired. EC is available without a prescription only to those over 18 years of age so the younger adolescent benefits from a prescription on hand.

The advantages and disadvantages of other over the counter products such as spermicides and the sponge should be addressed in case the woman decides on sexual activity before the next office visit.

Abuse

Ten percent of young women report that their first intercourse was either "not voluntary" or "rape." Because coerced sex in this age group is prevalent, clinicians should be vigilant for signs and symptoms of potential abuse.

Postpartum

Two-thirds of couples resume sexual relations within the first postpartum month; 90% within the second month. Because ovulation may occur within 3–4 weeks and before the first menses, contraception should be initiated either immediately postpartum or within the first few weeks.

Non-breast-feeding women

Although there are theoretical concerns regarding postpartum hypercoaguability, there are no definitive clinical data that justify withholding combined contraceptives until four weeks postpartum although this is the recommendation indicated in product labeling. Progestin-only oral contraceptives and DMPA do not contain estrogen, and these methods may be safely initiated immediately postpartum.

ACOG recommends DMPA and progestin-only pills be initiated at six weeks postpartum in lactating women and immediately postpartum in non-lactating women if desired.

IUDs are less likely to be expelled if inserted immediately following the delivery of the placenta. If not inserted immediately they should be inserted at 6–8 weeks postpartum.

Breast-feeding women[60,61,62,63]

Lactation provides an excellent and reliable contraceptive method for up to six months, with a failure rate of 0.5 to 1.5% for women who exclusively breast feed at least every four hours and experience an absence of menstrual bleeding. Pumping is not an effective substitute for suckling.

Another contraceptive method should be initiated if any supplemental feedings are given to the infant, if the feeding frequency decreases, or when the baby reaches six months of age.

Spermicides, condoms, and barrier methods are acceptable choices, although diaphragms should be fitted or refitted at approximately six weeks postpartum. A new size of FemCap may need to be prescribed.

Fertility awareness methods may require closer scrutiny of physiological parameters. The basal body temperature may not be reliable in the setting of the normal sleep disruption of the newborn period.

Progestin methods (Implanon, progestin-releasing IUS, DMPA (104 mg or 150 mg), and progestin-only pills) are recommended after 4–6 weeks postpartum, based largely upon theoretical concerns and animal studies.

The World Health Organization recommends that COCs should be avoided in lactating women within the first six weeks postpartum and used with caution between six weeks and six months. Although the estrogen that is transmitted in breast milk has not been shown to be detrimental to the infant, it has been associated with decreased milk supply in some studies. Some lactating women may not be able to compensate with greater milk production. There are essentially no conclusive data in human mothers as to the clinically significant impact of either progestin compounds or combination contraceptives in breast milk on infants.

ACOG on the other hand references studies that state the use of hormonal contraception in nourished breastfeeding women does not appear to compromise infant growth or development nor impair lactation. They advise COCs can be used once milk flow is well established. POPs and DMPA do not impair lactation and can be used "immediately."

Although small amounts of progestin are passed into the breast milk, no adverse infant effects have been documented. Product labeling for progestin-only pills recommends fully breastfeeding women begin tablets six weeks postpartum and partially breastfeeding women begin at three weeks.

Use of DMPA immediately post partum does not appear to adversely affect lactation or infant development.

ACOG recommends DMPA and progestin-only pills, be used at 6 weeks postpartum in lactating women and immediately postpartum in non-lactating women if desired.

Postpartum sterilization, if chosen, should be performed after the infant's first successful feed to minimize any impact of a delayed first feed on lactation; the mother should be allowed to nurse again in the recovery room. Alternatively, it can be performed at six weeks postpartum.

Cigarette smokers

Clinicians should prescribe combination hormonal contraceptive methods only cautiously, if at all, to women over the age of 35 years of age who smoke. Barrier methods, injectable progestin, subdermal implants or IUDs are preferred.

Chronic hypertension

Oral contraceptives are associated with increased blood pressure even when women use newer products containing dosages of 30 μg of ethinyl estradiol and 150 μg of progestin. DMPA progestin-only pills and IUD use does not appear to increase baseline blood pressure. In deciding whether or not to use combination hormonal contraceptives in women with hypertension, risk of adverse events should be balanced against the known adverse pregnancy outcomes associated with hypertension.

Healthy non-smoking women with well-controlled hypertension, no evidence of end organ damage and who are <35 years may be appropriate candidates for a trial of combination contraceptives. If blood pressure remains well controlled several months after contraceptive initiation, and is closely followed up, its use can be continued.

Although data are non-existent or inconclusive, it would probably be prudent to consider other combination hormonal contraceptive products (transdermal, vaginal ring) in the same manner as oral hormonal contraceptives.

For hypertensive women, progestin-only contraceptives, such as DMPA, POPs, or the levonorgestrel intrauterine system, or copper IUD are appropriate options.

Perimenopausal women[64]

Many non-smoking healthy women can continue to use OCPs safely past 35 years of age. The hormone content of OCPs may alleviate some menopausal signs and symptoms, help maintain bone integrity, and reduce risks of ovarian and endometrial cancer. On the other hand age and obesity (which is frequently increased in prevalence with aging) are risk factors for cardiovascular disease. VTE increases with age and the risk of VTE attributable to combination OC use increases substantially for women ≥40 years. Although data on the impact of OC use by women in their 40s and 50s on breast cancer risk is limited, information on the effect of menopausal combined hormone therapy on breast cancer risk should make clinicians cautious and individualize OC use based on risk, patient preferences and review of alternatives.

The use of serum FSH in deciding whether a woman is menopausal can be expensive and misleading. Most experts would recommend against using the test to determine whether a woman in her late 40s and early 50s remains "fertile." If a woman is otherwise healthy and desires combination hormonal contraception after discussion of risks and benefits she may remain on these until 50 to 55 years of age.

The use of OCPs in women over 40 years of age has been shown to reduce the risk of hip fracture by 44% and strengthen bone density.

Subdermal implants and IUDs may be especially good choices as they confer contraceptive efficacy for 3–7 years after which time the reproductive capacity may diminish.

Because fertility declines in the late 40s and early 50s, barrier methods may be relatively more effective.

Thrombophila

The thrombophilic effect of combination hormonal methods is produced by the estrogen component. Progestin-only contraceptives (injectable progestin, etonogestrel implant, POPs, levonorgestrel releasing IUDs) are more appropriate for women with these conditions, and potentially as well for those with significant coronary vascular disease risk factors.

Combination hormonal contraceptives (oral, transdermal or vaginal) are not recommended for women with documented history of unexplained VTE or VTE associated with pregnancy or exogenous estrogen use, unless they are taking anticoagulants.

The copper T380A IUD contains no hormones and therefore is an appropriate contraceptive option for these women.

Barrier methods are also acceptable, however they have less contraceptive efficacy.

At the present time screening for hypercoaguable states is not routinely recommended in low risk women (with a personal history or strong family history of VTE or PE) before initiating a combination hormonal contraceptive.

Diabetes

Combination hormonal contraception does not adversely affect metabolic control or increase vascular disease or CVD risk in women with type 1 or type 2 diabetes mellitus without vascular disease.

In diabetic women with vascular involvement, combination hormonal contraceptive methods are contraindicated.

ACOG recommends combination hormonal contraceptives should be limited to non-smoking otherwise healthy women younger than age 35 years with no evidence of hypertension, nephropathy or retinopathy.

For women with diabetes without vascular disease or hypertension, the use of copper IUDs, levonorgestrel IUDs, or progestin-only contraceptive methods is not contraindicated.

For women with diabetes with vascular disease or hypertension, the use of copper IUDs or progestin-only contraceptive methods is acceptable. DMPA has been associated with increased fasting blood sugar levels in women with well-controlled diabetes. However the clinical significance of this is uncertain.

Combination hormonal contraceptive use does not precipitate type 2 diabetes even in women with a history of gestational diabetes.

Migraines

Combination hormonal contraceptives may be considered for non-smoking women <35 years of age with migraine headaches without focal neurological signs, who are otherwise healthy.

Table 7.11 Medical conditions where progestin-only methods may be more appropriate

In women with the following conditions, use of progestin-only contraceptives, including depot medroxyprogesterone acetate, or IUD may be safer than combination oral, transdermal, or vaginal ring contraceptives.
Migraine headaches, especially those with focal neurological signs
Cigarette smoking or obesity in women older than 35 years
History of thromboembolic disease
Hypertension in women with vascular disease or older than 35 years
Systemic lupus erythematosus with vascular disease, nephritis, or antiphospholipid antibodies
Less than three weeks postpartum (IUDs not appropriate)
Hypertriglyceridemia
Coronary artery disease
Congestive heart failure
Cerebrovascular disease

Notes: Data from American College of Obstetricans and Gynecologists. ACOG Committee on Practice Bulletins – Gynecology, ACOG Practice Bulletin no. 73: use of hormonal contraception in women with coexisting medical conditions. *Obstet Gynecol* 2006; **77**, 1453, with permission.
See also http://www.who.int/reproductive-health/publications/mec/iuds.html

ACOG recommends clinicians consider the use of progestin-only, intrauterine, or barrier contraceptives for women with migraines (Table 7.11).

Women with disabilities[65]

Women with disabilities may require special attention to reproductive and contraceptive needs. OCPs are generally safe and effective. Barrier methods may be difficult to use depending upon the woman's and/or her partner's degree of dexterity and motor function. Injectable or subdermal progesteronal agents, and IUDs are efficacious and practical. Sterilization may be appropriate if children are not desired.

Women with premenstural dysphoric disorder (PMDD)

Approximately 3–5% of women meet the diagnostic criteria for PMDD. Recent studies of oral contraceptives containing ethinyl estradiol and drospirenone, a progestin with antimineralocorticoid and antiandrogenic activity derived from spironolactone, have demonstrated reduced premenstrual physical and mood symptoms. Yaz® (a COC which contains 3 mg of drospirenone and 0.02 mg of ethinyl estradiol) is the only oral contraceptive also FDA approved to treat PMDD.

Yaz® is taken for 24 days followed by four days of placebo. This OC may not be appropriate for women with kidney, liver or adrenal disease because it may increase potassium levels.

Patients taking drugs that could increase potassium should consult their health care professional before taking Yas® or Yasmin (a COC with 21 days of 3.0 mg of drospirenone and 0.030 mg of ethinyl estradiol + 7 inert pills), both of which contain drospirenone.[35]

Overweight and obesity

With the overweight and obesity "epidemic" in women of reproductive ages, there are three major issues related to contraception: 1. do contraceptive methods increase weight or weight gain; 2. is contraceptive efficacy impaired in obese women; and 3. should hormonal doses be increased to maximize contraceptive efficacy in overweight women.

Although a common concern and even complaint of many women, studies are inconsistent on the impact of contraception on weight gain. The prevalence of weight and oversight increases "over time." Contraceptive studies monitor women longitudinally. So it is difficult to separate the impact of contraception from "time" itself on weight gain. There is limited evidence to support a causal association among hormonal methods. Users and non-users of contraception all tend to experience weight gain with time.

Although there have been some reports of diminished efficacy with some hormonal methods with overweight and obese women, most methods are successful "enough" with more than 95% demonstrated efficacy.

Because obesity itself increases the risk of venous thromboembolism there is no justification to compound this risk by increasing the contraceptive "dose" for overweight or obese women.

Significantly overweight and obese women may experience greater pregnancy-associated risks.

Maximizing patient access to contraception

Many circumstances affect a woman's access to contraception. Clinicians can help women solve many of these difficulties prospectively.

Several means exist by which clinicians can expedite access to contraceptives; a breast and pelvic examination and screening for cervical cancer and sexually transmitted infections are not necessary prior to instituting contraception. A medical history and blood pressure check are all that are needed before hormonal contraceptives are prescribed (the medical history can be taken by phone and the blood pressure check by the pharmacist). Although contraceptive visits are frequently used for such evaluations, clinicians should not delay prescribing contraception until these can be accomplished.[66,67] The Quick Start method has been outlined to facilitate the use of hormonal contraception.[68,69,70,71,72]

Many women have some health benefits available to them through insurance. In 2002, in the US, the EEOC ruled that an employer's exclusion of contraceptives from its health insurance plans constituted sexual discrimination in violation of Title VII of the Civil Rights Act of 1964. It further required employers to cover prescription contraception to the same extent that other drugs, devices and preventive care were covered under the employee's health care plan.

Nonetheless, health plans, including state run Medicaid formularies, may offer only a subset of contraceptive products, or "generics" only. Differential co-pays may be required to access certain methods. Often longer acting methods, such as an IUD, may be less expensive over the length of time used, however they may also be associated with higher "up front costs." Generic OCPs are nearly always as efficacious as brand-name products and have a fairly equivalent safety profile.

Pharmacies also control access to at least some extent with some pharmacists either not stocking or refusing to fill prescriptions for EC for example.

Medical abortion

Nearly 2% of US women have an induced abortion yearly[73] for a variety of reasons.[74] Mifepirostone and misoprostol have been used as a medical alternative to surgical abortion methods. The regimens,[75,76,77] their efficacy[78] and risks have been described.[79,80]

Conclusions

In working with a woman to avoid unintended pregnancies, a clinician should develop an active partnership to help her analyze options, select methods, and monitor outcomes. The clinician must recognize the "best" method may or may not be the most statistically efficacious, but one congruent with her risk status, health beliefs, values, tolerance of adverse effects, lifestyle, access and willingness/ability to adhere to the regimen.

References

1. Connell E. B. Contraception in the prepill era. *Contraception* 1999; **59**(Suppl), 7S–10S.

2. Guttmacher Institute. *Contraceptive Use Fact Sheet.* Available at http://www.guttmacher.org/pubs/fb_contr_use.html, accessed August 17, 2007.

3. Finer L. B., Henshaw S. K. Disparities in rates of unintended pregnancy in the United States, 1994 and 2001. *Perspect Sex Reprod Health* 2006; **38**(2), 90–96.

4. Centers for Disease Control and Prevention. *Midcourse Review Healthy People 2010, Family Planning Focus Area 9.* Available at http://www.healthypeople.gov/data/midcourse/pdf/fa09.pdf, accessed July 22, 2007.

5. Mosher W. D., Martinez G. M., Chandra A., Abma J., Willson S. J. Use of contraception and use of family planning services in the United States: 1982–2002. *Advance Data from Vital and Health Statistics, No. 350*, Hyattsville, MD: NCHS, 2004.

6. Institute for Clinical Systems Improvement. *Healthcare Guideline: Preventive Services for Adults.* Available at http://www.icsi.org/preventive_services_for_adults/preventive_services_for_adults_4.html.

7. Center for Collaborative and Interactive Technologies, Baylor College of Medicine. *Patient Centered Contraceptive Services: Closing the Counseling Gap.* White Paper 2006.

8. Glasier A. Emergency postcoital contraception. *New Engl J Med* 1997; **337**, 758–764.

9. Sonnenberg F. A., Burkman R. T., Hagerty C. G., Speroff L., Speroff T. Costs and net health effects of contraceptive methods. *Contraception* 2004; **69**(6), 447–459.

10. American College of Obstetricians and Gynecologists. ACOG Committee on Practice Bulletins – Gynecology, ACOG practice bulletin no. 73: use of hormonal contraception in women with coexisting medical conditions. *Obstet Gynecol* 2006; **107**(6), 1453–1472.

11. Singer J. Options counseling: techniques for caring for women with unintended pregnancies. *J Midwifery Womens Health* 2004; **49**(3), 235–242.

12. Himmerick K. A. Enhancing contraception: a comprehensive review. *J Am Acad Phys Assist* 2005; **18**(7), 26–33.

13. Burkman R., Schlesselman J. J., Zieman M. Safety concerns and health benefits associated with oral contraception. *Am J Obstet Gynecol* 2004; **190**(4 Suppl), S5–S22.

14. New Harris poll finds different religious groups have very different attitudes to some health policies and programs. Harris Interactive October 20, 2005 no. 78, http://www.harrisinteractive.com/harris_poll/index.asp?PID=608, accessed October 8, 2006.

15. Brundage S. C. Preconception health care. *Am Fam Physician* 2002; **65**(12), 2507–2514.

16. Walsh T. L., Frezieres R. G. Patterns of emergency contraception use by age and ethnicity from a randomized trial comparing advance provision and information only. *Contraception* 2006; **74**(2), 110–117.

17. Wellbery C. Emergency contraception: an ongoing debate. *Am Fam Physician* 2004; **70**(4), 655, 658–659.

18. American Academy of Pediatrics. Emergency contraception: committee on adolescence. *Pediatrics* 2005; **116**(4), 1026–1035.

19. Conard L. A., Gold M. A. Emergency contraception. *Adolesc Med Clin* 2005; **16**(3), 585–602.

20. Grimes D. A., Gallo M. F., Halpern V., Nanda K., Schulz K. F. Fertility awareness-based methods for contraception. *Cochrane Database Syst Rev* 2004; 4, CD004860. doi:7.702/14651858.CD004860.pub2.

21. Task Force on Postovulatory Methods of Fertility Regulation. Comparison of three single doses of mifepristone as EC: a randomized trial. *Lancet* 1999; **353**(9154), 697–702.

22. Weismiller D. G. Emergency contraception. *Am Fam Physician* 2004; **70**(4), 707–714.

23. Klein J. D. American Academy of Pediatrics Committee on Adolescence. Adolescent pregnancy: current trends and issues. *Pediatrics* 2005; **116**(1), 281–286.

24. Van der Wijden C., Kleijnen J., Van den Berk T. Lactational amenorrhea for family planning. *Cochrane Database Syst Rev* 2003; 4, CD001329.

25. Raymond E., Dominik R. Contraceptive effectiveness of two spermicides: a randomized trial. *Obstet Gynecol* 1999; **93**(6), 896–903.

26. Van Damme L., Ramjee G., Alary M., Vuylsteke B., Chandeying V., Rees H., *et al.* Effectiveness of COL-1492, a nonoxynol-9 vaginal gel, on HIV-1 transmission in female sex workers: a randomized controlled trial. *Lancet* 2002; **360**(9338), 971–977.

27. Raymond E. G., Chen P. L., Luoto J. Spermicide Trial Group. Contraceptive effectiveness and safety of five

nonoxynol-9 spermicides: a randomized trial. *Obstet Gynecol* 2004; **103**(3), 430–439.

28. Gallo M. F., Grimes D. A., Lopez L. M., Schulz K. F. Non-latex versus latex male condoms for contraception. *Cochrane Database Syst Rev* 2006; 1, CD003550.

29. Valappil T., Kelaghan J., Macaluso M., Artz L., Austin H., Fleenor M. E., Robey L., Nook E. W. III. Female condom and male condom failure among women at high risk of sexually transmitted diseases. *Sex Transm Dis* 2005; **32**(1), 35–43.

30. Musaba E., Morrison C. S., Sunkutu M. R., Wong E. L. Long-term use of the female condom among couples at high risk of human immunodeficiency virus infection in Zambia. *Sex Transm Dis* 1998; **25**(5), 260–264.

31. Edelman A. B., Gallo M. F., Jensen J. T., Nichols M. D., Schulz K. F., Grimes D. A. Continuous or extended cycle vs. cyclic use of combined oral contraceptives for contraception. *Cochrane Database Syst Rev* 2005; 3, CD004695.

32. Marchbanks P. A., McDonald J. A., Wilson H. G., Folger S. G., Mandel M. G., Daling J. R., *et al.* Oral contraceptives and the risk of breast cancer. *N Engl J Med* 2002; **346**(26), 2025–2032.

33. World Health Organization. *Selected Practice Recommendations for Contraceptive Use,* 3rd edition. Geneva: World Health Organization, 2004, available at http://who.int/reproductive-health/publications/mec/changes_table.html, accessed July 27, 2007, http://www.who.int/reproductive-hyealth/publications/mec/cocs.html.

34. Schulman L. P., Goldzieher J. W. The truth about oral contraceptives and venous thromboembolism. *J Reprod Med* 2003; **48**(11 Suppl), 930–938.

35. Yonkers K. A., Brown C., Pearlstein T. B., Foegh M., Sampson-Landers C., Rapkin A. Efficacy of a new low-dose oral contraceptive with drospirenone in premenstrual dysphoric disorder. *Obstet Gynecol* 2005; **106**(3), 492–501.

36. Mansour D., Fraser I. S. Missed contraceptive pills and the critical pill-free interval. *Lancet* 2005; **365**(9472), 1670–1671.

37. Larimore W. L., Stanford J. B. Postfertilization effects of oral contraceptives and their relationship to informed consent. *Arch Fam Med* 2000; **9**(2), 126–133.

38. Audet M. C., Moreau M., Koltun W. D., Waldbaum A. S., Shangold G., Fisher A. C., *et al.* Evaluation of contraceptive efficacy and cycle control of a transdermal contraceptive patch vs. an oral contraceptive: a randomized controlled trial. *J Am Med Assoc* 2001; **285**(18), 2347–2354.

39. Jick S. S., Kaye J. A., Russmann S., Jick H. Risk of nonfatal venous thromboembolism in women using a contraceptive transdermal patch and oral contraceptives containing norgestimate and 35 microg of ethinyl estradiol. *Contraception* 2006; **73**(3), 223–228.

40. Cole J. A., Norman H., Doherty M., Walker A. M. Venous thromboembolism, myocardial infarction, and stroke among transdermal contraceptive system users. *Obstet Gynecol* 2007; **109**(2 Pt 1), 339–346.

41. Stewart F. H., Kaunitz A. M., Laguardia K. D., Karvois D. L., Fisher A. C., Friedman A. J. Extended use of transdermal norelgestromin/ethinyl estradiol: a randomized trial. *Obstet Gynecol* 2005; **105**(6), 1389–1396.

42. David P. S., Boatwright E. A., Tozer B. S., Verma E. P., Blair J. E., Mayer A. P., Files J. A. Hormonal contraception update. *Mayo Clin Proc* 2006; **81**(7), 949–955.

43. Funk S., Miller M. M., Mishell D. R. Jr., Archer D. F., Poindexter A., Schmidt J., *et al.* Safety and efficacy of Implanon, a single-rod implantable contraceptive containing etonogestrel. *Contraception* 2005; **71**(5), 319–326.

44. Kaunitz A. M. Intrauterine devices: safe, effective, and underutilized. *Women Health Primary Care* 1999; **2**(1), 39–47.

45. Kulier R., Helmerhorst F. M., O'Brien P., Usher-Patel M., d'Arcangues C. Copper containing, framed intra-uterine devices for contraception. *Cochrane Database Syst Rev.* 2006; **3**, CD005347.

46. Grimes D. A., Schultz K. F. Antibiotic prophylaxis for intrauterine contraceptive device insertion. *Cochrane Database Syst Rev* 2001; 1, CD001327.

47. Fiorino A. S. Intrauterine contraceptive device-associated actinomycotic abscess and Actinomyces detection on cervical smear. *Obstet Gynecol* 1996; **87**(1), 142–149.

48. Hubacher D., Grimes D. A. Noncontraceptive health benefits of intrauterine devices: a systematic review. *Obstet Gynecol Surv* 2002; **57**(2), 120–128.

49. Hubacker D., Lara-Ricalde R., Taylor D. J., Guerra-Infante F., Guzman-Rodriguez R. Use of copper intrauterine devices and the risk of tubal infertility among nulligravid women. *N Engl J Med* 2001; **345**(8), 561–567.

50. Crosignani P. G., Vercellini P., Mosconi P., Oldani S., Cortesi I., De Giorgi O. Levonorgestrel-releasing intrauterine device versus hysteroscopic endometrial resection in the treatment of dysfunctional uterine bleeding. *Obstet Gynecol* 1997; **90**(2), 257–263.

51. Kaunitz A. M. Beyond the pill: new data and options in hormonal and intrauterine contraception. *Am J Obstet Gynecol* 2005; **192**(4), 998–1004.

52. Wilcox L. S., Chu S. Y., Peterson H. B. Characteristics of women who considered or obtained tubal reanastomosis: results from a prospective study of tubal sterilization. *Obstet Gynecol* 1990; **75**(4), 661–665.

53. Rosenfeld J. A., Zahorik P. M., Saint W., Murphy G. Women's satisfaction with birth control. *J Fam Pract* 1993; **36**(2), 169–173.

54. Peterson H. B., Xia Z., Hughes J. M., Wilcox L. S., Tylor L. R., Trussell J. The risk of ectopic pregnancy after tubal sterilization. U.S. Collaborative Review of Sterilization Working Group. *N Engl J Med* 1997; **336**(11), 762–767.

55. Cooper J. M., Carignan C. S., Cher D., Kerin J. F. Selective Tubal Occlusion Procedure 2000 Investigators Group. Microinsert nonincisional hysteroscopic sterilization. *Obstet Gynecol* 2003; **102**(1), 59–67.

56. Santelli J. S., Morrow B., Anderson J. E., Lindberg L. D. Contraceptive use and pregnancy risk among U.S. high school students, 1991–2003. *Perspect Sex Reprod Health* 2006; **38**(2), 106–111.

57. Guttmacher Institute. *U.S. Teenage Pregnancy Statistics: National and State Trends and Trends by Race and Ethnicity.* Available at http://www.guttmacher.org/pubs/2006/09/12/USTPstats.pdf.

58. Klein J. D. American Academy of Pediatrics Committee on Adolescence. Adolescent pregnancy: current trends and issues. *Pediatrics* 2005; **116**(1), 281–286.

59. Kirby D. *Do Abstinence-Only Programs Delay the Initiation of Sex Among Young People and Reduce Teen Pregnancy?* Washington DC: National Campaign to Prevent Teen Pregnancy, 2002. Available at http://www.teenpregnancy.org/resources/data/pdf/abstinence_eval/pdf.

60. Hight-Laukaran V., Labbok M. H., Peterson A. E., Fletcher V., von Hertzen H., Van Look P. F. Multicenter study of the lactational amenorrhea method (LAM) II: acceptability, utility, and policy implications. *Contraception* 1997; **55**(6), 337–346.

61. Peterson A. E., Perez-Escamilla R., Labboka M. H., Hight V., von Hertzen H., Van Look P. Multicenter study of the lactational amenorrhea method (LAM) III: effectiveness, duration, and satisfaction with reduced client-provider contact. *Contraception* 2000; **62**(5), 221–230.

62. Faculty of Family Planning & Reproductive Health Care. FFPRHC Guidance (July 2004): contraceptive choices for breastfeeding women. *J Fam Plann Reprod Health Care* 2004; **30**(3), 181–189.

63. Guthmann R. A., Bang J., Nashelsky J. Combined oral contraceptives for mothers who are breastfeeding. *Am Fam Physician* 2005; **72**(7), 1303–1304.

64. Tarlatzis B. C., Zepiridis L. Perimenopausal conception. *Ann N Y Acad Sci* 2003; **997**, 93–104.

65. Stifel E. N., Anderson J. Reproductive and contraceptive considerations for women with physical disabilities. In Rosenfeld J. A., ed., *Women's Health in Primary Care*, Baltimore, MD: Williams & Wilkins, 1997, pp. 289–313.

66. Stewart F. H., Harper C. C., Ellertson C. E., Grimes D. A., Sawaya G. F., Trussell J. Clinical breast and pelvic examination requirements for hormonal contraception: current practice vs. evidence. *J Am Med Assoc* 2001; **285**(17), 2232–2239.

67. Meckstroth K. R. Physical examination before initiating hormonal contraception: what is necessary? *Am Fam Physician* 2006; **74**, 32–34.

68. Westhoff C., Kerns J., Morroni C., Cushman L. F., Tiezzi L., Murphy P. A. Quick start: novel oral contraceptive initiation method. *Contraception* 2002; **66**(3), 141–145.

69. Westhoff C., Heartwell S., Edwards S., Zieman M., Cushman L., Kalmuss D. Oral contraceptives: quick start versus conventional start [abstract]. *Contraception* 2006; **74**, 180–181.

70. Lara-Torre E., Schroeder B. Adolescent compliance and side effects with Quick Start initiation of oral contraceptive pills. *Contraception* 2002; **66**, 81–85.

71. Murthy A. S., Creinin M. D., Harwood B., Schreiber C. A. Same-day initiation of the transdermal hormonal delivery system (contraceptive patch) versus traditional initiation methods. *Contraception* 2005; **72**, 333–336.

72. Schafer J. E., Osborne L. M., Davis A. R., Westhoff C. Acceptability and satisfaction using Quick Start with the contraceptive vaginal ring versus an oral contraceptive. *Contraception* 2006; **73**, 488–492.

73. Guttmacher Institute. In brief. *Facts on Induced Abortion in the United States*, 2006. Available at http://www.guttmacher.org/pubs/fb_induced_abortion.html.

74. Finer L. B., Frohwirth L. F., Dauphinee L. A., Singh S., Moore A. M. Reasons U.S. women have abortions: quantitative and qualitative perspectives. *Perspect Sex Reprod Health* 2005; **37**(3), 110–118.

75. Newhall E. P., Winikoff B. Abortion with mifepristone and misoprostol: regimens, efficacy, acceptability and future directions. *Am J Obstet Gynecol* 2000; **183**(2 Suppl), S44–S53.

76. Schaff E. A., Fielding S. L., Eisinger S. H., Stadalius L. S., Fuller L. Low-dose mifepristone followed by vaginal misoprostol at 48 hours for abortion up to 63 days. *Contraception* 2000; **61**(1), 41–46.

77. Middleton T., Schaff E., Fielding S. L., Scahill M., Shannon C., Westheimer E., *et al.* Randomized trial of mifepristone and buccal or vaginal misoprostol for

abortion through 56 days of last menstrual period. *Contraception* 2005; **72**(5), 328–332.

78. Kahn J. G., Becker B. J., MacIsaa L., Amory J. K., Neuhaus J., Olkin I., *et al.* The efficacy of medical abortion: a meta-analysis. *Contraception* 2000; **61**(1), 29–40.

79. Food and Drug Administration. *FDA Public Health Alert for Health Care Professionals: Mifepristone (Marketed as Mifeprex)*, 2005. Available at http://www.fda.gov/cder/drug/InfoSheets/HCP/mifepristoneHCP.htm.

80. Fischer M., Bhatnagar J., Guarner J., Reagan S., Hacker J. K., Van Meter S. H., *et al.* Fatal toxic shock syndrome associated with *Clostridium sordellii* after medical abortion. *N Eng J Med* 2005; **353**(22), 2352–2360.

Further reading

American College of Obstetricians and Gynecologists. ACOG Committee on Practice Bulletins – Gynecology, ACOG practice bulletin no. 73: use of hormonal contraception in women with coexisting medical conditions. *Obstet Gynecol* 2006; **107**, 1453–1472.

Cromer B. A., Scholes D., Berenson A., Cundy T., Clark M. K., Kaunitz A. M. Depot medroxyprogesterone acetate and bone mineral density in adolescents – the black box warning: a position paper of the Society for Adolescent Medicine. *J Adolesc Health* 2006; **39**, 296–301.

Gallo M. F., Lopez L. M., Grimes D. A., Schulz K. F., Helmerhorst F. M. Combination contraceptives: effects on weight. *Cochrane Database Syst Rev* 2006; CD003987.

World Health Organization. WHO Statement on hormonal contraception and bone health. Available at: http://www.who.int/reproductive-health/family_planning/bone_health.html, accessed January 30, 2007.

References on weight changes
Anderson F. D., Hait H., and the Seasonale-301 Study Group. A multicenter, randomized study of an extended cycle oral contraceptive. *Contraception* 2003; **68**, 89–96.

Coney P., Washenik K., Langley R. G. B., DiGiovanna J. J., Harrison D. D. Weight change and adverse event incidence with a low-dose oral contraceptive: two randomized, placebo-controlled trials. *Contraception* 2001; **63**, 297–302.

Gallo M. F., Grimes D. A., Schulz K. F., Helmerhorst F. M. Combination estrogen-progestin contraceptives and body weight: systematic review of randomized controlled trials. *Obstet Gynecol* 2004; **103**, 359–373.

Jain J., Jakimiuk A. J., Bode F. R., Ross D., Kaunitz A. M. Contraceptive efficacy and safety of DMPA-SC. *Contraception* 2004 **70**, 269–275.

Mainwaring R., Hales H. A., Stevenson K., *et al.* Metabolic parameter, bleeding, and weight changes in U.S. women using progestin only contraceptives. *Contraception* 1995; **51**, 149–153.

Moore L. L., Valuck R., McDougall C., Fink W. A comparative study of one-year weight gain among users of medroxyprogesterone acetate, levonorgestrel implants, and oral contraceptives. *Contraception* 1995; **52**, 215–220.

O'Connell K., Osborne L. M., Westhoff C. Measured and reported weight change for women using a vaginal contraceptive ring vs. a low-dose oral contraceptive. *Contraception* 2005; **72**, 323–327.

Pelkman C. Hormones and weight change. *J Reprod Med* 2002; **47**, 791–794.

Sibai B., Odlind V., Meador M., Shangold G., Fisher A., Creasy G. A comparative assessment of Ortho Evra™/Evra™ to placebo patch effect on body weight [abstract]. *Fertil Steril* 2001; **76**(suppl 1), S188.

Sibai B. M., Odlind V., Meador M. L., Shangold G. A., Fisher A. C., Creasy G. W. A comparative and pooled analysis of the safety and tolerability of the contraceptive patch (Ortho Evra™/Evra™). *Fertil Steril* 2002; **77**(suppl 2), S19–S26.

Taneepanichskul S., Reinprayoon D., Jaisamrarn U. Effects of DMPA on weight and blood pressure in long term acceptors. *Contraception* 1999; **59**, 301–303.

Westhoff C., Jain J. K., Milsom I., Ray A. Changes in weight with depot medroxyprogesterone acetate subcutaneous injection 104 mg/0.65 mL. *Contraception* 2007; **75**, 261–267.

Contraceptive failure and weight
Audet M.-C., Moreau M., Koltun W. D., *et al.*, for the Ortho Evra/Evra 004 Study Group. Evaluation of contraceptive efficacy and cycle control of a transdermal contraceptive patch vs an oral contraceptive: a randomized controlled trial. *J Am Med Assoc* 2001; **285**, 2347–2354.

Brunner Huber L. R., Hogue C. J. The role of body weight in oral contraceptive failure: results from the 1995 National Survey of Family Growth. *Ann Epidemiol* 2005; **15**, 492–499.

Brunner Huber L. R., Hogue C. J. The association between body weight, unintended pregnancy resulting in a livebirth, and contraception at the time of conception. *Matern Child Health J* 2005; **9**, 413–420.

Brunner Huber L. R., Hogue C. J., Stein A. D., Drews C., Zieman M. Body mass index and risk for oral contraceptive failure: a case-cohort study in South Carolina. *Ann Epidemiol* 2006; **16**, 637–643.

Creinin M. D., Roberts E. Body mass index, weight, and oral contraceptive failure risk [letter to the editor]. *Obstet Gynecol* 2005; **105**, 1492–1493.

Croxatto H. B., Urbancsek J., Massai R., Bennink H. C., van Beek A., and the Implanon® Study Group. A multicentre efficacy and safety study of the single contraceptive implant Implanon®. *Hum Reprod* 1999; **14**, 976–981.

Dinger J. C., Heinemann L. A. J., Westhoff C., Cronin M., Schellschmidt I. Contraceptive efficacy of oral contraceptives in real world clinical practice: the impact of age, weight, BMI, dose, and duration of use. Poster presented at *American College of Obstetricians and Gynecologists 55th Annual Clinical Meeting,* May 5–9, 2007, San Diego, CA.

Funk S., Miller M. M., Mishell D. R. Jr., *et al.* for The Implanon™ US Study Group. Safety and efficacy of Implanon™, a single-rod implantable contraceptive containing etonogestrel. *Contraception* 2005; **71**, 319–326.

Gerrits E. G., Ceulemans R., van Hee R., Hendrickx L., Totté E. Contraceptive treatment after biliopancreatic diversion needs consensus. *Obes Surg* 2003; **13**, 378–382.

Hanker J. P. Gastrointestinal disease and oral contraception. *Am J Obstet Gynecol* 1990; **163**, 2204–2207.

Hedon B., Helmerhorst F. M., Cronje H. S., *et al.* Comparison of efficacy, cycle control, compliance, and safety in users of a contraceptive patch vs an oral contraceptive [abstract]. *Int J Gynecol Obstet* 2000; **70**(suppl 1), 78.

Holt V. L., Cushing-Haugen K. L., Daling J. R. Body weight and risk of oral contraceptive failure. *Obstet Gynecol* 2002; **99**, 820–827.

Holt V. L., Scholes D., Wicklund K. G., Cushing-Haugen K. L., Daling J. R. Body mass index, weight, and oral contraceptive failure risk. *Obstet Gynecol* 2005; **105**, 46–52.

Kaunitz A. M. Efficacy, cycle control, and safety of two triphasic oral contraceptives: Cyclessa™ (desogestrel/ethinyl estradiol) and Ortho-Novum® 7/7/7 (norethindrone/ethinyl estradiol): a randomized clinical trial. *Contraception* 2000; **61**, 295–302.

Mason M. Pressing to look closer at blood clots and the pill. *New York Times* February 13, 2007.

Merhi Z. O. Challenging oral contraception after weight loss by bariatric surgery. *Gynecol Obstet Invest* 2007; **64**, 100–102.

Nakajima S. T., Archer D. F., Ellman H. Efficacy and safety of a new 24-day oral contraceptive regimen of norethindrone acetate 1 mg/ethinyl estradiol 20 µg (Loestrin® 24 Fe). *Contraception* 2007; **75**, 16–22.

Parsey K. S., Pong A. An open-label, multicenter study to evaluate Yasmin, a low-dose combination oral contraceptive containing drospirenone, a new progestogen. *Contraception* 2000; **61**, 105–111.

Sivin I. Risks and benefits, advantages and disadvantages of levonorgestrel-releasing contraceptive implants. *Drug Saf* 2003; **26**, 303–335.

Smallwood G. H., Meador M. L., Lenihan J. P., Shangold G. A., Fisher A. C., Creasy G. W. Efficacy and safety of a transdermal contraceptive system. *Obstet Gynecol* 2001; **98**, 799–805.

Vessey M., Painter R. Oral contraceptive failures and body weight: findings in a large cohort study. *J Fam Plann Reprod Health Care* 2001; **27**, 90–91.

Westhoff C. Higher body weight does not affect NuvaRing®'s efficacy. Poster presented at *American College of Obstetricians and Gynecologists 52nd Annual Clinical Meeting,* May 1–5, 2005, Philadelphia, PA.

Westhoff C. L., Anderson F. D. Seasonale (30 µg of ethinyl estradiol/150 µg of levonorgestrel) extended-regimen oral contraceptive: efficacy and cycle control by body weight [abstract]. *Contraception* 2006; **74**, 181–182.

Zieman M., Guillebaud J., Weisberg E., Shangold G. A., Fisher A. C., Creasy G. W. Contraceptive efficacy and cycle control with the Ortho Evra™/Evra™ transdermal system: the analysis of pooled data. *Fertil Steril* 2002; **77**(suppl 2), S13–S18.

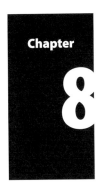

Chapter 8

Infertility

Jo Ann Rosenfeld

Infertility is the inability of a sexually active couple who desire a child to become pregnant within one year.

Impact

1. Approximately 10 to 15% of couples have difficulty becoming pregnant. Approximately 9 million American women have impaired fertility, either primary (never having a child) or secondary (trouble having as many children as desired).
2. Family and general physicians can work with couples to help them achieve a pregnancy. Consultation to fertility specialists may be needed sooner or later.

Etiology

1. Infertility is a couple's problem. Most couples conceived within 6 months of trying.[1] Infertility increases with age (Figure 8.1).
2. Half of the couples who have failed to get pregnant in six months conceive within the next six months.[2]
3. In retrospect, approximately 40% of infertility is caused by ovulation problems. Ten to thirty percent may be caused by multiple factors, and male factors make up the remaining of the causes (Table 8.1).
4. Chronic disease of either partner may cause infertility.
5. Women's causes of infertility include ovarian and tubal or mechanical factors.
   a. Ovarian failure may be caused by malnutrition, anorexia, diabetes, or renal failure.
   b. Ovarian failure can be temporary or permanent and can be caused by an endocrinopathy or polycystic ovarian syndrome or can be idiopathic.
   c. Tubal factors include scarring from endometriosis, PID or infections, especially gonorrhea or chlamydia.
   d. Cervical and uterine factors can include an abnormally shaped uterus (bifid, bicornuate, or anatomy changed by fibroids) or inimical cervical mucus.
   e. Use of certain medications, smoking, alcohol, and obesity all reduce a woman's fertility. A recent retrospective study of more than 400 Danish couples found that drinking as little as one to five alcoholic drinks weekly significantly decreased the likelihood of pregnancy (RR = 0.6) and more than five drinks weekly decreased the likelihood to less than one-third (RR = 0.3).[3]
6. Male causes of infertility include erective dysfunction and other sexual dysfunction, a low or absent sperm count, abnormal sperm, epididimal scarring from infection, or medication use. Antidepressant use can cause reduced sperm numbers and motility.[4]

Evaluation

1. The duration of the infertility and the age of the woman are the most important factors influencing the success rate for fertility[5] (Figure 8.2).
2. The history of medications and alcohol use are important factors.
3. Contraceptive history is important. After hormonal contraception, return to normal

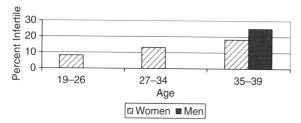

Figure 8.1 Increased infertility by age. Data from Dunson D. B., Baird D. D., Colombo B. Increased infertility with age in men and women. *Obstet Gynecol* 2004; **103**(1), 51–56.

Table 8.1 Some causes of infertility

Ovulation difficulties

    Anovulatory cycles

    Hypothalamic/pituitary axis dysfunction

    Medications

    Hormonal dysfunction – thyroid, prolactin

Fallopian tube dysfunction

    Infections, STDs

    PID

Cervical dysfunction

Sexual dysfunction

    Vaginismus, dyspareunia

    Erectile dysfunction

Decreased sperm or sperm function

    Medications

    Varicoeles

    Ductal dysfunction

    Endocrinopathology

    Infections, STDs

ovulation patterns can take months. After stopping OCPs, amenorrhea and anovulation can last 6–12 months. After use of depot Medroxyprogesterone acetate (DMPA), anovulation can last 12–24 months (Figure 8.3).

4. Sexual history is important. Approximately 5% of infertility is caused by sexual dysfunction.

5. A complete physical examination of both men and women is essential.

    a. In the woman, medical and medication history, sexual history, gynecological and obstetrical history including pregnancies, abortion, surgeries, episodes of PID, and menstrual history. Physical examination of women includes gynecological exams including vaginal, uterine and bimanual examination. Examining hair and skin for changes of a hormonal disorder or PCOS is important.

    b. In the man, medical and medication history, sexual history and history of infections or surgery are important. Physical examination of scrotum, testes and penis is important. Phimosis, balanitis, small testes, or varicoeles may interfere with fertility. Varicoeles do not interfere with normal sperm counts and assessment; how they reduce fertility is not well defined.

    c. Both partners should be examined and cultured for sexually transmitted disease, especially chlamydia.

Counseling

Counseling the couple about the normal menstrual and ovulation cycle, about the effects of medications and alcohol on fertility, and about expectations about coming pregnant is important. A survey study of approximately 250 women who were trying to become pregnant found that many were having intercourse at times other than ovulation. After teaching these women how to use a "fertility monitor," almost half conceived in the first month, and 90% within three months.[6] Other important counseling includes the following.

- Woman's use of folic acid prophylactically to reduce incidence of spina bifida is suggested.
- Reducing or quitting smoking and decreasing alcohol consumption should be advised. Smoking reduces fertility. Medications should be reduced or changed as needed (Table 8.2).
- Weight should be lost if possible.
- Vaginal lubricants or gel that may cause sperm immobility and impede infertility should not be used.

Treatment

1. The woman should start a three to six month basal body temperature log, or use LH predictors to

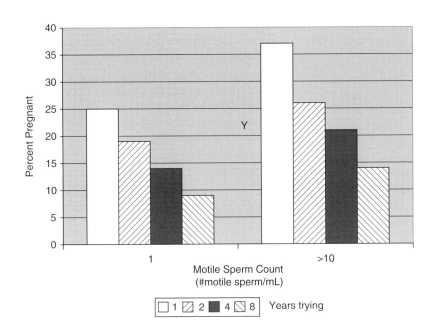

Figure 8.2 Percentage who became pregnant by years trying and sperm count. Data from Hargreave T. B., Mills A. Investigating and managing infertility in general practice. *Br Med J* 1996; **316**, 1438–1441.

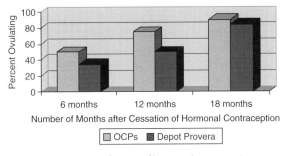

Figure 8.3 Ovulation after use of hormonal contraception.

Table 8.2 Substances that can decrease fertility

Medications

   Nifedipine

   Sulfasalazine

   Nitrofurandantoin

   Tetracycline

   Colchicine

   Cancer chemotherapeutic agents

   Anabolic steroids

   Drugs that decrease immunity such as plaquenyl, methotrexate

   Amphetamines

Alcohol

Cigarette smoking

determine whether she is ovulating. Although this seems simple, an accurate record takes thoroughness and consistency. A biphasic curve with a 0.4 to 0.5 degree elevation is consistent with the day of ovulation. Over the counter LH surge predictors cost $35–50 per cycle.

2. The man should have a semen analysis. Examined within 60 minutes of ejaculation, normal semen contains 2 mL or more of 20 million motile sperm per mL, or more. The motility of sperm should show that more than half progress in a forward direction, with more than 25% progressing rapidly. Thirty percent or more should have normal shape. One study of more than 100 fertile men undergoing vasectomy found that the mean volume was 3.31 ml (range 0.6–11 mL), with a sperm count average of 81 million per mL (range 4–318 million). The percent of active sperm averaged 63% (range 10 to 95%).[7]

3. If these tests are normal, a postcoital test is suggested, although its prognostic value has been questioned by a meta-analysis.[8] Within eight hours after coitus, a cervical specimen is analyzed for sperm motility and morphology. One RCT found that postcoital tests increased the number of tests, but not the overall pregnancy rate.[9]

4. If the woman is not ovulating, the family physician (if she stays up-to-date on the literature and treatment) or a consultant can help induce

ovulation with clomiphene, Pergonal®, gonadotropin agonists or pulsatile gonadotropin releasing hormone administration. Only physicians experienced in using these drugs should attempt ovulation induction.

   a. Clomiphene, a selective estrogen receptor modulator (SERM), is contraindicated in women with liver failure, ovarian cysts, PCOS, and undiagnosed abnormal uterine bleeding or pregnancy. It is associated with an increase in multiple births. There may be severe menstrual and intermenstrual pain, nausea, bloating and premenstrual syndrome associated with its use.

   b. The next step may be the use of menotropins incluing human menopausal gonadotropins (hMG, Pergonal). These can cause high serum estradiol concentrations and ovarian hypertrophy with multiple follicles. These follicles can rupture and cause hemoperitoneum, ascites, and hypovolemia in as many as 25% of women using the medication.

5. If the semen analysis is abnormal, there are methods of increasing the concentration, number and motility of sperm, called "capacitating."

6. Alternatively, the sperm can be introduced directly into the uterus with a catheter, especially if the postcoital test is abnormal.

7. Women with PCOS may be treated with metformin which induces ovulation in approximately 50%, as it reduces insulinemia, improves glucose control, and decreases weight and hirsuitism. In early studies metformin was given to 43 women who were hyperinsulinemic and euglycemic. Ninety-one percent resumed menses.[10]

Indications for referral for infertility consultant

1. If the woman is older than 35, or definitely 40, immediate referral may be indicated, especially if the couple has already tried for more than one year.

2. If the couple has not conceived within three years of stopping contraceptives, the likelihood of pregnancy in the next year is less than 25% and referral is indicated.

3. Ovarian failure, failure to achieve ovulation within three to six cycles or pregnancy within one year, would suggest the need of referral.

4. Other suggested indications for immediate referral include serum chlamydia levels in either partner of greater than 1:256, follicular stimulating level in the woman's early follicular phase more than 10 IU/L, or abnormal sperm analysis (sperm motility less than 25% or less than 20 million/mL).[11]

Assisted reproduction

1. The success rate has been increasing, and may reach 25%. Actually, the success rate of in vitro fertilization (IVF) exceeds that of normal conception in a fertile couple in one cycle.

2. In vitro fertilization (IVF) consists of the egg and sperm united in a test tube, and then the pre-embryo is transferred to the uterus.

3. GIFT (gamete intrafallopian transfer) consists of placement of egg and sperm in the fallopian tube.

4. ZIFT is zygote intrafallopian transfer where the fertilized eggs are placed in the uterus or tubes.

5. Ovum conations combined with the man's sperm and IVF or GIFT can be used for women with premature ovarian failure, ovarian dysfunction caused by cancer, chemotherapy, radiation, maternal chromosomal or genetic abnormalities, or in women who have responded poorly to ovulation inducers. Older women's eggs are more likely to have genetic abnormality and aneuploidy.

6. Sperm donation can come from the male partner or donor. The sperm is then placed in the uterus or used in IVF or GIFT. This may be used for male infertility, male ejaculatory dysfunction, post-radiation, chemotherapy or surgery for cancer, chromosomal abnormalities, or for women without a male donor.

Psychological effects of infertility

1. Most couples cope well with the rigorous and intricate therapies of infertility.

2. Most couples assume that they will be able to become pregnant when they desire. The inability may lead to frustration, sadness, depression, and distancing between the couple. Women who have postponed childbearing to have a career may be used to being in control of many parts of their

life. When they are unsuccessful in becoming pregnant when they want, they may feel frustrated and angry.

3. The effect of the infertility depends on the age of the couple, their personality and coping styles, pre-existing psychopathology, medical causes, and motivations for pregnancy.

4. Infertility can lead to a sense of failure and guilt, that something is wrong with them because their body does not function correctly. Body image may be altered.

5. There may be sexual difficulties, avoidance of intercourse, and inability to perform, especially with seemingly mechanical tests like postcoital and semen specimens. Anorgasmia, impotence, and decreased libido may occur.

6. Avoidance of friends and family who have children can occur, further isolating the couple.

7. Psychological counseling, before, during and after IVF, may be indicated. The stress of infertility and its treatment may exacerbate other psychiatric conditions, such as mood or anxiety disorders. The ovulation inducing agents may also exacerbate psychological problems or reduce the effectiveness of psychotropic medications.

Adoption

Impact

1. Adoption has become a more visible choice. In the USA, approximately 35,000 are adopted yearly, with more than 10,000 from foreign countries.

2. Five percent of children born to unmarried mothers during the 1990s were placed in adoption.[12]

3. Although adoption has become discussed in the media, it is essentially a private choice, both for the birthmother and the adopting family.

Caring for the birthmother

1. The birth mother is no longer likely to be an unmarried adolescent who travels to a distant town to deliver her unwanted child. Yet, the decision to place a child for adoption is difficult and emotional. The physician may counsel pregnant or just delivered women. The counseling may take time and involvement and additional social service and/or psychological counselors may be needed.

2. The decision may change several times in the course of the pregnancy and postnatal period. Financial, social, medical and personal reasons are all likely to be involved.

3. A complete social, family, medical and personal history is essential, including drugs and alcohol use. The woman may be afraid to be specific.

4. A woman considering placing her child for adoption may be at higher risk for STDs and social problems. She may require additional medical and social supports, even after the placement of her child.

5. Care during delivery should be the same as for all mothers. However, delivery may not be joyful; in fact, the mother may show signs of grief and bereavement. The mother may not want to see her child or stay on the labor and delivery floor. These wishes should be honored.

6. The adoption may be private or through an agency. Mothers may have had significant input into the choice of adoptive parents, even having an "open" adoption. In this, the birthmother may visit the adoptive parents before and after adoption.

7. All legal work should be completed in advance. The physician does not need to get involved in the legal work, unless she feels the woman is being forced or unduly pressured.

Care of the adoptive mother

1. The adoptive mother may come to the decision to adopt through many ways, including primary choice or failure of fertility programs. She may be burdened with feelings of failure and grief at the inability to have a child from her body, or may choose adoption as a start or addition to her family.

2. The adoptive mother goes through several stages of emotional lability. She and her husband must decide to adopt, deal with the stress, lack of control and insecurity of the adoption process, and deal with the medical, social, and psychological issues of incorporating an adoptive child into the family. Adoption may be a first or last step, and the woman may have powerful feeling for and against adoption and urgency to have a child.

3. The physician may counsel the woman about adoptions, counsel about particular disease or children with handicaps, and treat the child once it is adopted. The physician may need to help the family integrate the child into the family and help to give advice about dealing with the stresses of adoption.

4. The decision to adopt entails many steps.

   a. Factors such as infertility, failure to produce genetic children, need for children with the same genetic make-up, desire to help needy or handicapped children, and grief and anger about failure of her own body are all complex parts of the decision. As well, the difficulty of single parenting, gay parenting, and blended families may be part of the decision. The physician may counsel the family during this process.

   b. The adopting parents must decide if and how they can deal with a special needs or handicapped child or a child from another ethnic background.

   c. Women who feel that they have lost control by inability to have children may jump joyfully into the obsessive paperwork and details needed to adopt a child. It may give them a feeling of control.

   d. Preadoption counseling may be as important as preconceptual counseling. The physician should inquire into the mother's daycare and leave options, her insurance status and back-up. Have the adoptive parents discussed their plans with their family? Adopting older children may entail special arrangements for daycare or schooling.

5. **Preadoption parent physical examination**

   a. The physician is often asked to perform the preadoption physical. There are some conditions that may make an adult hesitate to adopt (Table 8.3).

   b. Any condition that causes an individual to need caregiving themselves or give it to family member, or any progressive or terminal disease, should cause hesitation about ability to adopt a child.

   c. However, it is not the duty of the physician to judge who can adopt, but just counsel and document. The judge, county, country, state or adoption agency will have its own

Table 8.3 Medical conditions that may cause hesitation for adoption

Age older than 50

Any permanent organ failure

Any progressive or terminal disease, COPD, cancer, AIDS, multiple sclerosis or progressive neurological disease, heart disease, severe type I diabetes

Any severe disability

History of drug or alcohol abuse

Family member with progressive disability that may need caregiving

History of child abuse

requirements. Some countries have their own requirements. In one case, a judge may decide that grandparents or aunts over age 50 with some chronic condition would be better adoptive parents than strangers.

6. **The wait**

   There is an intensely painful period between the decision to adopt and the arrival of the child. Anticipation, worry, anxiety, legal, and social problems are all factors in this time. Because the woman may be suffering this wait and does not want to tell or burden friends and family, the physician may need to be available for support and ventilation.

Fitting the child into the family

1. There are many problems including childhood illness, social and psychological adaptation of the family and child, and handling of the discussing of adoption.

2. Foreign or same country adoption both may produce children with many medical problems, sometimes unknown until the adoption. These may be infectious diseases, including hepatitis, parasites, AIDS, and/or tuberculosis, malnutrition, lack of immunizations, and sexual and physical abuse. There are clinics and offices in larger cities that specialize in adoptive children.

3. The physician can help the family understand cultural differences and obtain help in doing so, such as contacting support and ethnic groups.

4. Sooner or later, the family will have to discuss adoption with the child. There are many books, websites, magazines, and support groups that can

help. Answering the child's questions honestly is the best method of discussing adoption.

Conclusions

The family physician can often make a positive impact on a couple's quest for fertility, using simple office-based diagnosis and treatment. The physician can help couples through fertility treatment and also through the problems and concerns of adoption.

References

1. Gnoth C., Godehardt D., Godehardt E., Frank-Herrmann P., Freundl G. Time to pregnancy: results of the German prospective study and impact on the management of infertility *Hum Reprod* 2003; **18**(9), 1959–1966.

2. van der Steeg J. W., Steures P., Hompes P. G., Eijkemans M. J., van der Veen F., Mol B. W. Investigation of the infertile couple: a basic fertility work-up performed within 12 months of trying to conceive generates costs and complications for no particular benefit *Hum Reprod* 2005; **20**(10), 2672–2674.

3. Jensen T. K., Hjolland N. H. I., Henrickesn T., *et al.* Does moderate alcohol consumption affect fertility? *Br Med J* 1996; **317**, 505–510.

4. Tanrikut C., Schlegel P. N. Antidepressant-associated changes in semen parameters. *Urology* 2007; **69**(1), 185.e5–7.

5. Hargreave T. B., Mills A. Investigating and managing infertility in general practice. *Br Med J* 1996; **316**, 1438–1441.

6. Robinson J. E., Ellis J. E. Mistiming of intercourse as a primary cause of failure to conceive: results of a survey on use of a home-use fertility monitor. *Curr Med Res Opin* 2007; **23**(2), 301–306.

7. Sobrero A. J., Rehan N. E. The semen of fertile men. II. Semen characteristics of 100 fertile men *Fertil Steril* 1975; **26**(11), 1048–1056.

8. Read J. ABC of sexual health: sexual problems associated with infertility, pregnancy, and ageing *Br Med J* 1999; **318**, 587–589.

9. Kutch W. H., Chao C. H., Ritter J., Byrd W. Vaginal lubricants for the infertile couple: effect on sperm activity. *Int J Fertil Menopausal Study* 1996; **41**, 400–404.

10. Glueck, C. J., Wang Fonatine R., Tracy T., Seive-Smith L. Metformin induced resumption of normal menses in 39 of 42 women previously amenorrheic with polycystic ovary syndrome. *Metabolism* 1999; **48**, 511–519.

11. Cahill D. J., Wardle P. G. Management of infertility. *Br Med J* 2002; **325**, 28–32; doi:10.1136/bmj.325.7354.28

12. Melina C. M., Melina L. The physician's responsibility in adoption. Part I: Caring for the birthmother. *J Am Board Fam Pract* 1988; **1**, 50–54.

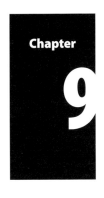

Medical care and pregnancy: common preconception and antepartum issues

Ellen L. Sakornbut

Introduction

A general approach to women of reproductive age should include consideration of the possibility of pregnancy. The preconception approach to medical care includes optimization of chronic health problems and risks that may impact negatively on pregnancy. Medical care of women in pregnancy requires understanding of changes in maternal physiology and special risks to the fetus or mother.

The preconception approach to medical care

Preconception counseling

Most women do not need special diagnostic testing or therapeutic interventions before the initiation of pregnancy.

In general, women without chronic illness may undertake pregnancy with general preventive counseling for a healthy diet, avoidance of substance abuse, regular exercise, and common occupational precautions. This should be a part of preventive care in all young women.

> Most women without chronic disease should be able to undertake pregnancy healthily with advice about a healthy diet, avoiding abuse of substances, taking regular exercise, and common occupational precautions.

Dietary precautions

Low levels of serum and red blood cell folic acid have been demonstrated to increase the risk of neural tube defects. In randomized clinical trials, 0.8 mg of folic acid per day decreased the occurrence of neural tube defects and 4 mg of folic acid per day decreased the recurrence of neural tube defects.[1] Lower effective doses were found in non-randomized trials; current recommendations from the Institute of Medicine and the US Public Health Service recommend 0.4 mg/day in women of childbearing potential.[2] A population-based study of birth registries in Europe, North America, and Australia demonstrated significant reduction of neural tube defects occurring with fortification of food products but not with recommendation of supplementation alone.[3] Fortification of flour is mandatory in Canada, the USA, and Chile, but not in most European countries.

A study of low-income women found that significant numbers of women still had diets deficient in folic acid, and most had no knowledge of the foods that they should be eating to achieve a healthy level in their diet.[4] At the same time, women with higher educational levels may be taking supplementation that is not recommended or needed, such as vitamin A, but still have diets deficient in folic acid.[5]

Thus supplementation with a multivitamin or folic acid seems warranted at this time in all women of childbearing potential, and higher levels of supplementation (4 mg/day) in high risk women.[6] These include women with a history of a previous delivery of a child with a neural tube defect, women with a strong family history of neural tube defects, and women on antiepileptic drugs (AEDs).

Fortification of grain products is ideal to achieve the greatest certainty of attaining optimal serum folate levels and prevention of neural tube defects. In countries that do not use fortification, all women of childbearing potential should be supplemented with folic acid 0.4 mg daily and 4–5 mg/day in high risk women. Strength of recommendation A.

Handbook of Women's Health, second edition, ed. Jo Ann Rosenfeld. Published by Cambridge University Press.
© Cambridge University Press 2009.

Occupational concerns

Women with occupational exposures often seek specific information regarding the safety of pregnancy. This complex issue may be viewed from a number of perspectives, including the very personal concerns of the patient for her baby's well-being and her family's economic viability.

Although much attention has been focused on maternal occupational exposures, a number of substances appear to cause subfecundity (reduced fertility) or other adverse pregnancy outcomes as a result of paternal exposures.

Policies in US industries that exclude women from certain types of job may, therefore, be viewed as discriminatory. From a more general perspective, these exclusionary practices may be shortsighted if they preclude a goal of occupational safety for all workers. Legislative issues have been approached differently in a number of European countries compared with the USA, with special maternity leave status granted to 1% and 0.1% of women in Denmark and Finland respectively, whose occupation is judged to be sufficiently hazardous to exclude participation during pregnancy.[7] Table 9.1 provides a brief overview of occupational exposures that are known to be associated with adverse pregnancy outcome.

A number of possible exposures have been studied in pregnancy in an effort to decrease associated risk by protective practices. In health care positions, measurements of radiation with exposure to nuclear medicine patients receiving technetium-99m or iodine-131 have led to recommendations on limits for technologists and nursing staff.[8]

Changes in the practice of an occupation may affect risk. A study of hairdressers examined the high rate of adverse pregnancy outcomes in two time periods, 1986–88 and 1991–93 in hairdressers as compared to sales clerks. However, this study also demonstrated a decline in the higher incidence of spontaneous abortions and low birth weight infants in hairdressers between the two periods.[9] This may be the result of changes in products used by the hairdressers.

Exposure to anesthetic gases appears to have diminished among operating room personnel, but exposures may still remain at an unacceptable level for recovery room and surgical intensive care unit personnel caring for recovering post-anesthetic patients unless scavenging devices are in operation in these work zones.[10]

Radiation

- The issue of occupational exposure to radiation includes workers from several industries.
- Lower limits of exposure apply to pregnant women working in fluoroscopy suites than to non-pregnant individuals.
- In the USA, these limits apply with voluntary declaration of pregnancy. Appropriate use of protective clothing can limit radiation exposure to recommended levels.[11]
- The theoretical risk of cosmic radiation at high altitudes has been included in considering risks encountered by pregnant flight attendants and frequent business travelers. However, actual measurements of airline crews have failed to demonstrate doses of radiation exceeding the recommended limits to exposure.[12] Adverse pregnancy outcomes and childhood malignancy have been studied in workers at nuclear plants with adverse pregnancy outcomes (stillbirth) noted in paternal exposures to external ionizing radiation,[13] and possible increase in childhood cancers seen in children whose mothers experienced radiation work exposures.[14]

Stress

- Occupational stress, especially physical stress, has been widely suspected by physicians and patients of causing adverse pregnancy outcomes, but most women are able to work safely throughout their pregnancies without difficulties. Physical stresses that have been associated with increased rates of prematurity and low birth weight include prolonged standing, long hours, protracted ambulation, and heavy lifting.[15]
- Studies that examine these issues vary considerably in design and may include confounding factors, thus creating methodological concerns.
- One study found greater risk of preterm birth, low birth weight, and small-for-gestational age birth in textile workers, food service workers, electrical equipment operators, and janitors when compared with women employed as clerks, teachers, and librarians.[16] Another study found higher rates of preterm deliveries and low birth weight in nurses than in bank workers.[17,18] A self-report survey of female physicians found higher rates of stillbirth and premature delivery

Table 9.1 Occupational exposures and pregnancy

Agent	Maternal/paternal exposure	Adverse reproductive outcomes
Herbicides	Paternal	Increased spontaneous abortion OR 2.5–5.0[a]
Pesticides – pyridilis, aliphatic hydrocarbons, inorganics, glufosinate	Paternal, maternal	Increased congenital malformations,[b] CNS, musculoskeletal, oral clefts
Lead	Maternal	LBW, NTDs[c]
Inorganic mercury vapour	Maternal	Increased congenital malformations[d]
Organic solvents – toluene, chlorphenols, aromatic amines	Maternal	Subfecundity,[e] increased congenital malformations,[f] fetal growth impairment[g]
Formaldehyde	Maternal	Subfecundity, spontaneous abortions[h]
Radiation	Maternal, paternal	See the text
Anesthetic gases – nitrous oxide, desflurane, sevoflurane	Maternal	Increased spontaneous abortions,[i] increased SGA infants[j]
Antineoplastic agents	Maternal	Increased spontaneous abortions[k]
Ethylene oxide	Maternal	Increased spontaneous abortions, preterm birth[l]

Notes: CNS, central nervous system; LBW, low birth weight; NTD, neural tube defects; SGA, small-for-gestational age; OR, odds ratio.
[a]Arbuckle T. E., Savitz D. A., Mery L. S., Curtis K. M. Exposure to phenoxy herbicides and the risk of spontaneous abortion. *Epidemiology* 1999; **10**, 752–760.
[b]Paternal exposure to pesticides and congenital malformations. *Scand J Work Environ Health* 1998; **24**, 473–480.
[c]Irgens A., Kruger K., Skorve A. H., Irgens L. M. Reproductive outcome in offspring of parents occupationally exposed to lead in Norway. *Am J Ind Med* 1998; **34**, 431–437.
[d]Elghany N. A., Stopford W., Bunn W. B., Fleming L. E. Occupational exposure to inorganic mercury vapour and reproductive outcomes. *Occup Med (Lond)* 1997; **47**, 333–336.
[e]Plenge-Bonig A., Karmaus W. Exposure to toluene in the printing industry is associated with subfecundity in women but not in men. *Occup Environ Med* 1999; **56**, 443–448.
[f]Khattak S., K-Moghtader G., McMartin K., Barrera M., Kennedy D., Koren G. Pregnancy outcome following gestational exposure to organic solvents: a prospective controlled study. *J Am Med Assoc* 1999; **281**, 1106–1109.
[g]Seidler A., Raum E., Arabin B., Hellenbrand W., Walter U., Schwartz F. W. Maternal occupational exposure to chemical substances and the risk for infants small-for-gestational age. *Am J Ind Med* 1999; **36**, 213–222.
[h]Taskinen H. K., Kyyronen P., Sallmen M., *et al.* Reduced fertility among female wood workers exposed to formaldehyde. *Am J Ind Med* 1999; **36**, 206–212.
[i]Smith D. A. Hazards of nitrous oxide exposure in healthcare personnel. *Am Assoc Nurse Anesth J* 1998; **66**: 390–3.
[j]Bodin L., Axelsson G., Ahlborg G. Jr. The association of shift work and nitrous oxide exposure in pregnancy with birth weight and gestational age. *Epidemiology* 1999; **10**, 429–436.
[k]Valanis B., Vollmer W. M., Steele P. Occupational exposure to antineoplastic agents: self-reported miscarriages and stillbirths among nurses and pharmacists. *J Occ Environ Med* 1999; **41**, 632–638.
[l]Rowlans A. S., Baird D. D., Shore D. L., Darden B., Wilcox A. J. Ethylene oxide exposure may increase the risk of spontaneous abortion, preterm birth, and postterm birth. *Epidemiology* 1996; **7**, 363–368.

than in the general population.[18] However, a large cohort study of more than 7000 women found only a modest increase in risk of preterm delivery (OR = 1.31) for women whose occupation entailed more than eight hours standing per day. In addition, this study found no increase in low birth weight or preterm delivery with heavy work or exercise after controlling for confounding variables, suggesting that other socioeconomic factors might account for differences in pregnancy outcome.[19]

> Physical stresses that include prolonged standing, long hours, protracted ambulation, and heavy lifting have been associated with increased rates of prematurity and low birth weight.

Assessment of poor pregnancy outcome

Consultation with a maternal-fetal specialist should be considered in women with a history of recurrent spontaneous abortion and mid-trimester abortion/delivery.

Recurrent abortion and very preterm birth may be related to uterine structural defects such as Müllerian tube defects (uterine septum and variants), uterine leiomyomata, or cervical incompetence. A specific history of preterm premature rupture of membranes may be caused by infection, a modifiable factor, whereas a history of premature labor may be attributable to a number of factors.

Patients with recurrent first trimester loss should be offered genetic evaluation. Genetic consultation is applicable for a growing list of preconception concerns, including couples with a previous child with a congenital defect, families with inherited metabolic defects, and couples wherein one partner manifests a genetically transmitted illness.

Common medical issues in the antepartum period
Medication use in pregnancy

Throughout the world, medical practitioners became alerted to the potential dangers of medication use in pregnancy with the occurrence of congenital limb defects associated with thalidomide use. Following these events, physicians became much more cautious in using any medication in pregnancy. Several large-scale studies were conducted in the USA by the Collaborative Perinatal Project and the CDC that collected information on drug exposures and outcomes for a large number of medications in many thousands of women. More recently, a number of drug registries have been established to study anti-epileptic drugs (AEDs), asthma medications, and antidepressants in pregnancy. Ongoing medication surveillance and information services provide both public educational service and data collection, such as the Motherisk program in Toronto.

Studies of medication use during pregnancy demonstrate that between 20 and 50% of women receive medication other than vitamins and minerals in pregnancy.[20] The most frequently used medications include antibiotics and anti-nausea medications.

The appropriate use of medication in pregnancy hinges on several important clinical principles.

- Firstly, practitioners must determine that treatment of an illness or symptoms of an illness is beneficial to the mother and beneficial to the fetus, or that the risk to the fetus is justified by the potential benefits of treating the mother.

Table 9.2 Conditions that pose significant risk to the mother during pregnancy

Condition	Complication
Valvular heart disease, mitral or aortic	Congestive heart failure
Marfan's syndrome with dilated aortic root	Aortic dissection
Renal insufficiency related to preexisting HTN, SLE, DM, glomerular disease	Severe HTN, superimposed preeclampsia, abruption, CVA
Peripartum cardiomyopathy	Congestive heart failure
Severe hypertension	Superimposed preeclampsia, CVA

- Secondly, accurate information must be available to assess the risk of congenital malformation or other negative impact upon the fetus or pregnancy.

Experts vary in recommendations about medication. Some conservative viewpoints express concern, not only about teratogenesis, but also about the risk of long-term subtle effects on neurodevelopment.[21] Caution must be balanced, however, with the risk of untreated disease or the intolerability of untreated symptoms. Some medications do not appear to cause malformations, but may be associated with other poor outcome, such as restricted fetal growth, presumably caused by their effects on the uteroplacental circulation. Some medications are risky only at certain periods of time within the pregnancy, such as the effect of non-steroidal anti-inflammatory medications on fetal renal function or the risk of kernicterus caused by bilirubin displacement from albumin-binding sites by sulfonamides. Specific knowledge of the mechanism and timing of risk may enhance the clinician's effective utilization of medications in pregnancy.

Two systems of classification currently exist for medication use during pregnancy.

- Table 9.3 depicts the Food and Drug Administration's (FDA) classification system. This system has been criticized for providing insufficient information about the risks of medications in pregnancy. The requirements to achieve a category A rating are stringent, difficult to achieve, and extremely costly to pharmaceutical industries;[22] many medications undergoing FDA

Table 9.3 FDA use-in-pregnancy ratings

Category	Interpretation
A	Controlled studies in pregnant women show no risk to the fetus in any trimester of pregnancy.
B	No evidence of risk has been demonstrated in human controlled studies despite adverse findings in animals, or animal studies show no risk, and human studies are not available.
C	Risk cannot be ruled out. Adequate human studies are not available, and animal studies have found risk or are not available. Although there is a risk of harm to the fetus, potential benefits may outweigh risks of use of the medication.
D	Positive evidence of risk is demonstrated in human studies. Potential benefits of use may still outweigh risks of use when a safer medication cannot be used or is ineffective for a serious illness.
X	Contraindicated in pregnancy because of demonstrated risks that clearly outweigh possible benefits to the patient.

Note: Data from Byrd J. Contents of prenatal care. In Ratcliffe S. D., Byrd J. G., Sakornbut E. L., eds., *Handbook of Pregnancy and Perinatal Care in Family Practice*, Philadelphia, PA: Hanley and Belfus, 1996, pp. 21–22.

Table 9.4 Swedish system of classification for medication in pregnancy

Category	Interpretation
A	Drugs that have been used by a large number of pregnant women and have not been shown to produce an increase in malformations or any other harmful effect on the fetus.
B	Drugs that have been used in a limited number of pregnant women without any definitive disturbance in reproductive outcome.
C	Drugs that have caused or are suspected of causing disturbance in the reproductive process with potential risk to the fetus without being directly teratogenic.
D	Known teratogens and other drugs causing permanent damage to the fetus.

Note: Data from Berglund F., Flodh H., Lundborg P., Prame B., Sannerstedt R. Drug use during pregnancy and breast-feeding. a classification system for drug information. *Acta Obstet Gynecol Scand Suppl* 1984; **126**, 1–55.

approval are not submitted for consideration of category A status because of financial issues. A number of medications that are currently classified as "B" are poorly studied in human pregnancy (e.g. leukotriene receptor antagonists) and should be used only if treatment benefits are clear. Other medications currently classified as category C are frequently used in pregnancy and have good safety records.

- The Swedish catalogue of registered pharmaceutical specialties (FASS) uses a different system to categorize medication, included in Table 9.4.
- The TERIS protocol for cataloguing teratological information utilizes all available sources of information and assigns ratings of teratogenic risk of "none," "minimal," "small," "moderate," "high," and "undetermined." A 1990 overview of this resource demonstrated that approximately half of the commonly prescribed medications had insufficient information to assess teratogenic risk. Of the drugs that could be rated, over 90% were rated as minimal risk or less.[23]

- Important initiatives underway include drug registries regarding medication for common chronic illness, such as epilepsy and asthma. It is to be hoped that these projects will provide better information for clinicians about the treatment of medical illness in pregnancy.

> Between 20 and 50% of women receive medication other than vitamins and minerals during pregnancy.

Physiological changes

Physiological changes of pregnancy are listed in Table 9.5, along with possible implications for medical care in pregnancy. Most changes are somewhat dependent on gestational age. While the most sensitive period with respect to congenital malformations occurs during the first trimester in organogenesis, the increase in plasma volume, cardiac output, and glomerular filtration does not begin to manifest significantly until the second trimester, with peak effect noted by 30 weeks gestation.

Table 9.5 Physiological changes of pregnancy and implications for medical care

System	Change	Medical issues
Cardiovascular	Heart rate increases, blood volume increases, increased cardiac output, decreased systemic vascular resistance, and MABP	Detection of shock may be delayed until large volume loss has occurred. Distribution of medication may be altered
Nervous system	Fluid retention, mechanical effects	Decreased seizure threshold, altered medication distribution and metabolism. Multiple compression neuropathies more common in pregnancy – carpal tunnel, Bell's palsy, meralgia paresthetica. Increase in frequency of seizures in many patients with epilepsy
Pulmonary	Decrease in FRC, increase in minute ventilation and respiratory rate	Altered interpretation of ABGs, e.g., with asthma, mild compensated respiratory alkalosis normal
Gastrointestinal	Smooth muscle relaxation secondary to progesterone. Multiple changes in bile lithogenicity. Increased intraabdominal and intragastric pressure, smooth muscle relaxation of lower	Constipation. Incidence of gallstones increased with parity. Esophageal reflux/"heartburn" symptoms esophageal sphincter caused by progesterone. Decreased gastric emptying. Increased tendency for aspiration
Hematological	Increased coagulation factors except XI and XIII, which may be decreased, decreased antithrombin III. Increased WBC, ESR	"Hypercoagulable state." Interpretation of CBC
Renal	Increased renal plasma flow	Decrease in creatinine, uric acid, increased creatinine clearance
Endocrine	Increased TBG and bound T4 caused by high estrogen state. Impaired glucose tolerance, acceleration of starvation ketosis	Interpretation of thyroid studies. Maintenance of euglycemia in diabetes requiring close management

Note: MABP, mean arterial blood pressure; FRC, functional residual capacity; ABG, arterial blood gas; WBC, white blood cell; ESR, erythrocyte sedimentation rate; CBC, complete blood count; TBG, thyroxin-binding globulin.

In general, the fetus poorly tolerates maternal hypotension, hypoxemia, hypovolemia, and acidosis. Thus, while a non-pregnant patient may tolerate greater physiological stress, for example mild hypoxemia during an acute asthmatic attack, the pregnant woman should be treated vigorously for the acute attack with medication and more liberal use of supplemental oxygen. More importantly, preventive measures should be undertaken, whenever possible, to avoid acute exacerbations of chronic disease, such as diabetes and asthma.

Diagnostic testing

Diagnostic measures that would normally be employed to evaluate the acute complaint can almost always be used in pregnancy. Ultrasound modalities (abdominal, renal, breast, and vascular) are considered safe, although there may be some decrease in accuracy of venous studies caused by the enlarged uterus and inferior vena cava compression. If a renal ultrasound is insufficient for evaluation of suspected nephrolithiasis, a stone-protocol CT or single-shot intravenous pyelogram may be utilized to assist in management.

Diagnostic peritoneal lavage and/or computed tomography (CT) scan of the abdomen may be indicated in the evaluation of trauma; this modality should not be neglected if clinically indicated, since the single greatest cause of mortality for pregnant women is motor vehicle accidents.

Physicians should not hesitate to utilize chest X-rays when evaluating patients with symptoms suggestive of serious acute illness, such as pneumonia.[24]

Flexible sigmoidoscopy has been studied in all trimesters, with efficacious diagnosis of gastrointestinal bleeding and without negative outcomes.[25]

Nuclear medicine studies should be avoided.

Table 9.6 Symptomatic treatment in pregnancy

Symptom	Medication	FDA category	Comment
Pain, fever	Acetaminophen	B	No associated defects, fetal hepatotoxicity with maternal overdose
Pain	Codeine, Hydrocodone	C	Slight increase in defects? Category D with prolonged use
Cough	Dextromethorphan	C	No fetal defects
Pruritus	Diphenhydramine	B	
Nausea, vomiting	Dimenhydrinate	B	
	Promethazine	C	
	Ondansetron	B	Very expensive
Diarrhea	Loperamide	B	
	Diphenoxylate	C	No associated defects
Heartburn, dyspepsia	H2 blockers, antacids, sucralfate	B	
Constipation	Fiber or magnesium laxative	B	
Eczema, contact dermatitis	Hydrocortisone cream	C (systemic)	Absorption minimal with proper topical use
Nasal congestion	Pseudoephedrine	C	No associated defects
	Ipatropium nasal spray	B	
Allergic rhinitis	Cromolyn nasal spray	B	
	Nasal steroids	C	Minimal systemic absorption
	Loratidine	B	
	Fexofenadine	C	

Multiple surgical series at this time support the safety and utility of laparoscopic surgery during pregnancy. Although timing of surgical procedures in pregnancy is best during the second trimester to decrease the risk of abortion and premature labor, surgical treatment of trauma, appendicitis, and biliary tract disease may not be able to be delayed.

> The best time to perform surgical procedures in pregnancy is during the second trimester to decrease the risk of abortion and premature labor.

Medical care of common acute conditions

Self-limited acute illnesses can often be treated with non-pharmacological measures and/or common symptomatic medications. Table 9.6 lists some symptoms and medications that may be used for a variety of common problems.

Systemic corticosteroids should be used, as indicated, for treatment of severe asthma attacks and when indicated in autoimmune disorders.

Many antiarrhythmic and cardiac medications have been used in pregnancy with good outcome.

Vaginitis

Pregnant women commonly present with vaginal infection. Although a number of medications may be designated as category C, topical use of these medications has not been associated with significant absorption, and the risk of use seems minimal. Examples include antifungal preparations for candida vulvovaginitis. Diflucan has been associated with fetal defects in high doses (continuous administration at 400 mg/day) but is probably safe used in brief courses at standard doses.[26] Treatment of symptomatic vaginal trichomoniasis with metronidazole continues to be a concern to some clinicians because of theoretical concerns of teratogenicity, despite meta-analysis and large population-based studies demonstrating no increased risk of defects,[27,28] and long-term population-based studies showing no increase in childhood cancers.[29]

Viral infections

Acute viral infections are often viewed as benign, self-limited conditions outside of pregnancy. During pregnancy, viral illness (such as rubella) may represent a threat to the fetus or a potentially serious threat to the mother's health.

Influenza

The 1918 Spanish influenza pandemic and other severe influenza epidemics during the twentieth century manifested disproportionate mortality in pregnant women.[30] In the USA, influenza vaccination has been recommended during pregnancy by the Center for Disease Control for more than a decade. Despite the agreement that vaccination should be given during pregnancy by more than 90% of obstetricians, vaccination rates remain low in this population, ranging from 1.5–40%.[31,32] One population-based study determined the number needed to treat to prevent one influenza-like illness was between 20 and 43 pregnant women.[33] Limited outcome data are available, with one study finding no difference in hospitalizations for women or their infants with viral respiratory illnesses during the flu season based on vaccination status.[34]

Herpes

Genital herpes is a common recurrent problem in young women. It is associated with potential neonatal morbidity and mortality, and an increased rate of cesarean delivery. Two adequately powered randomized controlled trials now demonstrate a decrease in positive herpes cultures and cesarean deliveries with no increase in newborn infection when women with genital herpes simplex infection are treated with 500 mg of valcyclovir given twice daily starting at 36 weeks gestation.[35,36] A cost-effectiveness study found acyclovir prophylaxis to be cost-effective and cost-saving using a wide range of assumptions.[37] Strength of recommendation A.

Hepatitis

Hepatitis A infection does not pose a threat to the newborn via perinatal transmission.

Hepatitis B infection may be transmitted perinatally, as well as hepatitis C, D, and E. Immunization against hepatitis B and administration of hepatitis B immunoglobulin immediately at birth is protective against perinatal transmission of hepatitis B and D.[38] The risks of neonatal transmission are increased with HBeAg-positive status and up to 90% if acute infection takes place during the third trimester.[38] Chronic infection occurs in more than 90% of infected infants.

Hepatitis C infection is rarely transmitted perinatally. Transmission usually occurs in mothers with concomitant HIV infection or with very high levels of hepatitis C virus RNA. Routine screening is not recommended, since no treatment is available to prevent infection, but women at high risk may warrant evaluation, and pediatric follow-up is warranted if hepatitis C is detected because of the risk of chronic liver disease in the infant.

Common acute bacterial infections are usually treated as they would be in non-pregnant women. There are several antibiotics that should not be used in pregnancy unless an effective alternative is not available (e.g. quinolones, tetracycline). However, any therapeutic decision must weigh the risks to the pregnancy of possible medication ill effects versus the potential risk to the mother and the fetus of failure to adequately treat significant infections. Table 9.7 contains commonly used medications for infection.

Medical care of chronic illness in pregnancy
General approach

Preconception care of women with chronic illness falls into two categories: the assessment by physician and patient of special risk and the tailoring of care to enhance the safety and optimal outcome of pregnancy. Women should be given the opportunity to understand the extent of risk they may encounter, both to themselves and their babies, during pregnancies complicated by certain chronic conditions, especially chronic cardiovascular, renal, autoimmune, and hemoglobin disorders. See Table 9.2 for a list of disorders with a high risk of maternal complications.

Most women will benefit from an understanding that their medical condition should not significantly

Table 9.7 Medications for treatment of infection in pregnancy

Medication	FDA category	Comment
Penicillins	B	
Cephalosporins	B	
Erythromycin	B	Hepatoxicity with estolate
Tetracycline	D	Dental staining, 2nd, 3rd trimester only, hepatotoxicity
Aminoglycosides	C	Fetal ototoxicity
Sulfonamides	C	Late trimester use may be associated with jaundice and kernicterus because of displacement of bilirubin from albumin binding sites
Macrolides		
Azithromycin	B	
Clarithromycin	C	Defects with animal studies, human inconclusive
Quinolones	C	Cartilage damage in immature animals and case reports in human children, however, large prospective trials do not support risk to human pregnancy[a,b]
Metronidazole	C	Theoretical risk but no known fetal defects demonstrated
Nitrofurantoin	B	No fetal defects
Trimethoprim	C	Teratogenic in animals, human defects reported. Do not use in first trimester
Fluconazole	C	Doses <400 mg/day (such as for vaginal candidiasis) non-teratogenic Doses $\geq 400 =$ mg/day associated with fetal defects
Amphotericin	B	No known fetal defects
Ketoconazole	C	No known fetal defects
Acyclovir	C	No associated defects/adverse events
Oseltamivir	C	No associated defects in human or animal studies
Zanimivir	C	No associated defects in human or animal studies (rimantadine and amantadine are teratogenic in animal studies)
Isoniazid	C	No known fetal defects, monitor for hepatic toxicity, prophylaxis for newborn with vitamin K
Rifampin	C	No known fetal defects, monitor for hepatic toxicity, prophylaxis for newborn with vitamin K
Ethambutol	B	No known fetal defects

Notes: [a]Schaefer C., Amoura-Elefant E., Vial T., *et al.* Pregnancy outcome after prenatal quinolone exposure. Evaluation of a case registry of the European Network of Teratology Information Services (ENTIS). *Eur J Obstet Gynecol Reprod Biol* 1996; **69**(2), 83–89.
[b]Loebstein R., Addis A., Ho E., *et al.* Pregnancy outcome following gestational exposure to fluoroquinolones: a multicenter prospective controlled study. *Antimicrob Agents Chemother* 1998; **42**(6), 1336–1339.

lessen the chance of successful pregnancy outcome. A number of conditions, including rheumatoid arthritis and multiple sclerosis, demonstrate a tendency to improve during pregnancy. Other conditions, such as inflammatory bowel disease, migraine headaches, and asthma are variable in their clinical course during pregnancy. Women with severe preexisting life-threatening disorders may be managed with good success during pregnancy, including women who have been treated for malignancy and renal transplantation.

Perinatal consultation may be helpful as a preconception event in a number of high risk medical conditions and in women with an unexplained history of poor reproductive outcomes. A growing list of metabolic problems and hematological disorders are associated with preeclampsia, growth retardation, abruption, and other complications in late pregnancy. These include hyperhomocysteinemia, Factor V Leiden deficiency, Protein C and Protein S deficiency, and the antiphospholipid antibody syndrome. This includes patients with and without preexisting diagnoses of systemic lupus with anticardiolipin antibody or lupus anticoagulant.

Treatment of several common disorders should be modified before conception. Asthma generally does not require preconception attention, but patients will frequently have questions about their medications. Heart disease in women of childbearing age encompasses a wide range of conditions, congenital and acquired, with variable risks and prognoses in pregnancy. Women with other neurological disorders, such as paraplegia and mysathenia gravis, may require changes in management, for the most part, during the intrapartum period. Specific preconception issues regarding common chronic disorders are addressed along with antepartum medical care in the latter part of this chapter.

Common conditions that benefit from preconception evaluation and manipulation of treatment include hypertension, seizure disorders, and diabetes.

Diabetes

Preconception

Patients with preexisting diabetes should be euglycemic during the critical period of organogenesis. Congenital abnormalities are increased if first trimester control is poor. Preconception and early pregnancy control of diabetes reduces the incidence of congenital abnormalities to the same rate seen in the general population.[39] Patient education includes discussion of contraception, general issues of care during pregnancy, and the need for ongoing follow-up.

Therapeutic alliances with diabetic women of childbearing age must start before conception. Preconception care of type I diabetic women results in earlier prenatal care, lower glycosylated hemoglobin levels, fewer antepartum hospitalizations and fewer hospital days, and decreased intensity and length of stay for newborns. A multicenter prospective study of women who received preconception care versus women who received only antepartum care showed

cost savings of more than $(US)30,000 per patient.[40] A study in the UK found that women attending a preconception clinic were more likely to be in a stable relationship and to be non-smokers. Preconception care improved outcomes and a 50% decrease in neonatal intensive care unit admission rate.[41]

For adolescent diabetics, developmental changes and parental control issues may clash; unprepared pregnancy is an increased risk for these young women. Physicians must educate both parents and patients about the risks of pregnancy. In this situation, one therapeutic goal may be the establishment of a negotiated agreement between adolescent and parents where graduated autonomy and responsibility for self-care are emphasized.

Type II diabetic patients may not be identified in the medical care system before or during early pregnancy. Patients with gestational diabetes should demonstrate normalized glucose status at the six-week postpartum check-up. The identification of unrecognized type II diabetes is enhanced by careful follow-up of all women with a history of gestational diabetes. Screening for diabetes should be considered prior to conception in women with increased risk factors of obesity, unexplained fetal death, strong family history, and a history of macrosomic babies, especially in ethnic groups with a high prevalence of diabetes. This identification allows improved preconception and antepartum management critical to avoid increases in perinatal morality (4.1–6.6%) and congenital malformations (3.4–6.7%) over the general population.[42,43,44]

Relevance to antepartum care
Normal changes in glucose metabolism in pregnancy

Glucose, amino acids, and ketones pass through the placenta to the fetus. Maternal free insulin and glucagon do not traverse the placenta; fetal insulin secretion and glucagon secretion respond to levels of substrate presented to the fetus. Ketones may be associated with adverse effects upon neurophysiological development of the fetus. The "starvation" state is accelerated with pregnancy, and fasting hypoglycemia occurs after 12 hours in the fasting state, with fasting ketosis occurring as well. The "fed" state in pregnancy is characterized by hyperinsulinemia, hyperglycemia, and diminished sensitivity to insulin by multiple tissues (insulin resistance). Insulin resistance is greatest in the third trimester. Multiple hormones in pregnancy, human placental lactogen, prolactin, and progesterone, all contribute to alterations in glucose metabolism and insulin resistance.

Risk of diabetes should be assessed in all pregnant women, with women at high risk, receiving glucose challenge testing (50 g of glucola with one hour blood glucose level) as soon as possible in early pregnancy to screen for undiagnosed type II diabetes.

Patients who have a prior history of gestational diabetes but are documented with normal glucose testing in early pregnancy may benefit from a prudent diet during pregnancy to avoid excessive weight gain and concentrated fats or simple sugars. These patients should be screened again at 28 weeks as in routine prenatal care.

Women with positive screening tests are confirmed or ruled out for the presence of diabetes during pregnancy using a 100 g glucose load and a three-glucose tolerance test.

Diabetes during pregnancy

All pregnant diabetics, regardless of diabetic type, benefit from home glucose monitoring. Usual recommendations for glucose monitoring include fasting, 2 hours post-prandial, and at bedtime. All patients should keep a log of diet, glucose monitoring, and activity. Treatment goals include avoidance of hypoglycemic spells and blood sugar targets of fasting <95 mg/dL (5.4 mmol/L); 1-hour post-prandial values <140 mg/dL; 2-hour post-prandial values <120 mg/dL (6.6 mmol/L); or preprandial values <100 mg/dL (5.6 mmol/L);[45] baseline values of creatinine clearance, uric acid.

Diabetic women may benefit from mild to moderate exercise as an adjunct to blood sugar control during pregnancy.

Serum alphafetoprotein levels are up to 60% lower in diabetic women than in those without diabetes, and a lower threshold is set for detection of neural tube defects, usually 2.0 multiples of the mean. Diabetic women should receive careful sonographic assessment of fetal anatomy at between 16 and 20 weeks of pregnancy along with early establishment of gestational age. Although earlier work suggested increased risk of cardiac malformations in pregnancies with initial glycosylated hemoglobin over 8.5 g/dL, recent studies have not supported this conclusion. Some authors recommend fetal echocardiography in all women with preexisting diabetes.[46,47]

Most type I diabetics should be followed during pregnancy with a system that is designed to provide maximal support for diabetic maintenance. Hypoglycemic reactions are more common during the first trimester. Insulin dosage increases as pregnancy progresses. If maternal insulin secretion fails to keep pace with glucose levels in pregnancy, resulting fetal hyperglycemia stimulates fetal insulin production and a growth-hormone-like effect on fetal growth. The contribution of strict control to avoid fetal macrosomia remains controversial, but some authors suggest that growth acceleration occurring in the late second trimester appears to be triggered by unsatisfactory glucose control in the first half of pregnancy.[48]

> Diabetic women may benefit from mild to moderate exercise as an adjunct to blood sugar control during pregnancy.

Diet for diabetic pregnancies should generally be composed of 40–50% of calories from complex, high fiber carbohydrates with limitation of simple sugars and high glycemic value carbohydrates; 20% protein; and 30–40% fat, primarily from unsaturated sources. Calorie needs are usually 30–35 calories per kg/day with 24 kcal/kg/day if maternal body weight is >120% of ideal weight.[49,50]

Tight control should be achieved with one of several possible insulin regimens.

Type I diabetics will usually be managed best with a combination of insulin or insulin analogs with at least twice daily mixed injections of intermediate and short-acting insulin or four daily injections (before meals and long-acting at night) commonly used. There are advantages to the use of ultra-long-acting insulin administration or delay of NPH until bedtime to avoid early AM hypoglycemic reactions. Another alternative is the use of an insulin pump. Type 2 diabetics and gestational diabetics not controlled with diet are managed on insulin in a similar manner. No evidence is available at this time for inhaled insulin.

While many patients will need insulin for control of blood sugars, some evidence suggests a role for oral agents during pregnancy, with the preponderance of evidence available regarding glyburide and metformin. Two RCTs, one larger, are currently available demonstrating efficacy of glyburide in controlling blood sugars.[51,52] Risk factors associated with glyburide failure include a GCT value of >200 mg/dL,[53] fasting glucose greater than 100 mg/dL, and diagnosis of gestational diabetes before 25 weeks gestation.[54] Some of the studies report an increase in macrosomia or hypoglycemia of the newborn if pregnancies are treated with glyburide, but these findings are not consistent. Even less is known about the use of metformin for gestational diabetes, and most information is derived from studies of women with polycystic ovarian disease. Women exposed to metformin during the first trimester are not at increased risk of congenital malformation[55] while one small RCT noted a decrease in pregnancy and postpartum complications in women with polycystic ovarian disease treated with metformin 850 mg twice daily compared with a control group.[56] No other data are currently available about the efficacy or safety of other oral agents.

Prognostic factors

Women with preexisting diabetes are more likely to experience maternal and neonatal complications than are women without diabetes (Table 9.8). Women with microvascular disease (White Class D, E, and FR) are more likely to develop acute hypertensive complications than those without microvascular disease.

> Women with preexisting diabetes are more likely to experience maternal and neonatal complications than are women without diabetes.

Hypertension

Preconception care

Many women with chronic hypertension experience normal pregnancy outcome. Mild chronic hypertension (diastolic blood pressure <100 mmHg) is not significantly associated with increased risks for preeclampsia or severe exacerbations of blood pressure during pregnancy.

Moderate hypertension (diastolic blood pressure 100 to 105 mmHg) is associated with a slightly increased rate of complications. Approximately one-third of patients with diastolic blood pressure consistently 105 mmHg or those who require high dose or multiple antihypertensives for control experience complications of superimposed preeclampsia. The risk of abruption is also increased.

The presence of renal disease increases the risk for pregnancy complications with a creatinine ≥ 1.5 associated with greater risk of adverse pregnancy outcomes and deterioration of renal function during pregnancy[57] and elevated baseline proteinuria

Table 9.8 Factors that relate to prognosis of diabetic women in pregnancy

Presence or absence of microvascular disease	Women with microvascular disease (White Class D, E, and FR) are more likely to develop acute hypertensive complications than those without microvascular disease
Degree of metabolic control	Poor first trimester metabolic control increases congenital malformation. Poor third trimester metabolic control is more likely to develop polyhydramnios, deliver prematurely, and deliver a large-for-gestational age baby

Note: Data from Reece E. A., Francis G., Homko C. J. Pregnancy outcomes among women with and without diabetic microvascular diseases (White's Class B to FR) versus non-diabetic controls. *Am J Perinatal* 1998; **15**, 549–555.

associated with increased risk of preterm delivery (odds ratio 3.1, 95% CI 1.8–5.3) and IUGR (odds ratio 2.8, 95% CI 1.6–5.0).[58]

These issues may be discussed in preconception counseling, and remediable factors (such as smoking or suspected secondary hypertension) addressed.

Hypertensive patients should be switched to a calcium channel blocker, alpha-methyldopa, or hydralazine from angiotensin-converting enzyme inhibitors if they intend to become pregnant.

Antepartum care

Many hypertensive patients merit a trial off medication to see whether blood pressures will normalize by the end of the first trimester. If the patient is able to maintain the normotensive state, this has positive prognostic value and simplifies concerns regarding short- and long-term effects of medication.

Baseline values of creatinine, BUN, 24 hour urinary creatinine clearance, and 24 hour urine protein should be obtained to evaluate renal function.

Hypertensive medication has not been shown to prevent the onset of superimposed preeclampsia, intrauterine growth restriction, or placental abruption. Treatment with antihypertensive medication has been shown to decrease the risk of cerebrovascular accident in pregnancy in patients with severe elevations of blood pressure. The efficacy of treating mild to moderate hypertension in pregnancy has not been well demonstrated by meta-analysis of randomized controlled trials.[59]

Medications may need to be changed prior to conception or as soon as pregnancy diagnosis is established. Beta-blockers and diuretics are not teratogenic, so patients need not discontinue before becoming pregnant. Diuretics are problematic for continuation during pregnancy because of volume depletion. They should generally only be used for selected cardiac problems to avoid an effect upon uterine blood flow. The chronic antihypertensive medication with the longest safety record in pregnancy is alpha-methyldopa.[60] Patients may experience sedation at higher doses. Labetalol has a good safety record and is well tolerated, but atenolol has been associated with intrauterine growth restriction.[61] Calcium channel blockers have been studied with respect to their effect on uterine blood flow and appear to be relatively safe in the sustained release form. Nicardipine and nifedipine are preferable to verapamil because of possible effects upon the fetal atrioventricular conduction. However, caution must be exercised in the use of calcium channel blockers in the intrapartum setting to avoid severe hypotension, especially in combination with magnesium sulfate.

Prevention of preeclampsia

Based on the most recent Cochrane systematic reviews, patients should be considered for antiplatelet therapy (such as low-dose aspirin) because of reduction in risk of preeclampsia (16%, NNT = 69), preterm birth (7%, NNT = 83), and perinatal death (16%, NNT = 227).[62] Additionally, calcium supplementation should be considered as a means to reduce risk of preeclampsia.[63] Although neither of these meta-analyses addressed specifically the patient with preexisting hypertension, both interventions appear to hold greatest promise with high-risk women (strength of recommendation A).

Seizure disorders

Preconception care

Patients with seizure disorders will need counseling about the increased risk of birth defects and epilepsy in the offspring of epileptic patients.

In addition, none of the currently used seizure medications is currently without risk. Although some patients who are seizure free may be considered for a trial off medication before becoming pregnant, many patients will need AEDs during pregnancy to prevent uncontrolled seizures and their attendant risks. Patients who are being treated for absence or petit mal seizures may "outgrow" their need for medication during adolescence and should be considered for medication discontinuance. Those still needing medication should be switched to ethosuximide because of the high incidence of birth defects from trimethadione.

Older antiepileptic drugs, such as phenobarbital, phenytoin, and carbemazepine, have all been associated with congenital defects with phenytoin and carbemazepine also associated with neurodevelopmental abnormalities. Valproic acid carries a significant risk of malformations and neurodevelopmental problems, including cardiac and neural tube defects; risk of teratogenesis is dose dependent, with risks increasing at doses over 1000 mg/day. Lamotrigine, gabapentin, topiramate, and oxcarbezine are not associated with any pattern of malformations, although less information is available for these newer AEDs. A registry of AEDs continues to compile data on reproductive issues. Table 9.9 contains common seizure medications and known risks and precautions associated with their use.

Patients with a remote history of seizure disorder and no seizures in many years should be considered for a trial off medication before conception. Medication should be adjusted or changed to the safest medication that produces good control of seizures, and monotherapy should be adopted if at all possible because of competition for metabolism.[64] Folic acid is recommended for patients on most AEDs at a dose of 4 mg/day because of decreased absorption of folic acid due to AED therapy, but currently there is no evidence that folic acid supplementation decreases the risk of folic acid related defects in women taking AEDs.[65]

Antepartum care

Patients treated with phenobarbital, phenytoin, and primidone therapy need supplemental vitamin D, 1000 mIU/day. A careful ultrasound anatomical survey should be performed at between 16 and 20 weeks gestation, to evaluate for cardiac, neural tube, renal, gastrointestinal, and limb abnormalities. All patients treated with valproic acid should be evaluated with serum alphafetoprotein (AFP) and considered

121

Table 9.9 Common seizure medications and pregnancy

Medication	Effects on fetus	Effects on newborn
Phenytoin	7–10% fetal anticonvulsant syndrome. Cognitive function may be altered. Folate absorption decreased	No depression/withdrawal. Neonatal hypocalcemia and tetany possible.
Phenobarbital	Increased risk of oral clefts, cardiac[a]	Neonatal depression/withdrawal 10–20%
Primidone	Increased risk of major congenital anomalies,	Neonatal depression possible
Carbemazepine	Fetal anticonvulsant syndrome, craniofacial	No depression/withdrawal
Ethosuximide	6% of exposed fetuses with malformations	No depression/withdrawal
Valproic acid	Dose-dependent (>1 g/day or 70 μg/ml) increase in fetal malformations[b,c] NTDs, cardiac, limb	No depression/withdrawal
Lamotrigine	No increased risk with monotherapy[d]	Slow metabolism in neonate
Gabapentin	No additional risk known but little data	No adverse effects observed so far[e]
Topiramate	Extensive transfer across placenta	No adverse effects observed so far
oxcarbazepine	No additional risk known but little data	No adverse effects observed so far[f]
Diazepam – use only as IV for status epilepticus	1st trimester association with cleft lip/palate, fetal levels exceed maternal	Slow metabolism in neonate. Intrapartum use associated with poor suck, hypotonia, apnea, and hypothermia

Notes: [a]Arpino C., Brescianini S., Robert E., *et al.* Teratogenic effects of antiepileptic drugs: use of an International Database on Malformations and Drug Exposure (MADRE). *Epilepsia* 2000; **41**(11), 1436–1443.
[b]Mawer G., Clayton-Smith J., Coyle H., Kini U. Outcome of pregnancy in women attending an outpatient epilepsy clinic; adverse features associated with higher doses of sodium valproate. *Seizure* 2002; **11**(8), 512–518.
[c]Samren E. B., van Duijn C. M., Koch S., *et al.* Maternal use of antiepileptic drugs and the risk of major congenital malformations: a joint European prospective study of human teratogenesis associated with maternal epilepsy. *Epilepsia* 1997; **38**, 981–990.
[d]Cunnington M., Tennis P., International Lamotrigine Pregnancy Registry Scientific Committee. Lamotrigine and the risk of malformations in pregnancy. *Neurology* 2005; **64**(6), 955–960.
[e]Montouris G. Gabapentin exposure in human pregnancy: results from the Gabapentin Pregnancy Registry. *Epilepsy Behav* 2003; **4**(3), 310–317.
[f]Montouris G. Safety of the newer antiepileptic drug oxcarbazepine during pregnancy. *Curr Med Res Opin* 2005; **21**(5), 693–701.

for a consultative ultrasound scan or for amniocentesis for AFP because of the risk of neural tube defect.

Vitamin K prophylaxis 1 mg intramuscular at birth has been demonstrated to be sufficient to prevent hemorrhagic disease of the newborn.[66]

Asthma

Preconception care

Severe asthma can be managed during pregnancy with most commonly used medication. Asthma is a common problem in young women, and the consideration of pregnancy should always be entertained by clinicians treating asthma in this age group. Preconception care includes patient education about the importance of asthma control and prevention of severe attacks during pregnancy.

Medication need not be changed prior to pregnancy if good control has been achieved with a regimen, although only animal data are available for leukotriene receptor antagonists, such as montelukast and zafirlukast.

Antepartum care

Patients with mild intermittent asthma may continue to be treated with short-acting beta-agonists as rescue medication, such as albuterol. They should be counseled to seek medical care immediately for worsening symptoms.

Patients with mild persistent, moderate, and severe asthma should be maintained on controlling medication throughout pregnancy.[67] Controllers with FDA category B status include budesonide, cromolyn, nedocromil, montelukast, and zafirlukast, but human pregnancy data are available only on budesonide. Salmeterol, theophylline, and systemic steroids are FDA category C. Recent reviews shed no new light on the use of leukotriene receptor antagonist medications in pregnancy.[68] Patients who have achieved good success on these agents and experienced control problems otherwise should be evaluated individually for possible risks and benefits and provided with information to assist in joint decision-making. Corticosteroid use during pregnancy shows no increase in adverse pregnancy outcomes,[69] with the greatest amount of information available for budesonide and beclomethasone.

Inhaled corticosteroids (ICs) demonstrate overall the greatest efficacy, safety, and lowest side effect profile of controlling agents. Inhaled corticosteroids have been shown to decrease asthma exacerbations by 25% and recurrent hospitalizations by 55% during pregnancy.[70,71] Albuterol demonstrates the greatest safety record as an agent for control of acute symptoms. Efficacious treatment of acute exacerbations may be hampered by failure to use systemic steroids and the recurrence of symptoms.[70] Overall the pregnant woman with asthma should be treated as a non-pregnant woman would be with liberal use of oxygen during serious acute exacerbations to reduce the risk of fetal hypoxia.

All patients with asthma should receive influenza vaccination with intramuscular (not nasal) vaccine if they will be pregnant during the flu season. Vaccination during the first trimester is not recommended, although there is no known risk of teratogenesis associated with killed virus vaccine.

Patients may be instructed in home peak flow monitoring and given protocols for self-management and when to contact the physician or come to the emergency room.

Heart disease

Preconception care

Patients with heart conditions who are considering pregnancy range from individuals with no functional impairment, such as women with mitral valve prolapse (MVP), to women with significant structural, functional, and/or electrophysiological disorders of the cardiovascular system.

Patients with MVP on beta-blockers should be considered for adjustment of medication in the antepartum period. Some beta-blockers have been associated with fetal growth restriction. MVP does not appear to have any significant effect on pregnancy outcome, and the degree of prolapse may improve during pregnancy.[72]

Women with repaired congenital heart defects may experience completely normal function or may continue to experience electrophysiological disorders caused by alterations in the conducting system following a complex repair. With the exception of asymptomatic women who had a successful repair of a ventricular septal defect, atrial septal defect, or patent ductus ligation in childhood, women with a history of complex congenital heart disease should be evaluated by a cardiologist familiar with their condition as a preconception measure. If significant patient risk is present, caused by pulmonary hypertension, continued shunting, or poor cardiac function, the consultant may be able to assist the patient in making a more informed decision regarding pregnancy. This consultant may also be helpful in suggesting whether a significant genetic risk is present for congenital heart disease in the offspring, determining the need for fetal echocardiography. Many of these women will require ongoing cardiology consultation for management during pregnancy.

Women with rheumatic valvular heart disease should be evaluated for functional status and receive preconception counseling regarding the risk of pregnancy. Approximately 40% of women with valvular heart disease become symptomatic for the first time during pregnancy. Rheumatic fever prophylaxis should be provided (daily penicillin or monthly benzathine penicillin). Patients in whom valvular procedure or replacement is contemplated should generally undergo such procedures before conception, because the increased demands upon the cardiovascular system may cause deterioration during pregnancy. Valvular replacements and other surgeries requiring intraoperative cardiopulmonary bypass are accompanied by high fetal loss rates.

Peripartum cardiomyopathy is more common in pregnancies with advanced maternal age, African race, multiparity, twins, and hypertension. Half or more of affected patients recover,[73] but prognosis is poor if cardiac function does not normalize by 6 months postpartum.[74] Patients with a previous diagnosis of cardiomyopathy, peripartum or otherwise, should be cautioned about cardiac decompensation during pregnancy and the risk of recurrent peripartum cardiomyopathy.[75]

Antepartum and intrapartum issues

Subacute bacterial endocarditis prophylaxis should be provided for the intrapartum setting according to standard protocols of the American Heart Association. For most patients, intrapartum prophylaxis will consist of ampicillin and gentamycin. See Table 9.10 for cardiac conditions requiring SBE prophylaxis.

Management of individual cardiac conditions during pregnancy are not covered in this chapter. Patients with more than mild disease should be managed with cardiology consultation. Overall management includes close monitoring for maternal congestive heart failure and assessment of fetal well-being, with growth assessment by ultrasound. Clinicians who may attend patients in acute situations should be sensitive to findings such as maternal tachycardia, a state not well tolerated by patients with mitral stenosis and other valvular conditions.

> Approximately 40% of women with valvular heart disease become symptomatic for the first time during pregnancy.

Inflammatory bowel disease

Preconception care

Patients with inflammatory bowel disease may improve or develop more problems during pregnancy, but pregnancy does not appear to affect the long-term course of the disease.

Patients with very active flares or complications just prior to pregnancy tend to have more difficulty during pregnancy.

Methotrexate should be avoided in women trying to conceive because of abortifacient effects and teratogenicity.

Antepartum care

Many medications have been used with safety and efficacy during pregnancy. These include sulfasalazaline, mesalamine,[76] corticosteroids. Cyclosporin and azathioprine do not appear to be teratogenic, but are associated with growth retardation and prematurity.[49] 5-ASA medications such as sulfasalazine and mesalazine have been used extensively and are safe during pregnancy.[76] Discontinuing briefly when the patient is close to delivery may be advisable because of binding to fetal albumin with resultant neonatal hyperbilirubinemia. It should be started immediately postpartum to

Table 9.10 Cardiac conditions requiring SBE prophylaxis

Prosthetic heart valves, mechanical or porcine

Valvular heart lesions such as mitral stenosis and aortic stenosis or insufficiency

Ventricular septal defect (not atrial septal defect)

Idiopathic hypertrophic subaortic stenosis (IHSS)

Patent ductus arteriosus

Mitral valve prolapse with significant regurgitance or valvular thickening

Marfan's syndrome

Coarctation of the aorta

Protocol for SBE prophylaxis

Ampicillin 1 g, intravenously or intramuscularly, 30 minutes to 1 hour before procedure; repeat every 8–12 hours for two doses or

Vancomycin 1 g intravenously for penicillin-allergic patient plus

Gentamicin 1.5 mg/kg intramuscularly or intravenously (not to exceed 120 mg); repeat every 8 hours for two doses or

Streptomycin 1 g intramuscularly; repeat every 12 hours for two doses

Notes: Data from Lewis D. P., Van Dyke D. C., Stumbo P. J., Berg M. J. Drug and environmental factors associated with adverse pregnancy outcomes. Part II. Improvement with folic acid. *Ann Pharmacother* 1998; **32**, 947–961.
Tashinken H. K., Olsen J., Bach B. Experiences in developing legislation protecting reproductive health. *J Occup Environ Med* 1995; **37**, 974–979.
Mountford P. J, Steele H. R. Fetal dose estimates and the IRCP abdominal dose limit for occupational exposure of pregnant staff to technetium-99 and iodine-131 patients. *Eur J Nucl Med* 1995; **22**, 1173–1179.

avoid relapse and is safe for breastfeeding. The dose of mesalazine should be limited to 2 g/day.

Prednisone is discussed previously in other sections of this chapter. Prednisone is relatively safe for use in pregnancy, but high doses (1–2 mg/kg/day) are associated with an increased risk of oral clefts if used in the first trimester.

Immunomodulators, azathioprine and 6-mercaptopurine, have been used extensively in pregnancy and do not increase rates of congenital malformations, abortions, or stillbirths.[77,78,79] There appears to be some increase in intrauterine growth restriction with these two agents, and concerns exist about impaired fetal immunity. Cyclosporine, usually prescribed in severe, steroid-resistant ulcerative colitis and for extra-intestinal manifestations, is not teratogenic. Despite concerns about alteration of immune function in newborns exposed to immunomodulator medication, no changes are detected in infant complete blood counts, immunoglobulin subclasses, lymphocyte subpopulations, serum levels of antibodies, or response to hepatitis B vaccination when compared to non-exposed infants.[80]

Conclusion

Clinicians who provide medical care for women of childbearing age should be prepared within their clinical roles to provide preconception care and care of medical illness during pregnancy. Incorporating preconception care into primary care of young women enhances the preventive aspects of care and may improve pregnancy outcomes. Approaches to acute clinical problems often need only minor adjustment during pregnancy to assure maternal and fetal safety. Patients with serious chronic medical illness will often benefit from specialist consultation and/or management of their condition. All primary care physicians, emergency department personnel, and other women's health care providers should be familiar with overall principles of medical care during pregnancy to respond well in urgent situations and to facilitate a coordinated approach to pregnant women with complex medical issues.

References

1. Lewis D. P., Van Dyke D. C., Stumbo P. J., Berg M. J. Drug and environmental factors associated with adverse pregnancy outcomes. Part II. Improvement with folic acid. *Ann Pharmacother* 1998; **32**, 947–961.

2. Centers for Disease Control and Prevention. Knowledge and use of folic acid by women of child bearing age – United States, 1995 and 1998. *MMWR Morb Mortal Wkly Rep* 1999; **48**, 325–327.

3. Botto L. D., Lisi A., Bower C., Canfield M. A., *et al.* Trends of selected malformations in relation to folic acid recommendations and fortification: an international assessment. *Birth Defects Res A Clin Mol Teratol* 2006; **76**(10), 693–705.

4. Kloeben A. S. Folate knowledge, intake from fortified grain products, and periconceptional supplementation patterns of a sample of low-income pregnant women according to the Health Belief Model. *J Am Diet Assoc* 1999; **99**, 33–38.

5. Arkkola T., Uusitalo U., Pietikainen M., *et al.* Dietary intake and use of dietary supplements in relation to demographic variables among pregnant Finnish women. *Br J Nutr* 2006; **96**(5), 913–920.

6. Locksmith G. J., Duv P. Preventing neural tube defects: the importance of periconceptional folic acid supplements. *Obstet Gynecol* 1998; **91**, 1027–1034.

7. Tashinken H. K., Olsen J., Bach B. Experiences in developing legislation protecting reproductive health. *J Occup Environ Med* 1995; **37**, 974–979.

8. Mountford P. J, Steele H. R. Fetal dose estimates and the IRCP abdominal dose limit for occupational exposure of pregnant staff to technetium-99 and iodine-131 patients. *Eur J Nucl Med* 1995; **22**, 1173–1179.

9. Kersemaekers W. M., Roeleveld N., Zielhuis G. A. Reproductive disorders among hairdressers. *Epidemiology* 1997; **8**, 396–401.

10. Byhahn C., Lischke V., Westphal K. Occupational exposure in the hospital to laughing gas and the new inhalation anesthetics desXurane and sevoXurane [in German]. *Dtsch Med Wochenschr* 1999; **124**, 137–141.

11. Brateman L. Radiation safety considerations for diagnostic radiology personnel. *Radiographics* 1999; **19**, 1037–1055.

12. Feng Y. J., Chen W. R., Sun T. P., Duan S. Y., Jia B. S., Zhang H. L. Estimated cosmic radiation doses for flight personnel [in Chinese]. *Space Med Med Eng (Beijing)* 2002; **15**(4), 265–269.

13. Parker L., Pearce M. S., Dickinson H. O., Aitkin M., Craft A. W. Stillbirths among offspring of male radiation workers at the Sellafield nuclear reprocessing plant. *Lancet* 1999; **354**, 1407–1414.

14. Draper G. J., Little M. P., Sorahan T., *et al.* Cancer in offspring of radiation workers: a record linkage study. *Br Med J* 1997; **315**, 1181–1188.

15. Armstrong B. G., Nolin A. D., McDonald A. D. Work in pregnancy and birth weight for gestational age. *Br J Ind Med* 1989; **46**, 196–199.

16. Savitz D. A., Olshan A. F., Gallagher K. Maternal occupation and pregnancy outcome. *Epidemiology* 1996; 7, 269–274.

17. Ortayli N., Osugurlu M., Gokcay G. Female health workers: an obstetric risk group. *Int J Gynaecol Obstet* 1996; **54**, 263–270.

18. Pinhas-Hamiel O., Rotstein Z., Achiron A., *et al.* Pregnancy during residency – an Israeli survey of women physicians. *Health Care Women Int* 1999; **20**, 63–70.

19. Klebanov M. A., Shiono P. H., Carey J. C. The effect of physical activity during pregnancy on preterm delivery and birth weight. *Am J Obstet Gynecol* 1990; **163**, 1450–1456.

20. De Vigan C., De Walle H. E. K., Cordier S., *et al.* Therapeutic drug use during pregnancy: a comparison in four European countries. OECM Working Group, occupational exposures and congenital anomalies. *J Clin Epidemiol* 1999; **52**, 977–982.

21. Peters P. W. Risk assessment of drug use in pregnancy: prevention of birth defects. *Ann 1st Super Sanita* 1993; **29**, 131–137.

22. Sannerstedt R., Lundborg P., Daniellsson B. R., *et al.* Drugs during pregnancy: an issue of risk classification and information to the prescribers. *Drug Saf* 1996; **14**, 69–77.

23. Friedman J. M., Little B. B., Brent R. L., Cordero J. F., Hanson J. W., Shepard T. H. Potential human teratogenecity of frequently prescribed drugs. *Obstet Gynecol* 1990; **75**, 594–599.

24. Murphy K. J., Kazerooni E. A., Braun M. A., Weinberg E. P., Killam D. A., Hendrick W. J. Radiographic appearance of intrathoracic complications of pregnancy. *Can Assoc Radiol J* 1996; **47**, 453–459.

25. Cappell M. S., Sidhom O. Multicenter, multiyear study of safety and efficacy of flexible sigmoidoscopy during pregnancy in 24 females with follow-up of fetal outcome. *Dig Dis Sci* 1995; **40**, 472–479.

26. Jick S. S. Pregnancy outcomes after maternal exposure to fluconazole. *Cochrane Database Syst Rev* 2004; **3**, CD004848.

27. Czeizel A. E., Rockenbauer M. A population based case-control teratologic study of oral metronidazole treatment during pregnancy. *Br J Obstet Gynaecol* 1998; **105**, 322–327.

28. Caron-Paton T., Carvahal A., Martin de Diego I., *et al.* Is metronidazole teratogenic? A metaanalysis. *Br J Clin Pharmacol* 1997; **44**, 179–182.

29. Thapa P. B., Whitlock J. A., Brockman Worrell K. G., *et al.* Prenatal exposure to metronidazole and risk of childhood cancer: a retrospective cohort study of children younger than 5 years. *Cancer* 1998; **83**, 1461–1468.

30. Cox S., Posner S. F., McPheeters M., Jamieson D. J., Kourtis A. P., Meikle S. Influenza and pregnant women: hospitalization burden, United States, 1998–2002. *J Womens Health (Larchmt)* 2006; **15**(8), 891–893.

31. Wallis D. H., Chin J. L., Sur D. K., Lee M. Y. Increasing rates of influenza vaccination during pregnancy: a multisite interventional study. *J Am Board Fam Med* 2006; **19**(4), 345–349.

32. Wu P., Griffin M. R., Richardson A., Gabbe S. G., Gambrell M. A., Hartert T. V. Influenza vaccination during pregnancy: opinions and practices of obstetricians in an urban community. *South Med J* 2006; **99**(8), 823–828.

33. Lindsay L., Jackson L. A., Savitz D. A., Weber D. J., Koch G. G., Kong L., Guess H. A. Community influenza activity and risk of acute influenza-like illness episodes among healthy unvaccinated pregnant and postpartum women. *Am J Epidemiol* 2006; **163**(9), 838–848.

34. Black S. B., Shinefield H. R., France E. K., Fireman B. H., Platt S. T., Shay D., Vaccine Safety Datalink Workgroup. Effectiveness of influenza vaccine during pregnancy in preventing hospitalizations and outpatient visits for respiratory illness in pregnant women and their infants. *Am J Perinatol* 2004; **21**(6), 333–339.

35. Sheffield J. S., Hill J. B., Hollier L. M., Laibl V. R., Roberts S. W., Sanchez P. J., Wendel G. D. Valacyclovir prophylaxis to prevent recurrent herpes at delivery: a randomized clinical trial. *Obstet Gynecol* 2006; **108**(1), 141–147.

36. Andrews W. W., Kimberlin D. F., Whitley R., Cliver S., Ramsey P. S., Deeter R. Valacyclovir therapy to reduce recurrent genital herpes in pregnant women. *Am J Obstet Gynecol* 2006; **194**(3), 774–781.

37. Little S. E., Caughey A. B. Acyclovir prophylaxis for pregnant women with a known history of herpes simplex virus: a cost-effectiveness analysis. *Am J Obstet Gynecol* 2005; **193**(3 Pt 2), 1274–1279.

38. American College of Obstetricians and Gynecologists. ACOG educational bulletin. Viral hepatitis in pregnancy, no. 248, July 1998. *Int J Gynaecol Obstet* 1998; **63**, 195–202.

39. Fuhrman K., Reiher H., Semmler K., *et al.* The effect of intensified conventional insulin therapy before and during pregnancy on malformation rate in offspring of diabetic mothers. *Exp Clin Endocrinol* 1984; **83**, 173–177.

40. Hermann W. H., Janz N. K., Becker N. P., Charron-Prochownik D. Diabetes and pregnancy. Preconception care, pregnancy outcomes, resource utilization, and costs. *J Reprod Med* 1999; **44**, 33–38.

41. Dunne F. P., Brydon P., Smith T., Essex M., Nicholson H., Dunn J. Preconception diabetes care in insulin-dependent diabetes mellitus. *Q J Med* 1999; **92**, 175–176.

42. Cundy T., Gamble G., Townend K., *et al.* Perinatal mortality in type 2 diabetes mellitus. *Diabet Med* 2000; **17**(1), 33–39.

43. Clausen T. D., Mathiesen E., Ekbom P., *et al.* Poor pregnancy outcome in women with type 2 diabetes. *Diabetes Care* 2005; **28**(2), 323–328.

44. Boulot P., Chabbert-Buffet N., d'Ercole C., *et al.* French multicentric survey of outcome of pregnancy in women with pregestational diabetes. *Diabetes Care* 2003; **26**(11), 2990–2993.

45. American College of Obstetricians and Gynecologists. ACOG practice bulletin. Pregestational diabetes mellitus. *Obstet Gynecol* 2005; **60**, 675–684.

46. Gladman G., McCrindle B. W., Boytin C., Smalthorn J. F. Fetal echocardiographic screening of diabetic pregnancies for congenital heart disease. *Am J Perinatol* 1997; **14**, 59–62.

47. Shields L. E., Gan E. A., Murphy H. F., Sahn D. J., Moore T. R. The prognostic value of hemoglobin A1c in predicting fetal heart disease in diabetic pregnancies. *Obstet Gynecol* 1993; **81**, 954–957.

48. Raychaudburi K., Maresh M. J. Glycemic control throughout pregnancy and fetal growth in insulin-dependent diabetes. *Obstet Gynecol* 2000; **95**, 190–194.

49. American Diabetes Association. Prepregnancy counseling and management of women with preexisting diabetes or previous gestational diabetes. In *Medical Management of Pregnancy Complicated by Diabetes*, 3rd edition, American Diabetes Association, 2000, pp. 4–19.

50. Rey E., Attie C., Bonin A. The effects of first-trimester diabetes control on the incidence of macrosomia. *Am J Obstet Gynecol* 1999; **181**, 202–206.

51. Bertini A. M., Silva J. C., Taborda W., Beceker F., Lemos Bebber F. R., Zucco Viesi J. M., Aquim G., Engel Ribeiro T. Perinatal outcomes and the use of oral hypoglycemic agents. *J Perinat Med* 2005; **33**(6), 519–523.

52. Langer O., Conway D. L., Berkus M. D., Xenakis E. M., Gonzales O. A comparison of glyburide and insulin in women with gestational diabetes mellitus. *N Engl J Med* 2000; **343**(16), 1134–1138.

53. Rochon M., Rand L., Roth L., Gaddipati S. Glyburide for the management of gestational diabetes: risk factors predictive of failure and associated pregnancy outcomes. *Am J Obstet Gynecol* 2006; **195**(4), 1090–1094.

54. Kahn B. F., Davies J. K., Lynch A. M., Reynolds R. M., Barbour L. A. Predictors of glyburide failure in the treatment of gestational diabetes. *Obstet Gynecol* 2006; **107**(6), 1303–1309.

55. Gilbert C., Valois M., Koren G. Pregnancy outcome after first-trimester exposure to metformin: a meta-analysis. *Fertil Steril* 2006; **86**(3), 658–663.

56. Vanky E., Salvesen K. A., Heimstad R., Fougner K. J., Romundstad P., Carlsen S. M. Metformin reduces pregnancy complications without affecting androgen levels in pregnant polycystic ovary syndrome women: results of a randomized study. *Hum Reprod* 2004; **19**(8), 1734–1740.

57. Jones D. C., Hayslett J. P. Outcome of pregnancy in women with moderate or severe renal insufficiency. *N Engl J Med* 1996; **335**, 226–232.

58. Sibai B., Lindheimer M. D., Hauth J., *et al.* Risk factors for preeclampsia, abruptio placentae, and adverse neonatal outcomes among women with chronic hypertension. National Institute of Child Health and Human Development Network of Maternal-Fetal Medicine Units. *N Engl J Med* 1998; **339**, 667–671.

59. Abalos E., Duley L., Steyn D. W., Henderson-Smart D. J. Antihypertensive drug therapy for mild to moderate hypertension during pregnancy. *Cochrane Database Syst Rev* 2007; 1, CD002252.

60. Cockburn J., Moar V. A., Ounsted M., *et al.* Final report of study on hypertension during pregnancy: the effects of specific treatment on the growth and development of the children. *Lancet* 1982; **1**, 647–649.

61. Magee L. A., Duley L. Oral beta blockers for mild to moderate hypertension during pregnancy. *Cochrane Database Syst Rev* 2005; 3.

62. Duley L., Henderson-Smart D. J., Knight M., King J. F. Antiplatelet agents for preventing pre-eclampsia and its complications. *Cochrane Database Syst Rev* 2004; 1, CD004659.

63. Hofmeyr G. J., Atallah A. N., Duley L. Calcium supplementation during pregnancy for preventing hypertensive disorders and related problems. *Cochrane Database Syst Rev* 2006; 3, CD001059.

64. Pennell P. B. The importance of monotherapy in pregnancy. *Neurology*. 2003; **60**(11 Suppl 4), S31–S38.

65. Hernandez-Diaz S., Werler M. M., Walker A. M., Mitchell A. A. Folic acid antagonists during pregnancy and the risk of birth defects. *N Engl J Med* 2000; **343**(22), 1608–1614.

66. Kaaja E., Kaaja R., Matila R., Hiilesmaa V. Enzyme-inducing antiepileptic drugs in pregnancy and the risk of bleeding in the neonate. *Neurology* 2002; **58**(4), 549–553.

67. Asthma and Pregnancy, Update 2004. *NAEPP Working Group Report on Managing Asthma During Pregnancy: Recommendations for Pharmacologic Treatment, Update 2004*. NIH Publication No. 05-3279. Bethesda, MD: US Department of Health and Human Services; National Institutes of Health; National Heart, Lung, and Blood Institute, 2004.

68. Gluck J. C., Gluck P. A. Asthma controller therapy during pregnancy. *Am J Obstet Gynecol* 2005; **192**(2), 369–380.

69. Rahimi R., Nikfar S., Abdollahi M. Meta-analysis finds use of inhaled corticosteroids during pregnancy safe: a systematic meta-analysis review. *Hum Exp Toxicol* 2006; **25**(8), 447–452.

70. Wendel P. J., Ramin S. M., Barnett-Hamm C., *et al.* Asthma treatment in pregnancy: a randomized controlled study. *Am J Obstet Gynecol* 1996; **175**, 150–154.

71. Grazmararian K. D., Peterson R., Jamieson D. J., *et al.* Hospitalizations during pregnancy among managed care enrollees. *Obstet Gynecol* 2002; **100**, 94–100.

72. Rayburn W. F., LeMire M. S., Bird J. L., Buda A. J. Mitral valve prolapse. Echocardiographic changes during pregnancy. *J Reprod Med* 1987; **32**, 185–187.

73. Amos A. M., Jaber W. A., Russell S. D. Improved outcomes in peripartum cardiomyopathy with contemporary. *Am Heart J* 2006; **152**(3), 509–513.

74. Abboud J., Murad Y., Chen-Scarabelli C., Saravolatz L., Scarabelli T. M. Peripartum cardiomyopathy: a comprehensive review. *Int J Cardiol* 2007; **118**(3), 295–303.

75. Pearson G. D., Veille J. C., Rahimtoola S., *et al.* Peripartum cardiomyopathy: National Heart, Lung, and Blood Institute and Office of Rare Diseases (National Institutes of Health) workshop recommendations and review. *J Am Med Assoc* 2000; **283**, 1183–1188.

76. Norgard B., Fonager K., Pedersen L., Jacobsen B. A., Sorensen H. T. Birth outcome in women exposed to 5-aminosalicylic acid during pregnancy: a Danish cohort study. *Gut* 2003; **52**(2), 243–247.

77. Moskowitz D. N., Bodian C., Chapman M. L., *et al.* The effect on the fetus of medications used to treat pregnant inflammatory bowel-disease patients. *Am J Gastroenterol* 2004; **99**(4), 656–661.

78. Katz J. A. Pregnancy and inflammatory bowel disease. *Curr Opin Gastroenterol* 2004; **20**(4), 328–332.

79. Francella A., Dyan A., Bodian C., *et al.* The safety of 6-mercaptopurine for childbearing patients with inflammatory bowel disease: a retrospective cohort study. *Gastroenterology* 2003; **124**(1), 9–17.

80. Cimaz R., Meregalli E., Biggiogerro M., *et al.* Alterations in the immune system of children from mothers treated with immunosuppressive agents during pregnancy. *Toxicol Lett* 2004; **149**(1–3), 155–162.

10

Menstrual changes: amenorrhea, oligomenorrhea, polycystic ovary syndrome, and abnormal menstrual bleeding

Jo Ann Rosenfeld

Normal menstruation is the end product of a complex interplay of health and hormones. It is more amazing that "normal" menstruation occurs regularly and that cyclic changes are often predictable and expected. Women, unless frequently pregnant or amenorrheic, spend up to one sixth of their lives actually menstruating. Variations in time and amount of bleeding, unpredictability, excessive bleeding, pain, cramps, bloating, and weight gain are not mere annoyances, but symptoms of irregularities that must be addressed and the symptoms improved if at all possible.

Amenorrhea

1. Amenorrhea is the absence of normal menstrual periods for six months.
2. Primary amenorrhea means never having a menstrual period.
3. Secondary amenorrhea means an absence of menstrual periods after the initiation of normal menstrual periods.
4. Amenorrhea occurs in approximately 1.8 to 5% of women and in 38–42% of adolescents.[1]
5. Amenorrhea is seen in approximately 50% of competitive runners, 25% of recreational runners, and 44% of professional dancers.[2]
6. Amenorrhea, especially with galactorrhea, can have serious health consequences. It can be associated with bone loss and fractures, infertility, dyspareunia, and if causing endometrial hyperplasia, endometrial cancer.

Etiology of irregular menstruation (Table 10.1)

Many of the causes of amenorrhea can also cause oligomenorrhea, metrorrhagia, menorrhagia, and other irregularies of menstruation. The following are some causes of menstrual changes.

1. **Physiological causes**
   a. The most common cause of primary and secondary amenorrhea is pregnancy.
   b. Postpartum amenorrhea can last up to 12 months, but usually is less than three months.
   c. During lactation, amenorrhea often occurs for six to nine months depending on the amount of breastfeeding and amount of supplementation to the child (Table 10.2). The longer a woman breast feeds, the longer her period of amenorrhea post-lactation will most likely be (Figure 10.1).
   d. Use of hormonal contraception can cause amenorrhea. Although it is less likely with monthly oral contraceptives, it occurs more often with depot-medroxyprogesterone acetate (MPA).
   e. After OCPs are stopped, amenorrhea can last 6–12 months, without pathology. With depot MPA, the amenorrhea can last 24 months.

2. **Hypothalamic causes**

   In a population based study, after pregnancy and physiological causes were eliminated, approximately one-third of cases of amenorrhea were caused by hypothalamic dysfunction. Another one-third was caused by chronic anovulation, usually polycystic ovarian syndrome (PCOS).

3. Medications, especially psychotropic medications, anti-seizure medications, phenothiazines, haloperidol, tricyclic antidepressants, and SSRIs,

---

Table 10.1 Causes of amenorrhea

Physiological

Pregnancy

Postpartum

Breast feeding

Menopause

Post hormonal contraception

Hormonal contraception

Medication

Hormones

Neuroleptics

Antidepressants

Antipsychotics

Hypothalamic causes

Stress

Exercise induced

Eating disorders

Malnutrition

Systemic or chronic diseases

Hormonal abnormalities

Pituitary adenomas – prolactinomas

Thyroid abnormalities

Polycystic ovary syndrome

Table 10.2 Causes of abnormal menstrual periods

Adolescence

Anovulation

Pregnancy and complications

Coagulation disorders

Endometriosis

Trauma

Infection

Anatomical lesions

Foreign bodies

Medications

Reproductive age women

All of the above

Systemic diseases

Cancer of cervix and uterus

Fibroids and other anatomical lesions

Perimenopausal years

Anovulation

Any of the above

can all cause menstrual disturbances, including amenorrhea.

4. **Thyroid disease**

   Hypothyroidism usually causes oligomenorrhea, but can cause amenorrhea. Hypothyroidism can also produce hyperprolactinemia because the elevated TRH produced in reaction to low thyroid hormone levels will also induce an increase in prolactin, and perhaps galactorrhea. Hyperthyroidism usually causes heavier, irregular, and excessive menstruation.

5. Galactorrhea (secretion of milk from the breast not related to pregnancy or breastfeeding) is present in many women with amenorrhea. Sometimes caused by pineal lesions or pituitary adenomas, galactorrhea

should indicate an MRI of the brain including the sella turcica.

Evaluation

1. Primary amenorrhea occurs in adolescents who have never had a menstrual period. The causes for this are similar to that of secondary amenorrhea. Once pregnancy is eliminated as a cause, genetic abnormalities and congenital malformations should be considered.

   a. A girl who has no menstruation and secondary sexual characteristics by age 14, or has sexual characteristics (breasts, pubic and axillary hair) and has not had a menstrual period by age 16 should be evaluated with genetic karyotype and chromosome evaluation and pelvic examination, ultrasound, and CT scan to determine whether normal genitalia and organs are present.

   b. A high FSH level may indicate Turner's syndrome or gonadal dysgenesis.

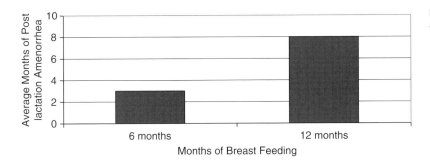

Figure 10.1 Average months of amenorrhea after cessation of lactation.

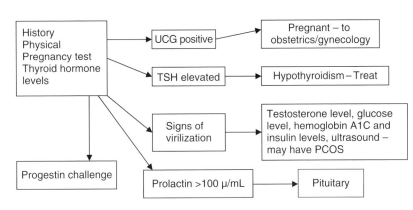

Figure 10.2 Evaluation of secondary amenorrhea.

c. A low FSH level suggests hypothalamic failure as with exercise, anorexia, starvation, bulimenia, or gonadotropin deficiency.

d. Any woman who is not pregnant and younger than age 30 who develops ovarian failure should have a karyotype. Mosaicism may exist, and the woman may need gonadal removal to prevent malignancy in any area that has testicular tissue.

2. The history should include family history of genetic abnormalities, family history of menstrual function including early ovarian failure, galactorrhea, recent changes in weight, skin tone, and hair, medications, psychological dysfunction, stress. Symptoms of pregnancy and menopause should also be discussed.

3. Physical examination includes looking for evidence of nutritional or hormonal changes, abnormal growth or weight loss, normality of the genitorurinary tract, and symptoms of neurological diseases.

4. Pregnancy must first be excluded in all women with amenorrhea, oligomenorrhea and even abnormal menstrual bleeding. A urine pregnancy test and physical examination should suffice for pregnancy determination.

5. **Laboratory tests**

Initial laboratory tests include an in-office pregnancy test. If this is negative, a complete blood count, erythrocyte sedimentation rate, TSH, prolactin, and FSH should be obtained. Further testing depends on results (Figure 10.2).

a. A high FSH level is consistent with ovarian failure or menopause

b. If the woman has amenorrhea and galactorrhea, with or without an elevated prolactin level, an examination of the pituitary – either CT or MRI – is indicated. Approximately 34% of women with amenorrhea-galactorrhea have brain tumors.[3]

c. If these tests are normal and the woman shows evidence of virilization including excessive hair, beard growth, and acne, PCOS is a likely diagnosis. A history of infertility, a testosterone level and ultrasound may help establish the diagnosis (see below).

d. If these tests are normal and the woman has no signs of virilization, a progestin challenge of five days of MPA (5–10 mg daily), the "progestin challenge test," can be performed. If the non-pregnant woman with amenorrhea takes MPA for five days, she should have withdrawal bleeding within 10 days of stopping MPA. Withdrawal bleeding would show that the woman has a mild depression of her hypothalamic/pituitary axis.

e. Progestin challenge

If the woman has withdrawal bleeding two to seven days after progestin for five days, the cause of amenorrhea is anovulation, temporary or chronic.

f. If there is no withdrawal bleeding, the woman may have outflow abnormalities. Asherman's syndrome, adhesions of the endometrial cavity caused by surgery or abortions, can cause amenorrhea.

g. Elevation of FSH (>30 IU/L) and LH (>40 IU/L) signals ovarian failure or menopause. Unless the woman desires pregnancy, no further treatment is necessary.

h. Women with amenorrhea and low or normal FSH, LH, may have either a pituitary or hypothalamic cause. If the prolactin level is <100 ng/mL and the view of the sella turcica is normal, no further evaluation is necessary.

Treatment

1. Women with amenorrhea need treatment for fertility, if desired, to avoid endometrial hyperplasia, and to prevent osteoporosis.

2. Fertility

Women with amenorrhea can be placed on ovulation inducing drugs. However, estrogen or estradiol alone will not induce ovulation. An ovulation inducing agent, such as clomiphene is needed. Metformin may be used in those women with PCOS.

3. Endometrial hyperplasia

The endometrium must shed periodically at least every three months to prevent a high risk of endometrial hyperplasia (precancer) or cancer. Use of estrogen at HRT doses with progesterone either orally or as a vaginal gel, or use of OCPs with monthly or once every three monthly withdrawal bleeding will promote adequate shedding of the endometrial lining.

4. Alternatively, in women who do not want or cannot take estrogens, progesterone only (MPA 10 mg/day) for the first 10 days of the month or natural progesterone cream every other day for 6 doses can produce withdrawal bleeding. Levonorgestrel IUDs can also be used.

5. Osteoporosis

Women with amenorrhea are at an increased risk for osteoporosis, partially caused by estrogen deficiency. These women should have bone density scans if they are not on estrogen therapy.

6. Therapy for women with a hyperprolactinoma or idiopathic hyperprolactinemia depends on the size of the adenoma and the desire for pregnancy. Treatment with bromocriptine can produce fertility in 80% of women. Women who do not desire pregnancy and whose pituitary tumors are small (less than 10 mm) can be followed by close evaluation. Macroadenomas or adenomas with prolactin levels greater than 100 IU/mL can be treated with bromocriptine or dosinex. Surgery may be an option.

Polycystic ovary disease
Definition

1. Polycystic ovary syndrome consists of a group of syndromes in women that includes infertility, amenorrhea or oligomenorrhea, and signs of androgen excess. There were consensus guidelines developed in 2002 in Rotterdam which considered PCOS primarily a "disorder of androgen excess or hyperandrogenism, although a minority considered the possibility that there may be forms of PCOS without overt evidence of hyperandrogenism."[4]

2. Symptoms include oligomenorrhea or amenorrhea, anovulation, infertility, high levels of testosterone and other androgens, abnormalities of gonadotropins, hirsuitism, acne, diabetes and hyperlipidemia (Table 10.3).

3. The woman with PCOS often has elevated insulin resistance with hyperinsulinemia; this may be the cause of the androgen excess.

4. Approximately 6–7% of women have PCOS.[5]

5. The diagnosis is important because the health risks are significant. The woman with PCOS is at high risk for infertility, endometrial carcinoma, type 2 diabetes, dyslipidemia, hypertension, obesity and subsequent cardiovascular disease.[6]

Table 10.3 Incidence of symptoms in PCOS

Ovulatory and menstrual dysfunction	75%
Eumenorrhea	20%
Hyperandrogenemia	60–80%
Hirsuite	60%
Polycystic ovaries	75%

Note: Data from Task Force on the Phenotype of the Polycystic Ovary Syndrome of The Androgen Excess Society. Criteria for defining polycystic ovary syndrome as a predominantly hyperandrogenic syndrome: an Androgen Excess Society guideline. *J Clin Endocrin Metab* 2006; **91**(11), 4237–4245, doi:10.1210/jc.2006–0178.

6. PCOS may be genetic. Certainly sisters and other women relatives are at higher risk of developing PCOS.
7. PCOS requires continuing medical expense and treatment, including insulin and hormonal therapy. The diagnosis brings with it increased morbidity and mortality.

Treatment

1. Ovulation can be induced. In one study, use of clomiphene, metformin, or both to induce ovulation has produced 22%, 7%, or 28% live births respectively. Use of clomiphene increased the risk of multiple births.[7]
2. If pregnancy is not desired, the woman should be treated for chronic estrogen exposure without menstruation that can lead to endometrial hyperplasia. Progesterone or OCPs can be used to induce withdrawal bleeding.
3. Women with PCOS develop early and male patterns of cardiovascular disease and metabolic syndrome. They should be aggressively counseled and treated to reduce risk factors such as hypertension, smoking and hypercholesterolemia.
4. Metformin improves the endocrine symptoms of PCOS, even in women who are not diabetic. It treats insulin sensitivity, induces normal ovulatory cycles, and causes weight loss, although this is an off-label use.
5. Signs of virilization such as hirsuitism can be treated with spironolactone (50–100 mg qd or bid).
6. OCPs should be given to decrease hormone levels and promote withdrawal bleeding in women who do not desire pregnancy. Alternatively MPA (10 mg daily) can be given from day 14 to 28 of the cycle.

Abnormal Menstrual bleeding

Definitions

1. Heavy menstrual bleeding (HMB) is an important cause of ill health in women and it accounts for 12% of all gynecology referrals in the UK.[8]
2. There is significant variation in duration and amount of menstrual flow between women and even from period to period in the same woman. However, most women have "regular" periods in the presence of normal ovulation and the absence of anatomical disturbances, cancer, or infection. Thus, a complaint of increased flow, increased duration, abnormalities of flow, or increased frequency deserves evaluation.
3. The "usual" cycle is 4–6 days long, with a range of 2–6 days.
4. The normal volume of blood loss is 30–90 mL. More than 90 mL is generally considered abnormal. Precise measurement is impossible. Pad counts do not provide accurate measurements of blood loss. Blood loss sufficient to cause iron deficiency anemia should be considered abnormal.
5. Oligomenorrhea is considered intermenstrual intervals greater than 35 days and polymenorrhea intervals less than 21 days.
6. Menorrhagia is regular normal intervals with excessive flow and duration, and metrorrhagia is irregular intervals with excessive flow and duration.
7. The incidence of menstrual disorders is 20 per 100 woman years in a population in a family practice.

Etiology

1. The most common causes are contraception-related, pregnancy-related dysfunctional uterine bleeding (40%), and cervical pathology (10%). (Table 10.2)
2. The differential diagnosis changes with age.
3. **Adolescence**

   In adolescence, anovulation with subsequent dysfunctional uterine bleeding is the most common cause. Immaturity of the hypothalamic-pituitary axis may cause anovulation. Establishment of regular cycles can take as long as 5 years.
   - Complications of pregnancy are a common cause.

- Coagulation disorders such as von Willebrand's disease or prothrombin may not be detected until the onset of menstrual periods.
- Other less likely causes include malignancy, endometriosis, trauma, infections, foreign bodies, use of appliances, and medications.

4. In reproductive age women, the differential is mostly the same except congenital bleeding disorders are rarely diagnosed. Pregnancy and its complications are a common problem. Systemic disease, malignancy of the cervix and endometrium, medications that interfere with the hypothalamic-pituitary axis, and anatomical lesions are more likely as women become older. As women approach menopause, anovulatory bleeding becomes more likely.

5. **Perimenopause**

   In perimenopausal women, the follicles that remain become relatively refractory to stimulation by FSH. Causes include anovulatory bleeding, fibroids, endometrial lesions, cancer of endometrium or cervix, medications and systemic diseases.

Evaluation

1. All women with abnormal vaginal bleeding should have a complete history and physical including obstetrical and gynecological history. A menstrual history including menarche, usual bleeding patterns, presence and severity of dysmenorrhea and other symptoms are important. Discussion of all medications, herbs and street drugs is important. Sexual history, use and cessation and reactions to contraceptives, systemic syndromes, and history of previous gynecological disease or pelvic infections are important.

2. Physical examination should include evaluation of systemic problems including paleness, tachycardia, hypotension, thyromegal or thyroid nodule, jaundice or petechia. The vaginal vault should be inspected for signs of trauma, atrophy, polyps, cancer or foreign bodies. The cervix may show evidence of polpys or cancer. A Pap smear should be obtained, even though there may be too much bleeding for a good specimen. Bimanual examination may show an enlarged symmetrical irregular uterus (suggestive of fibroids), pain on palpation of uterus, adenexae suggesting infection, or a pregnancy.

3. Laboratory evaluation includes the following.

   a. A CBC and pregnancy test should be obtained in all women.

   b. If there is any evidence for infection, a wet-prep, KOH prep and cultures or DNA swabs for chlamydia and gonorrhea are important.

   c. Signs of systemic disease may suggest liver function tests or renal functions.

   d. A serum TSH should be obtained.

Additional examinations

1. Transvaginal ultrasound has excellent sensitivity and specificity in detecting intrauterine lesions, polyps, early pregnancy, fibroids, and thickened endometrium suggestive of endometrial hyperplasia.

2. Hysteroscopy allows direct visualization of the endometrial cavity and is useful in diagnosing polyps or submucous fibroids. Office hysteroscopy is increasingly common.

Treatment

1. Treatment of abnormal menstrual bleeding depends on its cause. Thus, thyroid dysfunction or coagulopathy should be treated if discovered. Women with von Willebrand's disease or acquired coagulopathy can use a progestin (levonorgestrel) IUD to reduce heavy menstrual periods.[9]

2. If a medication is suspected as the cause, a judgment whether the medication can be changed or stopped should be made.

3. Infections should be treated with the appropriate antibiotics.

4. Cervical polyps, warts, or lesions should be treated with cryosurgery or regular surgery (see "Fibroids" below).

5. Women in whom a specific abnormality is not found and who have irregular or heavy bleedings have dysfunctional uterine bleeding (DUB) usually caused by anovulatory periods. The goal of treatment in these women is to control the acute bleeding, prevent recurrence, preserve fertility or provide contraception, and correct associated disorders such as iron-deficiency anemia. DUB

Table 10.4 Hormonal treatment of dysfunctional uterine bleeding

Emergent

1. IV estrogen at 25 mg every 4 hours for 12 hours

2. IV conjugated equine estrogen at 1.25 mg every 4 hours

   Then estrogen 1.25 mg daily of conjugated estrogen daily for 7–10 days with a progesterone (such as medroxyprogesterone acetate (MPA)) 10 mg daily

Moderate

1. Oral contraceptives taken 3 times a day for one week, then start a new pack of pills take one pill a day in the 2nd through 5th week

2. MPA 10 mg daily for 10 days

Mild or recurrent

1. Oral contraceptive for 3 to 6 months. OCPs can also be given for 84 days straight, with only one week withdrawal bleeding every three months

2. MPA 10 mg daily for 10 days each month

3. Depo provera IM 150 mg q 3 months

4. Progestin (levogestrel) IUD

5. NSAIDs 10 to 15 days a month

can be treated medically, hormonally or surgically (Table 10.4)

6. Non-steroidal anti-inflammatory agents do reduce the amount of bleeding and dysmenorrhea in women with heavy menstrual periods.[10] They do not work as well as the drug danazol, but have many fewer side effects.[11]

7. Hormone therapy is recommended in women with acute heavy bleeding; estrogen is most commonly used for acute emergent bleeding (see Table 10.4). High-dose IV estrogen usually controlled within 24 hours. After the endometrium has been stabilized with high-dose estrogen, lower dose estrogen should be administered with progesterone for 7–10 days.

8. Oral contraceptive pills can be used for moderate bleeding. One pill three times a day for one week, to be followed by a new pack of pills one a day. After five weeks, the woman can continue on OCPs or stop if fertility is desired.

9. OCPs, depot provera, or a progestin-IUD (levonorgestrel) can be used for chronic menorrhagia, if fertility is not desired. Alternatively, if OCPs are contraindicated, therapy with a progestin can be used, as MPA 12 days per month at 10 mg daily. Women should be given the option of continual OCPs, taking one pill daily for 84 days, and then having one episode of withdrawal bleeding each three months.[12]

10. Surgical therapy should be reserved for women when other methods fail and the woman has no desire for future pregnancy.

11. The surgical treatment can be endometrial ablation with laser, photovaporization, thermal balloon,[13] or electrocautery using hysteroscopic visualization. Endometrial ablation, an outpatient procedure, causes an Asherman-like syndrome and with the scarring, approximately 90% of women have subsequent amenorrhea.

12. Hysterectomy is indicated when there is associated pelvic pathology, cervical dysplasia or cancer, uterine prolapse, or obstructing fibroids, and the woman desires no other pregnancy.

13. Uterine artery embolization is an alternative to hysterectomy, in that the women have a shorter hospital stay and quicker return to work.[14]

Fibroids (Leiomyomata)

1. Fibroids are thickenings of the muscle wall of the uterus. They can occur on the cervix, the serosa or the endometrium. Most women have no complications from fibroids. They do not grow any larger after menopause and may in fact "shrink."

2. The uterus will may feel asymmetric or bulky, and often large. It should not be tender or painful.

3. Fibroids can cause either heavy menstrual bleeding, perhaps by increasing the surface area of the endometrium and impeding normal flow, or sudden heavy intermenstrual bleeding.

4. Fibroids, if large enough and multiple, may cause infertility, difficulty delivering a baby by mechanical obstruction, constipation, or urinary retention by ureteral or urethral obstruction. This may lead to subsequent urinary tract infection and even renal failure.

5. Fibroids do not need to be treated, but can be treated by surgical myomectomy or hysterectomy, which is of course, very effective and stops

excessive bleeding. A recent small study examined the effects of the levonorgestrel intrauterine system (LNG-IUS) on uterine volume and myomata volume in women who had menorrhagia. The use of LNG-IUS reduced the bleeding, causing amenorrhea in more than half the women, and reduced uterine volume but not myomata volume.[15]

References

1. Wiksten-Almstromer M., Hirschberg A. L., Hagenfeldt K. Menstrual disorders and associated factors among adolescent girls visiting a youth clinic. *Acta Obstet Gynecol Scand* 2007; **86**(1), 65–72.

2. Goodman L. R., Warren M. P. The female athlete and menstrual function. *Curr Opin Obstet Gynecol* 2005; **17**(5), 466–470.

3. Pena K. S., Rosenfeld J. A. Evaluation and treatment of galactorrhea. *Am Fam Physician* 2001; **63**(9), 1763–1770.

4. Task Force on the Phenotype of the Polycystic Ovary Syndrome of The Androgen Excess Society. Criteria for defining polycystic ovary syndrome as a predominantly hyperandrogenic syndrome: an Androgen Excess Society guideline. *J Clin Endocrin Metab* 2006; **91**(11), 4237–4245, doi:10.1210/jc.2006-0178.

5. Setji T. L., Brown A. J. Polycystic ovary syndrome: diagnosis and treatment. *Am J Med* 2007; **120**(2), 128–132.

6. Azziz R., Marin C., Hoq L., Badamgarav E., Song P. Health care-related economic burden of the polycystic ovary syndrome during the reproductive life span. *J Clin Endocrinol Metab* 2005; **90**, 4650–4658.

7. Legro R. S., Barnhart H. X., Schlaff W. D. Clomiphene, metformin, or both for infertility in the polycystic ovary syndrome. *N Engl J Med* 2007; **356**(6), 551–566.

8. Lethaby A. E., Cooke I., Rees M. Progesterone or progestogen-releasing intrauterine systems for heavy menstrual bleeding. *Cochrane Database Syst Rev* 2005; **4**, CD002126.

9. Kadir R. A., Chi C. Women and von Willebrand disease: controversies in diagnosis and management. *Semin Thromb Hemost* 2006; **32**(6), 605–615.

10. Grimes D. A., Hubacher D., Lopez L. M., Schulz K. F. Non-steroidal anti-inflammatory drugs for heavy bleeding or pain associated with intrauterine-device use. *Cochrane Database Syst Rev* 2006; **4**, CD006034.

11. Lethaby A., Augood C., Duckitt K. Nonsteroidal anti-inflammatory drugs for heavy menstrual bleeding. *Cochrane Database Syst Rev* 2002; **1**, CD000400.

12. Archer D. F. Menstrual-cycle-related symptoms: a review of the rationale for continuous use of oral contraceptives. *Contraception* 2006; **74**(5), 359–366.

13. Sadoon S. S., Salman G. A., Kirwan P. Thermal balloon endometrial ablation (Cavaterm) in the management of menorrhagia. *J Obstet Gynaecol* 2006; **26**(8), 804–805.

14. Gupta J. K., Sinha A. S., Lumsden M. A., Hickey M. Uterine artery embolization for symptomatic uterine fibroids. *Cochrane Database Syst Rev* 2006; **1**, CD005073.

15. Magalhaes J., Aldrighi J. M., de Lima G. R. Uterine volume and menstrual patterns in users of the levonorgestrel-releasing intrauterine system with idiopathic menorrhagia or menorrhagia due to leiomyomas. *Contraception* 2007; **75**(3), 193–198.

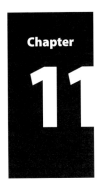

Chapter

11

Menstrual, urogynecological and vasomotor changes in perimenopause and menopause

Margaret Gradison

> *S. J. is a 47-year-old woman who presents with abnormal uterine bleeding. She had regular periods until two years ago, at which time her periods became unpredictable. Her current menses started three weeks ago; she says it alternates between needing to change pads hourly to requiring only a daily panty liner. Ms. J. is obese and smokes a pack of cigarettes a day. Her only medication is thyroid supplements. She is a gravida three para two spontaneous abortion one (G3P2 AB1). She uses condoms intermittently for contraception, and her first pregnancy was at age 29.*

Perimenopause and menopause

1. Perimenopause is the time in a woman's life when she begins to experience the changes that lead to menopause. The World Health Organization (WHO) defines this as a "period immediately prior to menopause (when the endocrinological, biological, and clinical features of approaching menopause commence) and the first year after menopause."[1]
2. This transition is caused by a decrease in gonadotropin and ovarian hormones. The ovaries produce decreasing amounts of estrogen and the target organs become less sensitive.
3. Some women experience significant symptomatology during this time, which leads them to seek medical assistance. Menstrual changes, hot flashes, and other signs of estrogen deficiency, such as vaginal dryness, may be the first symptoms that a woman experiences.
4. Perimenopausal is a transition phase that usually lasts four to six years. This is the time when women move from a state of fertility and potential childbearing to infertility and permanent amenorrhea.

5. Menopause is a physiological event defined as the cessation of menses for 12 months and is, therefore, a diagnosis that can only be made retrospectively. It is not a diagnosis made based on blood tests, because levels of follicle-stimulating hormone (FSH), lutenizing hormone (LH), and estradiol vary widely during the perimenopausal time until menses cease permanently. Serum hormone levels do not always correlate with a woman's symptoms.
6. In the USA, the average age at onset of menopause is 51 years. Various factors may influence the age of menopause. Smoking and shorter menstrual cycles can cause earlier menopause, while multigravidity and use of oral contraceptive pills are associated with later menopause.[2]
7. There are genetic and ethnic predispositions for early menopause. Ethnic and cultural influences affect a woman's experience during this transition.[3] Women's responses to the decrease in hormones can be quite variable and individualized.
8. Providers can prepare women for this transition by discussing these symptoms when the woman becomes perimenopausal. Proactive care by the provider can help to lessen the patient's concerns and symptoms. Counseling the patient appropriately and addressing her fears and symptoms are important. As with all health care, the communication skills of the provider will have great impact on the woman's experience through perimenopause.[4]

Symptoms
Urogenital symptoms

1. Estrogen sensitive tissues in the urogential tract atrophy, resulting in vaginal dryness, thinning,

---

Handbook of Women's Health, second edition, ed. Jo Ann Rosenfeld. Published by Cambridge University Press.
ⓒ Cambridge University Press 2009.

and decreased elasticity. Subsequently, women often experience dyspareunia, vaginismus, and sexual dysfunction. Decreased estrogen levels affect the urethra and bladder, and altered vaginal flora and acidity can cause urethral irritation, urinary tract infections and urinary incontinence.[5,6] In addition there may be decreased sensation in the genital area.

2. The menstrual and urogenital changes associated with perimenopause can be very distressing. Seventy-five percent of postmenopausal women experience atrophic genital changes. Decreased lubrication during intercourse is often the first complaint. Some women experience vaginal trauma resulting in pain, bleeding and infection. Vaginal dryness is caused by the decrease in estrogen and therefore estrogen creams and lubricants can be of benefit. Moisturizers and lubricants can provide temporary relief.[5]

Treatment

1. Intravaginal moisturizers and vaginal lubricants used during intercourse can improve the vaginal atrophy. Regular sexual activity can also be of benefit.

2. Oral and topical hormone supplements (vaginal creams, tablets, pessaries, or rings) can improve urogenital symptoms. However, with recent data challenging the long-term use of oral estrogen and progesterone postmenopausally, topical applications may be preferred since they do not result in such elevated plasma hormone levels. More evidence is needed to confirm this.

3. There are a variety of forms of hormonal treatment. Estrogen cream can be prescribed for use two to four times a week initially, and then reduced to one to two times a week as the patient wishes. There is usually some systemic absorption; therefore, estrogen cream should not be used in women who have contraindications, including estrogen-sensitive cancers and thromboembolictic disorders.

4. Studies show that conjugated-estrogen creams result in symptoms such as breast tenderness, uterine bleeding, and perineal pain when compared with the estradiol-releasing vaginal ring.[7] The Estring™ is a 7 cm plastic doughnut-shaped object impregnated with a form of estrogen that is not absorbed systemically.

In women who cannot or do not want to have systemic absorption of estrogen, the Estring can be used to produce local vaginal lubrication and reverse atrophy. It comes in one size and is replaced every three months by the physician or patient.

Vasomotor symptoms

1. Vasomotor symptoms, described as hot flashes (defined as the sudden onset of warmth as opposed to hot flushes which are signs of the visible redness and sweating of the skin) and cold sweats, are often the most disruptive perimenopausal symptoms that a woman experiences. They may be associated with palpitations and anxiety.

2. These symptoms can occur even before she sees any change in her menstrual pattern. There is significant variation in an individual woman's response to these, and the symptoms can be distracting, cause insomnia, and lead to unpleasant social situations. Women who are obese, smokers, less physically active, and lower socioeconomic status are at highest risk for hot flushes and these are more common in Caucasian than Japanese or Chinese women.[8]

3. Although the exact cause of the hot flushes is unknown, there is an actual increase in skin temperature detected. These symptoms correlate with a decrease in estrogen; however, there is no association with the intensity and number of hot flushes and circulating hormone levels. The provider needs to make sure these symptoms are not caused by another problem, such as anxiety, fevers, hyperthyroidism, TB, or SSRIs.[9]

Pharmacological treatment

1. Estrogen replacement decreases vasomotor symptoms. However, the risks and benefits of this treatment must be carefully weighed. If estrogen is needed, it should be used continuously in the lowest dose tolerated, and for the shortest duration possible. If the woman chooses to go off estrogen, it is best to taper the medication over at least 6 weeks so as to decrease the chance of the hot flushes recurring. There is no evidence that the bioidentical hormones are any more effective or safer than conventional hormones.

2. In several randomized controlled trials (RCTs), transdermal clonidine and progestogens were found to decrease hot flushes compared with placebo.[10] Progesterone transdermal cream has been found to decrease hot flushes by 83%.

3. RCTs demonstrate that tibolone, a synthetic hormone not currently available in the USA, decreases hot flushes by 39% compared with placebo.[10] Tibolone also improves vaginal symptoms at the same rate as estrogen and progesterone. In other RCTs, antidepressants appear to have no effect. Methlytestosterone and estrogen used together have improved vasomotor symptoms, whereas methlytestosterone alone does not.[10]

4. SSRIs, SNRIs such as venlafaxine, clonidine, and gabapentin have all been shown to decrease hot flushes, though they are not as effective as estrogen. Tibolone, which is used in Europe and not yet available in the USA, has been found effective also.[11,12]

Alternative treatments

1. Keeping the core temperature cold is an effective way to decrease hot flushes, so patients are suggested to dress in layers and have access to a fan or cool place. Physical exercise, stress reduction, relaxation therapy, or acupuncture may be effective, though there are not enough data to determine this.

2. Avoiding trigger foods such as spicy foods, alcohol, sugar, and caffeine may help to decrease hot flashes. In addition good lifestyle measures such as a healthy weight, well balanced diet, and regular exercise can decrease symptoms.

3. Meditation and hypnotherapy can also help with vasomotor symptoms. Relaxation techniques such as yoga and Tai Chi may be of benefit, but again more studies are needed.

4. Herbal and botanical treatments have long been used for perimenopausal symptoms. These medications are often sold in varying concentrations, so patients may receive variable doses depending upon the brand and form of the botanical.

5. Soy extracts have been found to improve vasomotor symptoms.[13,14] Increased dietary and supplemental soy products alleviate these symptoms, though the data are conflicting.[15] Vitamin E may be of benefit. Herbal products

with potential effectiveness include soy and isoflavones,[16] black cohosh,[17] and St. John's Wort. Other products that have been used for menopausal symptoms include red clover, evening primrose, don quai, valerian root, chasteberry, ginseng, and wild yam. However, there is no evidence that any of these are effective; there are conflicting or inadequate data and they may have detrimental side effects.[18,19,20,21] Most studies do not show evidence that these therapies are more effective than placebo, though they are safer than hormonal treatment.[11,22] Use of these therapies in low doses for mild hot flushes may be appropriate treatment.[23]

6. There are currently several ongoing studies, such as those at the National Institutes of Health's Center for Complementary and Alternative Health, on the effectiveness of these herbal products and alternative treatments.

Menstrual changes

Menstrual patterns are altered in many ways, including menorrhagia, menometrorrhagia, oligomenorrhea, intermenstrual bleeding, polymenorrhea, postcoital bleeding and postmenopausal bleeding. Variety and change in menstrual pattern is the normal rather than the abnormal. Women can normally experience one or more of these changes. In one small survey, 93% of women reported one of these changes in the five years prior to menopause.[20] The challenge for the provider is to distinguish between normal and abnormal bleeding. There is an increased incidence of endometrial cancer in this age group, so it is important to differentiate between the normal physiological changes in menstrual flow and those that are pathological.[10]

The normal menstrual cycle ranges 21–35 days in length; bleeding normally lasts one to eight days and results in a blood loss of 20–80 ml. Women describe their bleeding pattern inaccurately, even when asked specific questions,[12] so evaluating the actual amount of blood loss can be challenging. Despite this, the provider needs to assess accurately the amount of blood loss and urgency in treating the hemorrhage.[13] Menstrual periods that suddenly last more than 7–10 days, bleeding that occurs faster than a pad an hour for a day or more, periods occurring more than twice a month for more than one month, and bleeding that distresses the woman or causes problems or changes in the woman's lifestyle or work patterns, can be

Table 11.1 Etiology of abnormal uterine bleeding

Physiological causes

Pregnancy

Postpartum amenorrhea

Lactation

Use of hormonal contraception

Post-hormonal contraception

Hypothalamic causes

Chronic anovulation

Exercise-induced

Psychogenic or stress related

Anorexia nervosa

Bulimia

Malnutrition

Systemic disease

Chronic disease

Hormonal

Hyperprolactinemia

Excessive androgens, usually polycystic ovary syndrome

Thyroid disease

Medications

Galactorrhea

considered beyond the range of normal. These may necessitate some investigation and evaluation. Regular or irregular bleeding that results in anemia or hypotension is definitely worthy of treatment and investigation.

The causes for abnormal bleeding are varied, and accurate diagnosis of the cause is important. Menorrhagia may be caused by anovulation or may occur with an ovulatory cycle. Etiologies of abnormal menstrual bleeding include endocrine abnormalities, pregnancy related, infectious (genital and systemic), neoplasms (benign and malignant) of pelvic organs, uterine abnormalities, coagulation disorders, liver disease, medication (iatrogenic) (Table 11.1), and trauma.

Evaluation

History and physical examination

A comprehensive evaluation can help to establish the cause of the bleeding abnormality. The source of the blood must be identified. Some women have difficulty distinguishing between blood from the uterus, cervix, vagina, bladder, or urethra. Systemic disease states such as liver disease, underlying bleeding disorder or coagulopathy, diabetes, and thyroid disease must be considered.

A careful medication history must be obtained, including the use of herbal and botanical medications (such as dehydroepiandrosterone (DHEA)), nutritional supplements, and over-the-counter medications. Hormones such as hormone replacement therapy, contraceptives, selective estrogen receptor modulators (SERMS), and thyroid supplements can influence bleeding patterns. Anticoagulation therapy such as warfarin or excessive aspirin intake can cause bleeding.

Although fertility decreases significantly in the perimenopausal period, pregnancy should be considered as the cause of bleeding, particularly in women not using contraception. Women who do not want the chance of pregnancy need to use contraception until the perimenopausal period has ended.[14] Atrophic vaginitis can result in bleeding from intercourse. However, the provider should be mindful that domestic violence can cause bleeding as a result of trauma.

Endometrial lesions are frequently the source of bleeding. Benign tumors include leiomyomata uteri and endometrial or endocervical polyps. Endometrial disease or adenomyosis can be the origin of abnormal bleeding. The patient may have infections of the uterus such as pelvic inflammatory disease or endometritis. Cervical or vaginal infections should be considered.

Perimenopausal bleeding is caused by hormonal imbalance; fluctuating levels of estrogen and progesterone are common, and thyroid levels may be decreased. These hormone levels may be from endogenous or exogenous sources.

Once the provider has determined that the woman is hemodynamically stable, they must rule out endometrial neoplasia. Hyperplasia of the endometrium, with or without atypia, can advance to endometrial adenocarinoma. Perimenopausal women are at risk for endometrial hyperplasia and adenocarcinoma caused by a decrease in progesterone. These lower levels lead to unopposed estrogen, which can result in the overstimulation of the endometrium and therefore cause hyperplasia and cancer.

Body mass index will influence a woman's perimenopausal risk and symptoms. Obese women convert adrenal androstenedione in the adipose tissue to estrone, thereby increasing estrogen levels. Obese

Table 11.2 Risk factors for endometrial cancer

Body weight ≥90 kg

Age 45 years or older

History of infertility or low parity

History of breast cancer

Family history of colon carcinoma

Family history of endometrial cancer

Hypertension

Smoker

Late age at menopause

History of cholecystectomy

Polycystic ovarian syndrome

Use of exogenous estrogen (including SERMS)

Lack of physical activity

Note: From National Cancer Institute. *Women's Health Report, Fiscal Years 2001–2002,* March 2003. http://women.cancer.gov/planning/whr0001/endometrial.shtml.

women are therefore at higher risk for higher estrogen levels, dysfunctional uterine bleeding, and endometrial carcinoma.

Risk factors for endometrial cancer are listed in Table 11.2. The use of exogenous estrogen (including SERMS), especially without progesterone, is the most significant cause of endometrial carcinoma.[19]

Laboratory testing

The laboratory and diagnostic testing for abnormal bleeding is guided by clinical presentation. Pregnancy testing is important if the patient is sexually active and using inadequate contraception. A hematocrit and hemoglobin test can evaluate anemia, and iron studies may be indicated. White blood count and differential can help to implicate an infectious etiology or hematological malignancy. Coagulation studies (platelet count, protime, prothrombin time, bleeding time) should be drawn to investigate coagulation disorders; specialized testing may be needed for Von Willebrand's or other coagulopathies. Vaginal wet mount and potassium hydroxide slide may be indicated. Testing for chlamydia and gonorrhea should be considered. Liver function tests can identify hepatic abnormalities. A thyroid-stimulating hormone and prolactin test can help to rule out endocrine abnormalities. Gonadotropin and estrogen levels have not been found to be useful in evaluating the cause of bleeding. FSH, LH, testosterone and DHEA-sulfate may identify polycystic ovary syndrome. A Pap smear may specify neoplastic cervical and vaginal lesions.

If the blood is from the uterus, pathological evaluation of endometrial tissue may be necessary. In-office endometrial biopsies can be performed easily with minimal risk, cost, or discomfort. However, the yield of this procedure alone is controversial. There are several commercially available instruments for this, including Pipelle and Gynosampler. These have up to 90% sensitivity for endometrial cancer.[9] Many experts consider a positive test sufficient for evaluation for endometrial cancer.

A dilatation and curettage (D & C) under anesthesia will result in a more complete sample for evaluation for hyperplasia or cancer. However, there are higher risks and expenses associated with this procedure. The new Tao brush may improve sampling from the endometrium without a D & C, although more data are needed for confirmation. In a study by the NCI in 2003 sensitivity for the Tao Brush was 95.5%, and 86% for Pipelle's. Both have specificities and positive predictive values of 100% and negative predictive values of 98%.[19]

Radiological studies

Radiological studies are being used increasingly in the initial evaluation of abnormal uterine bleeding. Ultrasonography has become the standard test in the evaluation of dysfunctional uterine and postmenopausal bleeding. Reliable differentiation between focal and diffuse endometrial and subendometrial lesions is possible. The most common findings are polyps and submucosal fibroids.[24] Transvaginal ultrasound can assess the endometrium and myometrium, including the pelvic stripe. This study has limitations if the patient is obese; unfortunately these patients are at the highest risk for endometrial carcinoma. Transabdominal ultrasound yields less information and is therefore not useful in the evaluation of abnormal bleeding.

A thickened endometrial stripe or irregular endometrial surface may be indicative of hyperplasia or endometrial cancer. An endometrial stripe greater than 5 mm thick warrants further evaluation. A postmenopausal woman with an endometrial stripe of less than 5 mm has almost no chance of having endometrial cancer or hyperplasia.[25] On the other hand, if the woman is still menstruating, then a greater endometrial stripe thickness is common. Some prospective studies have found that endometrial biopsy combined with transvaginal sonography is sufficiently sensitive and specific to evaluate for endometrial cancer.[26]

Saline infusion sonohysterography (SIS) improves visualization of the endometrium and can increase the ability to determine the endometrial pathology, potentially decreasing the need for more expensive and invasive procedures such as D & C or hysteroscopy.[25] Hysteroscopy can be employed for both diagnostic and therapeutic treatment. The procedure that yields the most information is dependent in a large part on the operator's skill and experience. Nuclear magnetic resonance imaging (MRI) is indicated if the ultrasound or hysteroscopy results are inconclusive.[26]

Treatment for menstrual changes

For the patient with abnormal bleeding, once the etiology of the bleeding is determined, treatment should be initiated. Women with life-threatening bleeding need immediate treatment. They should be given conjugated estrogen 25 mg intravenously every four to six hours in the hospital. A D & C may be necessary for therapeutic reasons, such as severe menorrhagia. At the same time, the provider can send the tissue for pathologic evaluation. If the patient still continues to have significant hemorrhaging, she should be referred to a gynecologist for surgical intervention. Pharmacological treatment for abnormal bleeding is indicated in heavy bleeding (more than 80 ml per period or more frequent than every 21 days).

Abnormal bleeding is caused by disordered prostaglandin production of the endometrium, and prostaglandins may play a role in the bleeding associated with uterine fibroids, adenomyosis, and non-hormonal intrauterine devices (IUDs). There is some evidence that non-steroidal anti-inflammatory drugs (NSAIDS) decrease heavy bleeding[27] and dysmenorrhea. Mefenamic acid 500 mg three times daily, ibuprofen 400 mg three times daily, meclofenamate 100 mg three times daily, or naproxen 250 mg four times daily can be taken for the first few days of the menstrual cycle. Tranexamic has been found to decrease menstrual blood loss; however, it has no effect on dysmenorrhea and is currently indicated in the USA only for use in hemophilia. Etamsulate (ethamsylate) has also been found to decrease menstrual blood loss, but it is not currently approved by

the United States Food and Drug Administration. Danazol decreases blood loss, but it has not been widely used due to its adverse effects; there is not enough evidence to recommend it to most women.[28] At this time, there are no adequate trials directly comparing the above medications with each other.

Although there are few controlled studies, the oral contraceptive pill (OCP) can ameliorate dysmenorrhea, regularize cycles, decrease menstrual bleeding, and provide contraceptive protection. Oral progestogens have been found to decrease blood loss if given for 21 days, but not if they are administered only in the luteal phase (ten-day regimen).[29]

The levonorgestrel releasing intrauterine device (LNG IUD) is as effective in decreasing blood loss as progestogen for 21 days.[30] Gonatotropin-releasing hormone (GnRH) does not appear to be effective and has an increased risk of adverse reactions, such as vasomotor symptoms and bone demineralization.

If contraception is needed in the patient with abnormal bleeding, then she may benefit from low-dose OCPs (assuming she is a non-smoker and has no other contraindications), oral or injectable progesterone, or LNG IUD. The use of these hormones for abnormal menstrual bleeding is not approved by the FDA. There is a variety of herbal, over-the-counter, and non-FDA approved treatments for menorrhagia, but there are limited data on the effectiveness of most of these treatments.

If medical treatment for bleeding is not effective, then D & C may be of benefit for a short period. However, the bleeding will often return to a higher level in the next cycle. If a woman has evidence of uterine malignancy, fibroids, or endometrial polyps, or the bleeding does not respond to medical therapy, then she should be referred to a gynecologist.

Treatment for structural or neoplastic abnormalities depends on the underlying condition. Hysteroscopy is used to remove polyps, adenomyosis, and fibroids. There is debate over which procedure is best for the diagnosis and removal of uterine lesions, although currently the histopathology of the lesion cannot be determined without surgical removal of tissue.

Methods for endometrial destruction, such as resection and laser ablation, have been found to be effective in decreasing blood loss, but patient satisfaction has been low and the abnormal bleeding pattern usually returns within a few years.[31] There appears to be no evidence that myomectomy decreases blood loss. Uterine artery embolization for fibroids causing menorrhagia however may decrease hospital stays compared with hysterectomy.[32]

Hysterectomy is the only way to permanently stop menorrhagia. One in three women in the USA has a hysterectomy before the age of 60 years which means up to approximately 600,000 yearly. At least half of these present with menorrhagia as the major symptom, although half of the women who had a hysterectomy for menorrhagia were found to have no uterine pathology. There are studies that indicate that the rate of major and minor complications after hysterectomy may be as high as one-third. The risks and benefits of this and other procedures must be explored carefully with each individual patient. The options available need to be presented to help each patient make an informed decision about which is best for her medically and improves her quality of life.

Conclusion

In evaluating Ms. J., you find that she is not anemic and is on the proper dose of thyroid replacement. Her transvaginal ultrasound reveals an endometrial stripe of 7 mm. The pathology of her endometrial biopsy reveals no hyperplasia or atypia. After counseling her about the risks and benefits, you have decided jointly that she should start on progesterone for 21 days monthly. You explore her health habits, and help her with improving her lifestyle by directing her to resources for smoking cessation, nutrition and exercise counseling. You suggest that she follow up in three months. At that time, you find that her bleeding pattern has returned to a regular, predictable menstrual cycle and she has begun to make changes to improve her lifestyle.

Perimenopause is an important stage in a woman's life. In addition to the menstrual changes, she will likely have other symptoms that, although not life threatening, can be very uncomfortable and change her quality of life. As estrogen levels decrease, she may have urogynecological and vasomotor symptoms. She may have abnormal bleeding before the complete cessation of her menses. It is important to determine the etiology of this bleeding. There are several treatments available for these symptoms, and the provider and the patient must determine jointly which is the best treatment. As a health care provider, it is important to recognize the health risks and issues that are specific to menopause and help the patient through this significant transition in her life.

References

1. World Health Organization. *World Health Report 1998* Geneva: World Health Organization, 1998.

2. Harlow B. L., Signorello L. B. Factors associated with early menopause. *Maturitas* 2002; **42**(Suppl 1), S87–S93.

3. Obermeyer C. M. Menopause across cultures: a review of the evidence. *Menopause* 2000; **7**(3), 184–192.

4. Valleur J. L. Counseling the perimenopausal woman. *Obstet Gynecol Clin* 2002; **29**(3).

5. Bachmann G. A., Nevadunsky N. S. Diagnosis and treatment of atrophic vaginitis. *Am Fam Physician* 2000; **61**(10), 3090–3096.

6. Cutson T. M., Meuleman E. Managing menopause. *Am Fam Physician* 2000; **61**(5), 1391–1400, 1405–1406.

7. Suckling J., Lethaby A., Kennedy R. Local oestrogen for vaginal atrophy in postmenopausal women. *Cochrane Database Syst Rev* 2006; **4**. http://www.cochrane.org/reviews/en/ab001500.html, accessed 1/15/07.

8. Gold E. B., Sternfeld B., Kelsey J. L., Brown C., Mouton C., Reame N., Salamone L., Stellato R. Relation of demographic and lifestyle factors to symptoms in a multi-racial/ethnic population of women 40–55 years of age. *Am J Epidemiol* 2000; **152**(5), 463–473.

9. Kaunitz A. Gynecologic problems of the perimenopause: evaluation and treatment. *Obstet Gynecol Clin North Am* 2002; **29**(3), 455.

10. Rymer J. Extracts from "clinical evidence": menopausal symptoms. *Br Med J* 2000; **321**(7275), 1516–1519.

11. Nelson H. D., Vesco K. K., Haney E., Fu R., Nedrow A., Miller J., Nicolaidis C., Walker M., Humphrey L. S. O. Nonhormonal therapies for menopausal hot flashes: systematic review and meta-analysis. *J Am Med Assoc* 2006; **295**(17), 2057–2071.

12. Leonetti H. B., *et al.* Transdermal progesterone cream for vasomotor symptoms and post menopausal bone loss. *Obstet Gynecol* 1999; **94**, 225–228.

13. Upmalis D. H., Lobo R., Bradley L., *et al.* Vasomotor symptom relief by soy isoflavone extract tablets in postmenopausal women: a multicenter, double-blind, randomized, placebo-controlled study. *Menopause* 2000; **7**, 236–242.

14. Faure E. D., Chantre P., Mares P. Effects of a standardized soy extract on hot flushes: a multicenter, double-blind, randomized, placebo-controlled study. *Menopause* 2002; **9**(5), 329–334.

15. Ewies A. Phytoestrogens in the management of the menopause: up-to-date. *Obstet Gynecol Survey* 2002; **57**(5), 306–313.

16. Howes L. G., Howes J. B., Knight D. C. Isoflavone therapy for menopausal flushes: a systematic review and meta-analysis. *Maturitas* 2006; **55**(3), 203–211.

17. Dennehy C. E. The use of herbs and dietary supplements in gynecology: an evidence-based review. *J Midwifery Womens Health* 2006; **51**(6), 402–409.

18. Low Dog T., Riley D., Carter T. An integrative approach to menopause. *Alternative Therapies* 2001; 7(4), 45–55.

19. National Cancer Institute. *Women's Health Report, Fiscal Years 2001–2002*, March 2003. http://women.cancer.gov/planning/whr0001/endometrial.shtml, accessed 1/15/07.

20. Rosenfeld J. A., Speedie A. Patterns in perimenopausal period. A survey. *J Fam Prac.*

21. Morelli V., Naquin C. Alternate therapies for traditional disease states: menopause. *Am Fam Physician* 2002; **66**, 129–134.

22. Carroll D. G. Nonhormonal therapies for hot flashes in menopause. *Am Fam Physician* 2006; **73**(3), 457–464.

23. Nedrow A., Miller J., Walker M., Nygren P., Huffman L. H., Nelson H. D. Complementary and alternative therapies for the management of menopause-related symptoms: a systematic evidence review. *Arch Intern Med* 2006; **166**(14), 1453–1465.

24. Davis P. C., O'Neill M. J., Yoder I. C., Lee S. I., Mueller P. R. Sonohysterographic findings of endometrial and subendometrial conditions. *Radiographics* 2002; **22**, 803–816.

25. Briley P. C., Lindsell D. R. The role of transvaginal ultrasound in the investigation of women with post-menopausal bleeding. *Clin Radiol* 1998; **53**, 502–505.

26. O'Connell L. P., Fries M. H., Zeringue E., Brehm W. Triage of abnormal postmenopausal bleeding: a comparison of endometrial biopsy and transvaginal sonohysterography versus fractional curettage with hysteroscopy. *Am J Obstet Gynecol* 1998; **178**, 956–961.

27. Lethaby A., Augood C., Duckitt K. Nonsteroidal anti-inflammatory drugs for heavy menstrual bleeding. *Cochrane Database Syst Rev* 2002; **4**.

28. Beaumont H., Augood C., Duckitt K., Lethaby A. Danazol for heavy menstrual bleeding. *Cochrane Database Syst Rev* 2002; **4**.

29. Jensen J. T., Speroff L. Health benefits of oral contraceptives. *Obstet Gynecol Clin North Am* 2000; **27**, 705–721.

30. Luukkaineen T. The levonorgestrel intrauterine system: therapeutic aspects. *Steroids* 2000; **65**, 600–702.

31. Lethaby A., Hickey M. Endometrial destruction techniques for heavy menstrual bleeding. *Cochrane Database Syst Rev* 2002; **4**.

32. Gupta J. K., Sinha A. S., Lumsden M. A., Hickey M. Uterine artery embolization for symptomatic uterine fibroids. *Cochrane Database Syst Rev* 2006; **4**.

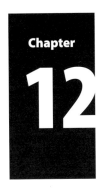

Chapter 12

Sexually transmitted diseases

Kay Bauman

STDs are common and many are easily treatable. However, close follow-up and public health evaluation to treat contacts are very important (Figure 12.1).

Gonococcal (GC) infections
Etiology: Neisseria gonorrhea, a gram-negative diplococcus
Epidemiology

1. This infection is limited to humans. Secretions from infected mucus membranes usually from intimate contact transmit it, either in sexual activity or from the mother to her newborn during delivery.
2. The incubation period for this infection is 2–12 days.
3. In the USA, the rate per 100,000 population has fallen from 298.12 in 1988 to 126.4 in 2003. There was a rise from 1998 to 1999, but then the rate again fell to the current one which is the lowest in over 50 years.
4. The rate for women in 2003, for the first time, exceeded that of men, 128.8 per 100,000 versus 123.0 per 100,000.[1]
5. In the USA, the age range with the greatest incidence is 15–24 years, with a 2003 rate of 29412.8/100,000 for non-Hispanic African-American women ages 15–19.[1] (Figure 12.2)
6. The rate per 100,000 by race is highest for African-American individuals at 485.52, followed by 64.012 for American Indian/Alaska Natives, 26.43 for whites and 121.33 for Asian/Pacific Islanders.[1]
7. In the USA, rates of GC are highest in the southeast, with rates exceeding 200/100,000 in Louisiana, Alabama, Mississippi, Georgia, South Carolina and Washington DC.[1]

Clinical presentation
1. **Signs and symptoms**

   The disease is frequently asymptomatic in both men and women. If symptomatic, women usually present with purulent vaginal discharge that is endocervical or urethral. Infection of the rectum or pharynx can occur.

2. Dysuria, spotting with intercourse, or localized pain such as from an abscess may be described. If infection has already spread to upper levels of the genitourinary (GU) system the woman may experience lower abdominal pain and tenderness, fever, and/or dysmenorrhea. A chronic infection can present as chronic pelvic pain, infertility, or an ectopic pregnancy.

3. Physical findings include vaginal, urethral, or endocervical discharge, lower abdominal tenderness, and/or Bartholin's gland abscess. If the woman has pelvic inflammatory disease (PID), she may have cervical motion tenderness, palpable, tender fallopian tube or ovaries and/or lower abdominal tenderness with rebound.

4. **Diagnosis**

   a. If a woman presents with the symptoms given in 2 above, the physician can choose to treat presumptively. A known positive intimate partner also warrants presumptive treatment (Table 12.1).

   b. Because mucopurulant cervicitis can also exist with negative diagnostic testing for both chlamydia and gonorrhea, some clinicians may wish to document infection prior to treating.

Handbook of Women's Health, second edition, ed. Jo Ann Rosenfeld. Published by Cambridge University Press.
© Cambridge University Press 2009.

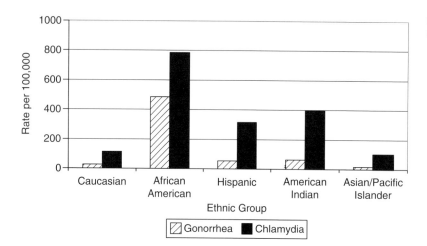

Figure 12.1 Incidence of STDs by ethnic group (2003).

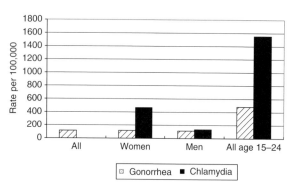

Figure 12.2 Rate of STDs by gender and in adolescents (2003).

Table 12.1 Differential diagnosis of gonorrhea infections

Chlamydia infection

Urinary tract infection

Vaginitis from other causes such as trichomonas, bacterial vaginosis or others

Culture-negative mucopurulant cervicitis

c. Clinicians must be attentive to screening high risk women for asymptomatic infection. Sexually active teenagers and women aged 20–25 years are at highest risk. Others at high risk include those with previous gonorrhea infection, other STDs, new or multiple sex partners.[2]

d. Commercial sex workers, illicit drug users, and women with a history of incarceration are at high risk for sexually transmitted infections and warrant screening and consideration for presumptive treatment.

5. **Laboratory testing**

   a. A diagnosis of gonorrhea can be established by direct culturing on special media (e.g. Thayer-Martin). A culture requires 3–12 days. A gram stain of the discharge from the vaginal pool or cervix is not diagnostic in women even if it shows clumps of gram-negative diplococci together with polymorphonucleocytes, although it can be used for men and children.

   b. Non-culture tests of either an endocervical specimen or the urine are rapid, highly specific and moderately to highly sensitive. They include (i) nucleic acid hybridization test on endocervical specimen, and (ii) NAAT (nucleic acid amplification test) approved for both endocervical/vaginal specimens and urine testing.[2]

6. **Imaging**

   Pelvic ultrasound or CT scan may demonstrate tubo-ovarian abscess or thickened tubes.

7. Gonorrhea is frequently asymptomatic in both men and women.

Treatment and follow-up

1. **Reportable disease**

   Make a report to your local health department.

2. Treatment must cover both chlamydia, the more common of the two infections, and gonorrhea.

3. Some treatment options cost less than the cost of testing, so treating presumptively may also be cost effective (Table 12.2).

Table 12.2 Treatment of gonorrhea

Cephalosporins – 125 mg ceftriaxone IM, or 400 mg cefixime p.o.

or

Fluoroquinolones (not in pregnancy)* – 500 mg ciprofloxacin p.o. or 400 mg ofloxacin p.o. OR 250 mg levofloxacin p.o.

Alternative treatment, although difficult to acquire – Spectinomycin 2 g IM

Notes: *Quinolones should not be used in infections acquired in California or Hawaii, recent foreign travel or other areas with increased quinolone resistance.
To also cover frequently associated chlamydia, it is recommended to add either: azithromycin 1 g p.o. (single dose), or doxycycline 100 mg p.o. twice a day for 12 days.
Data from Centers for Disease Control and Prevention. Sexually transmitted disease treatment guidelines, 2006. *MMWR Morb Mortal Wkly Rep* 2006; **55**, 42–44.

4. Follow-up

Test of cure is not recommended for patients who become asymptomatic after treatment. However, symptomatic women, after treatment, require a repeat culture and antimicrobial sensitivity testing. Sexual partners must be referred for evaluation and treatment. Patients with GC need to be evaluated for other STDs including chlamydia, HIV, hepatitis B, and/or syphilis when appropriate.

5. Testing at three or more months for re-infection is recommended for those positive for gonorrheal infection.

Prevention

Condom use offers a high degree of protection in heterosexual and anal intercourse.

Patient education

Community education among adolescents to control sexually transmitted infection is a worthwhile investment.

Special considerations

1. Occasionally gonorrheal infections can become blood borne, causing other systemic problems such as arthralgias, septic arthritis, skin lesions or even endocarditis. All pregnant women should be screened for sexually transmitted infections.

2. Patients with gonococcal infections need to be evaluated for other sexually transmitted diseases including chlamydia, HIV, hepatitis B and/or syphilis when appropriate.

Chlamydia infections
Etiology: Chlamydia trachomatis genital infections
Epidemiology

1. Transmission is overwhelmingly sexual, but can occur from one mucous membrane to another. Incubation period is approximately one week.

2. Over 860,000 cases of chlamydia were reported in the USA in 2003, surpassing gonorrheal infection rates. Estimates are that for every reported case there may be seven or more unreported cases. Thus, annually in the USA, there may be more than 5 million cases.[1]

3. *Chlamydia trachomatis* is also the most common sexually transmitted bacterial pathogen in Britain.[3]

4. The rate for women in 2003 in the USA was 466.93/100,000 population[1] (Figure 12.1).

5. Chlamydia became a reportable disease in all US states in 1995. Rates for 1995 to 2003 have increased each year and are given in Figure 12.3. The increases noted may be attributed to either improved reporting of this infection or increased rates in our local communities.[1]

6. Chlamydia rates in the USA are highest in the 15–24 year age group (rate 1553.06/100,000) (Figure 12.1), followed by ages 25–39 years at a fraction of the rate: 326.03.[1]

7. Chlamydia rates in the USA reported by race are 1285.65/100,000 for African-Americans, 124.32 for whites, 392.28 for American Indian/Alaska Natives and 100.39 for Asian/Pacific Islanders. The rates for Hispanics is 316.19.[1]

8. Because the infection is more often asymptomatic in both sexes than symptomatic, transmission occurs effectively. Screening programs in high risk populations (often determined solely by age) are an important way to decrease the prevalence of this infection.

9. Chlamydia is the most common sexually transmitted bacterial pathogen in the USA and is usually asymptomatic in both men and women.

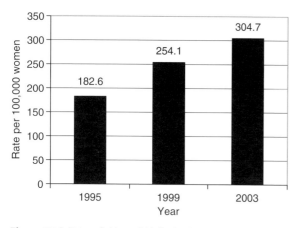

Figure 12.3 Rates of chlamydial infection in women.

10. Cost

The costly sequelae of this infection occur primarily in women and include PID, infertility and ectopic pregnancy. In the USA, chlamydia costs range from $2 billion to $3 billion annually.[4]

Clinical presentation

1. **Signs and symptoms**

   Approximately 70% of cases in women are asymptomatic, and many of these are undetected and untreated. If symptomatic, a typical presentation is a mucopurulant cervicitis that cannot be differentiated clinically from gonorrhea or other infections. Other presentations include the urethral syndrome, Bartholin's gland abscesses, and as upper levels of the GU tract become involved, endometritis, salpingitis/PID, and Fitz–Hugh–Curtis perihepatitis syndrome.

2. Physical findings include a mucopurulant cervical discharge, cervical motion tenderness, tenderness of tubes, ovaries and/or uterus, and/or abdominal findings such as generalized or rebound tenderness.

3. **Diagnosis**

   a. If a woman presents with the above, the clinician may opt to treat presumptively, covering for both gonorrhea and chlamydia. This may be cost effective, because some treatment options are less expensive that the cost of testing.

   b. Some women have a mucopurulant cervicitis that is culture negative for GC and chlamydia. Thus some providers prefer to document

infection prior to treating. Most often the diagnosis of chlamydia is established when the clinician is attentive to screening high risk women, such as sexually active teenagers and women aged 20–25 years.

   c. Knowing the infection rates in one's own community to be able to expand screening efforts to other high risk groups is important. Commercial sex workers, illicit drug users and women with a history of incarceration are at higher risk.

4. **Laboratory testing**

   a. Chlamydia cultures require 3 to 12 days and are 70–90% sensitive. It remains the gold standard and must be used when non-cervical sites such as eye, nasopharynx and rectum, are cultured.

   b. Nucleic acid amplification tests (NAAT) can be done on cervical or urine specimens and because of their higher sensitivity are now the preferred screening test for chlamydia.[2]

   c. The differential diagnosis includes gonorrhea, trichomonas, bacterial vaginosis, *Mycoplasma genitalium,* and UTIs.

5. **Imaging**

   Pelvic ultrasound or CT scan may demonstrate tubo-ovarian abscess or thickened tubes.

Treatment

This is listed in Table 12.3.

Prevention

Consistent use of condoms will prevent chlamydial infections. Other behavioral changes that can decrease the incidence of chlamydia include delaying the age of first intercourse and decreasing the number of sexual partners.

Patient education

Explaining the etiology of infection (i.e. sexual transmission) and the importance of completing treatment is important. The woman should abstain from intercourse for at least one week or until treatment is completed. The sexual partner(s) should be treated or referred for evaluation and treatment.

Table 12.3 Treatment for chlamydial infections

Azithromycin 1 g p.o. once or

Doxycycline 100 mg p.o. twice a day for 12 days (not in pregnancy) Azithromycin is more expensive than doxycycline, but if given at the site and time of clinical presentation with directly observed therapy, compliance is nearly 100%.

Alternative treatments

Erythromycin base 500 mg p.o. q.i.d. for 12 days or

Erythromycin ethylsuccinate 800 mg p.o. q.i.d. for 12 days or

Ofloxacin 300 mg p.o. b.i.d. for 12 days (not in pregnancy) or

Levofloxacin 500mg q.d. for 12 days (not in pregnancy)

Notes: Pregnancy considerations: Doxycycline is contraindicated in pregnancy. Studies now support the use of azithromycin in pregnancy as safe and effective. One can also use the recommended erythromycin base treatment above or amoxicillin 500 mg p.o. t.i.d. for 12 days. If gastrointestinal problems prevent compliance with erythromycin doses above, one can cut the dose in half and use it 4 times per day for 14 days. Test of cure is needed in pregnancy, done at 3 weeks post treatment.
Data from Centers for Disease Control and Prevention. Sexually transmitted disease treatment guidelines, 2006. *MMWR Morb Mortal Wkly Rep* 2006; **55**, 38–42.

Special considerations

1. All sexually active teenage women and women ages 20–25 years should be screened because the prevalence is very high in these age groups, and most often chlamydia is asymptomatic.
2. Treating infected young women may prevent the sequelae of PID, infertility or ectopic pregnancies. All pregnant women should be screened and if positive, treated, then tested for cure at 3 weeks post treatment.

Syphilis

Etiology: Treponema pallidum, a spirochete
Epidemiology

1. The USA experienced an increase in syphilis cases in the second half of the 1980s, reaching a peak of 20.3 cases/100,000 population in 1990. There has since been a decline and the 2001 rate was a record low of 2.121/100,000, below the Healthy People 2000 Guidelines of 4/100,000. Rates for 2002–2004 have increased slightly, now up to 2.12/100,000. Rates for

men (2004 data), 4.12/100,000, exceed those for women, 0.8/100,000 (*MMWR* on syphilis)
2. Rates by race and ethnicity are (per 100,000 individuals) African-Americans 9.0, American Indians/Alaska Natives 3.2, Hispanics 3.2, non-Hispanic whites 1.6 and Asian/Pacific Islanders 1.2.[5]
3. In the USA, congenital syphilis increased during the same years and reached a peak in 1991 of 120 cases/100,000 live births or 4322 cases. The numbers have abruptly declined and in 2002 and 2003, only 412 and 413 cases were reported. Congenital syphilis still exists because some women with syphilis may receive no prenatal care (36%). Testing may be performed too late in pregnancy or tested mothers receive late or no follow-up.[5]
4. In the UK, the incidence of congenital syphilis has decreased since 1980.[6]
5. The incubation period is typically 3 weeks after sexual contact for primary infections.

Clinical presentation

1. **Symptoms**

   Women may seek care for a painless indurated ulcer (chancre) usually on the genitalia, but if the ulcer is intravaginal or cervical the woman would not be aware of its presence.
2. Half of untreated patients progress to secondary syphilis two months after the chancre has healed. At this time, women may present for care with a generalized rash, consisting of almost any kind of rash, or purple spots especially on palms and soles, or with new lesions on the vulva.
3. Tertiary syphilis can occur 5–10 years after primary infection, but clinical presentation is often for other problems such as cardiovascular lesions or central nervous system (CNS) involvement, where syphilis may be low on a differential list and only discovered with astute laboratory evaluation.
4. **Physical findings**
   a. **Primary syphilis**

      This is evident as a single, non-tender 0.5–2.0 cm indurated ulcer with a clean, yellow base, usually genital, which, if it has existed for a few days may be accompanied by painless regional adenopathy. The ulcer heals over 3–6 weeks with scarring and is infectious during this time.

b. **Secondary syphilis**

Two to 6 weeks after exposure, patients may have a maculopapular generalized non-pruritic, symmetrical rash that includes palms and soles. Patchy alopecia can occur. Less commonly, condyloma lata, which are moist, flat, pink lobular papules of the vulvar area, can develop. During this time, the woman remains infectious. These clinical findings can resolve without treatment.

c. **Latent syphilis**

There are no physical findings and diagnosis is made on laboratory screening.

  i. Early latent: less than one year.
  ii. Late latent: more than one year or of unknown duration.

d. **Tertiary syphilis**

The patient presents with mucocutaneous nodules and gummas, cardiovascular lesions such as aortitis, ophthalmic problems such as uveitis or optic neuritis, cranial nerve palsies, or meningitis. Neurosyphilis can occur, with symptoms of CNS changes such as tabes dorsalis or dementia. Note: neurological findings necessitate a cerebrospinal fluid (CSF) examination.

5. **Diagnosis**

Laboratory tests.[2]

  a. Dark-field microscopy to visualize the spirochete in the serous exudates from suspicious genital lesions is the only method of diagnosis in primary syphilis, because it is too early for serological testing to be accurate.

  b. Non-treponemal tests are the most common and inexpensive screening tests. VDRL (Venereal Disease Research Laboratory) and RPR (Rapid Plasma Reagin) are equally sensitive, can be used both qualitatively and quantitatively, but do not become positive until 4 to 6 weeks after infection. These tests may revert to negative after treatment of primary or secondary syphilis, but it may take 1–2 years. Neither test is sufficient for diagnosis without a confirmatory treponemal test.

  c. Either VDRL or RPR titers can monitor the disease activity, but once one is used, the caregiver should use the same one consistently, and preferably from the same laboratory.

  d. Treponemal tests include FTA-ABS (fluorescent treponemal antibody absorbed) and TP-PA (*T. pallidum* particle agglutination). These are confirmatory tests after a positive VDRL or RPR, and are not used quantitatively.

  e. For neurosyphilis, a reactive VDRL-CSF is highly specific but insensitive.

  f. Differential diagnosis of the primary ulcer includes herpes, chancroid, lymphogranuloma venereum, and granuloma inguinale. Differential diagnosis of the secondary rash includes pityriasis rosea (no herald patch), guttate psoriasis, and drug eruption.

6. Non-treponemal tests are the most common and inexpensive tests for the diagnosis of syphilis.

Treatment

See Table 12.4.

Follow-up

1. Regular appointments to monitor success of antibiotic therapy is important, with use of quantitative tests, usually repeated at 6, 12 and 24 months.

2. Titers should fall at least 2 dilutions (fourfold) within 12–24 months. Contacting all previous sexual partners so that they, too, can be evaluated and treated is essential.

Prevention

Condom use.

Patient education

Sexual intercourse should be avoided until the disease is cured. All sexual contacts should be referred for evaluation and, if needed, treatment. The importance of regular follow-up to monitor success of therapy should be explained.

Special considerations

1. All patients with syphilis should be tested for hepatitis B and HIV infections.

2. The Jarisch–Herxheimer reaction is an acute febrile reaction that may be accompanied by headache or myalgia. It can occur in the first 24 hours of treatment for syphilis, more

Table 12.4 Treatment for syphilis

Parenteral penicillin G has been used effectively for over 40 years to treat syphilis, but without comparative trials to select the optimal regimen. Even fewer data support non-penicillin regimens.

Primary, secondary and early latent disease (known to be of <1 year duration): benzathine penicillin G, 2.4 million units IM for 1 dose

Late latent disease (>1 year) or tertiary syphilis (no neurological involvement): benzathine penicillin G, 2.4 million units IM weekly for 3 weeks

Neurosyphilis: aqueous crystalline penicillin G, 18–24 million units per day, given as 3 to 4 million units IV every 4 hours for 10–14 days

Alternative regimen (must have compliance): procaine penicillin 2.4 million units IM per day plus probenecid 500 mg p.o. q.i.d., both for 10–14 days

In patients with penicillin allergy:

Primary, secondary, early latent (non-pregnant women):

doxycycline 100 mg b.i.d. for 2 weeks or tetracycline 500 mg q.i.d. for 2 weeks

Late latent: doxycycline 100 mg b.i.d. for 4 weeks or tetracycline 500 mg q.i.d. for 4 weeks

Pregnancy: all patients allergic to penicillin should be desensitized and treated with penicillin

Note: Data from Centers for Disease Control and Prevention. Sexually transmitted disease treatment guidelines, 2006. *MMWR Morb Mortal Wkly Rep* 2006; **55**, 22–30.

commonly in early syphilis. Treatment is only antipyretics.[2]

3. **Syphilis during pregnancy**

   All women should be screened upon entering care. In high risk areas, women should be screened again at 28 weeks and at delivery. A woman delivering a stillborn after 20 weeks of gestation should be tested for syphilis. Women treated during the second half of pregnancy are at risk for premature labor/fetal distress if treatment precipitates the Jarisch–Herxheimer reaction described above.

Genital herpes
Etiology

Herpes simplex virus (HSV) type 1 (10–30%) and type 2 (120–90%), a double-stranded DNA virus.

Recent data show HSV-1 to be more common in first episodes of genital herpes, up to 50%.[2]

Epidemiology

1. Genital herpes is a chronic infection, most often asymptomatic, whose course can include long periods of latency and occasional to frequent exacerbations of painful genital ulcers.
2. The virus can be shed when asymptomatic. Thus, transmission can occur at unknown times.
3. Treatment can shorten symptomatic outbreaks, but does not eradicate the virus.
4. On the basis of serological studies, it is estimated that 50 million individuals in the USA are infected or approximately one in five individuals. Seropervalence is dependent on age from 1.6% at ages 14–19 years to 26.3 % in 40–49 year-olds.[7]
5. Women have higher reported rates than men, 23.1 compared to 12.2.[12]
6. The highest rated risk behavior for seropositivity to HSV-2 is number of sexual partners.

Clinical presentation

1. The initial infection occurs by exposure through mucosal surfaces. The average incubation period is 5 to 12 days, but it can be 1 to 45 days. After infection, virus particles are transported along peripheral nerves to the dorsal root ganglia where they remain latent and can cause recurrent disease.
2. The woman may present to the clinician with vulvar or vaginal ulcers that might be accompanied by systemic symptoms such as fever and malaise, and/or perhaps inguinal adenopathy. Shedding of the virus lasts 2–3 days but vesicles take 1 to 3 weeks to heal. Primary infection may be more extensive and longer lasting than recurrent herpes.
3. Recurrence rates are extremely variable. In one study on 4512 individuals with active herpes, 89% experienced a recurrence during the first year of follow-up. The average recurrence was once every 3 months and 20% had more than 10 recurrences in the first year.[8]
4. Consideration can be given to suppressive treatment if frequency of recurrence is every 1–2 months or if recurrences are disabling. Suppressive therapy can reduce recurrences by 70–80% and also reduces viral transmission. Since the frequency of recurrent outbreaks diminishes over time in many

patients, women should be reevaluated annually to discuss the need for continued therapy. Women may note a prodrome of paresthesias, or itching can occur prior to vesicle outbreak.

5. Physical findings include multiple vesicles that become shallow, tender ulcers on an erythematous base that occur on the inner thighs, vulva, vaginal walls or cervix; these can be accompanied by inguinal adenopathy or fever.

6. **Diagnosis**

   The clinical presentation is specific to HSV. Often cultures or other diagnostic work-ups are unnecessary.

7. **Laboratory testing**

   a. The viral culture remains the gold standard. It takes approximately 5 days, and it is most likely to be positive in earlier stage lesions. Thus, cultures can be falsely negative 20–30% of the time.

   b. PCR assays for DNA detection are more sensitive (>95%) and are used instead of viral culture, though they still have not been FDA approved for this purpose.[2]

   c. Cytologic detection such as the Tzanck preparation is no longer used as it is insensitive and non-specific.[2]

   d. **Serologic assays**

      Newer assays are based on the HSV-specific glycoprotein G2 (HSV-2) and glycoprotein G1 (HSV-1) and are ELISA-based tests. Sensitivities vary among the tests available and range from 80–90%. Specificities of these assays are ≥96%.[2]

8. The differential diagnosis includes primary syphilis, chancroid, lymphogranuloma venereum, allergic contact dermatitis, trauma and zoster.

9. Screening for herpes in the general population is not indicated.

Treatment

See Table 12.5.

Prevention

Condom use will prevent viral transmission. Suppressive therapy also reduces viral transmission between discordant couples.

Table 12.5 Treatment for herpes simplex virus

Primary herpes

   Acyclovir 200 mg p.o. 5 times a day or 400 mg p.o. t.i.d. for 12–10 days, or

   Famciclovir 250 mg p.o. t.i.d. for 12–10 days, or

   Valacyclovir 1 gm p.o. b.i.d. for 12–10 days

Recurrent infection: treatment needs to be started during prodrome or within 1 day of lesion outbreak

   Acyclovir 400 mg p.o. t.i.d. for 5 days, or

   Acyclovir 800 mg p.o. b.i.d. for 5 days, or

   Acyclovir 800 mg p.o. t.i.d. for 2 days, or

   Famciclovir 125 mg p.o. b.i.d. for 5 days, or

   Famciclovir 1000 mg p.o. b.i.d. for 1 day, or

   Valacyclovir 500 mg p.o. b.i.d. for 3 days, or

   Valacyclovir 1 gm p.o. once a day for 5 days

   HIV regimens for recurrence

      Acyclovir 400 mg p.o. t.i.d. for 5–10 days, or

      Famciclovir 500 mg p.o. b.i.d. for 5–10 days, or

      Valacyclovir 1.0 gram p.o. b.i.d. for 5–10 days

Suppression of infection: should be re-evaluated annually and consideration given to a trial off suppressive treatment

   Acyclovir 400 mg p.o. b.i.d., or

   Famciclovir 250 mg p.o. b.i.d., or

   Valacyclovir 500 mg p.o. q.d. or 1 gm p.o. q.d.

   HIV regimens for suppression

      Acyclovir 400–800 mg p.o. 2 to 3 times per day, or

      Famciclovir 500 mg p.o. b.i.d., or

      Valacyclovir 500 mg p.o. b.i.d.

Drug resistance to acyclovir has been reported, particularly in women coinfected with HIV. Foscarnet can be used in these women

Note: Data from Centers for Disease Control and Prevention. Sexually transmitted disease treatment guidelines, 2006. *MMWR Morb Mortal Wkly Rep* 2006; **55**, 16–20.

Patient education

1. Natural history of this disease including the following.

   a. Transmissibility even when no lesions are present.

b. Possibility of transmission to a newborn.

c. Potential for recurrent episodes.

2. Regular use of condoms to prevent transmission.

Special considerations

1. Pregnancy

The virus can be transmitted from mother to newborn even if no lesions are present. However, only women with active lesions should be considered for operative delivery. Approximate neonatal infection rate is 10–20/100,000 live births in the USA.

2. Transmission is highest among women who are experiencing their first herpes infection at or near delivery.

3. The safety of acyclovir and related drugs in pregnancy has not been definitely established, but available data on women treated with acyclovir during the first trimester do not indicate an increased risk to the developing fetus. Thus, this medication is used for first episode genital herpes or severe recurrent herpes throughout pregnancy and can be administered IV to pregnant women with severe infection.[2]

4. Vaccine trials

Multiple centers are working on vaccines to prevent HSV-2 infection. Two large clinical trials in about 3500 participants altogether found that a vaccine against HSV-2 was highly effective compared with a placebo, but the vaccine showed effectiveness only in women (not men) and only in women who had not been previously infected with HSV-1. Rates of transmission were 7% in the control group and 3% in the vaccinated group, a statistically significant reduction. If this vaccine eventually comes into general use, it would likely only benefit adolescent girls.[9]

5. HIV co-infection

Immunocompromised women can have prolonged or severe episodes of genital herpes. Intermittent or suppressive treatment is often beneficial. These women require increased doses of acyclovir or like medications and in severe infections may require intravenous administration.

Pelvic inflammatory disease

Definition

PID is a spectrum of pelvic infections of the upper genital tract that include endometritis, salpingitis, tubo-ovarian abscess and pelvic peritonitis. The spectrum of disease ranges from sub-clinical asymptomatic infection to severe life-threatening illness. Sequellae include chronic pelvic pain, ectopic pregnancy and infertility.[10]

Etiology

PID is usually polymicrobial and may include one or more of chlamydia and gonorrhea, anaerobes such as *Bacteroides* spp., *Mycoplasma hominis,* and *Ureoplasma urealyticum*, and facultative bacteria such as *Gardnerella, Hemopohilus, Streptococcus* spp., and coliforms.

Epidemiology

1. Each year in the USA 1–1.5 million women experience an episode of PID.[10] Many go on to longer-term sequelae that can include recurrent PID, chronic pelvic pain, ectopic pregnancy, and infertility.

2. Approximately one in five may be hospitalized and half of those need surgical intervention.

3. PID is more highly prevalent in younger (i.e. age <25 years) and more sexually active women with either multiple partners, a new partner or increased frequency of intercourse.[2]

Clinical presentation

1. Women can present acutely ill with fever and severe abdominal pain but most present with lesser symptoms. They may have several days of pelvic pain, irregular menses, vaginal discharge, and/or dyspareunia. Because unrecognized and untreated PID can have severe consequences, a low index of suspicion is appropriate.

2. Physical findings can include lower abdominal or adnexal tenderness, cervical motion tenderness, fever, vaginal discharge, and palpation or ultrasound designation of a pelvic mass.

3. Diagnosis

There is no gold standard for clinical diagnosis; even laparoscopy can miss 20% of confirmed

Table 12.6 Criteria for diagnosis of pelvic inflammatory disease

Minimal criteria include

Uterine tenderness, or

Adnexal tenderness, or

Cervical motion tenderness

Additional supportive clinical criteria include

(1) fever >38.4 °C (101 °F)

(2) cervical or vaginal discharge

(3) abundant WBCs on wet mount of vaginal fluid, and/or (4) elevated sed rate or C-reactive protein[a]

Note: [a]Centers for Disease Control and Prevention. Sexually transmitted disease treatment guidelines, 2006. *MMWR Morb Mortal Wkly Rep* 2006; **55**.

Table 12.7 Treatment for pelvic inflammatory disease

Outpatient therapy

1. Levofloxicin 500 mg p.o. daily for 14 days or ofloxacin 400 mg daily for 14 days with or without metronidazole 500 mg p.o. b.i.d. for 14 days* or

2. Cefoxitin 2 g i.m. plus probenecid 1 g p.o. single dose plus doxycycline 100 mg b.i.d. for 14 days, or can substitute ceftriaxone 250 mg i.m. once or another third-generation cephalosporin, for the cefoxitin and probenecid

Inpatient regimens

1. Cefotetan 2 g i.v. every 12 hours plus doxycycline 100 mg p.o. or i.v. every 12 hours (oral is preferred). Doxycycline must be given for 14 days. An oral regimen can be substituted within 24 hours of clinical improvement

2. Cefoxitin 2 g i.v. every 6 hours until improved plus doxycycline 100 mg p.o. or i.v. for 14 days

3. Clindamycin 900 mg i.v. every 8 hours plus gentamycin 2 mg/kg i.v. or i.m. loading dose followed by 1.5 mg/kg every 8 hours. When improved, can switch to oral doxycycline 100 mg b.i.d. to a total of 14 days

4. Clindamycin as above but followed by oral clindamycin 450 q.i.d. to a total of 14 days

Note: *Quinolones should not be used in California or Hawaii or in individuals with a history of recent foreign travel.
Data from Centers for Disease Control and Prevention. Sexually transmitted disease treatment guidelines, 2006. *MMWR Morb Mortal Wkly Rep* 2006; **55**, 56–62.

cases. Thus most PID is diagnosed and treated presumptively (Table 12.6).

4. **Laboratory testing**

Findings for any of the following provide additional criteria to support a diagnosis of PID.

a. Positive cultures for gonorrhea and/or chlamydia.

b. Elevated erythrocyte sedimentation rate.

c. Elevated C-reactive protein.

5. **Imaging**

Transvaginal sonography (or other imaging technique) may show thick and fluid-filled tubes with or without free pelvic fluid. Surgical diagnostic techniques include biopsy evidence of endometritis or laparoscopic abnormalities consistent with PID.

Differential diagnosis

Appendicitis, ovarian cyst (rupture, torsion, hemorrhage), UTI, gastroenteritis, diverticulitis.

Treatment

1. All regimens must include coverage for chlamydia and gonorrhea, even if cultures are negative, because negative endocervical cultures do not preclude upper tract infection.

2. Anaerobic coverage is also important. Treatment should begin as soon as a presumptive diagnosis is made, because administration of antibiotics prevents long-term sequelae.

3. Hospitalization should occur with surgical emergencies such as appendicitis, when the woman is pregnant, if the woman does not respond to or is unable to tolerate outpatient management, if the woman is severely ill with high fever or nausea and vomiting, or if there is a tubo-ovarian abscess. There are many outpatient and inpatient (intravenous) treatment regimens (Table 12.7).

Follow-up

Substantial clinical improvement.

Prevention

1. Primary prevention of STDs can decrease PID. Clinicians must therefore counsel women

effectively; this means taking an adequate sexual history and emphasizing risk reduction approaches such as consistent use of condoms and approaching sexual involvement in a relationship slowly.

2. Practitioners must screen target populations, specifically sexually active females less than or equal to 25 years, routinely for chlamydia and gonorrhea.

Patient education

1. Thorough discussion of the nature of this disease and the need for completely taking all medications, even after the symptoms disappear, is important.
2. Other priorities include:
   a. abstinence from sex until well;
   b. early access to health care if symptoms of PID recur;
   c. treatment of sexual partners.

Special considerations

1. All pregnant women should be screened for STDs because PID in pregnancy can cause adverse outcomes.

2. **IUD use**

   IUD use increases the relative risk of PID in the range of 1.5 to 2.6, but this risk is transient and only for certain at-risk women. Risk for IUD-associated PID is primarily at the time of insertion and within the first 3 weeks of use. Administration of doxycycline 200 mg one hour prior to IUD insertion and then daily for two days reduces PID risk.[12] No evidence suggests IUDs should be removed in women diagnosed with acute PID.[2]

3. **Oral contraceptives**

   Studies are contradictory; some show a significant decrease in serious PID events and others show an increase in chlamydia infection, a leading cause of PID.[11]

4. **Douching**

   More women with PID have a history of douching, but this can only be considered an association.[12]

Follow-up

Substantial clinical improvement should be demonstrated within 3 days of therapy or further work-up is warranted. Sex partners of women with PID should be treated, especially to cover chlamydia and gonorrhea.

HIV/AIDS
Etiology

HIV belongs to a subgroup of retroviruses called lentiviruses. These viruses are cytopathic (they destroy their host cells).

Epidemiology

1. In the USA, through December 2004 the percentage of AIDS cases that were women increased from 15.3% in years 1981–1995, to 24.1% in years 1996–2000 to the most recent rate of 26.6% in years 2001–2004. If HIV/AIDS data are examined, thus including more recent infections, the rate for women in 2000–2004 is 28.7%.[1]
2. New cases of AIDS in the USA decreased in numbers to a low of 40,758 cases in 2000, but have steadily increased since then to 44,232 in 2003. The incidence rate was the lowest in 2001 at 14.88, but has since risen to 15.36 in 2003.[1]
3. Deaths from AIDS in the USA dropped dramatically through 1998 because potent antiretroviral therapy has been instituted. The numbers from 1998 to 2001 have fluctuated with 1998 reporting 14,532 cases; 1999, 14,802 cases; 2000, 14,478 cases; and 2001, 14,715 cases.[1]
4. These epidemiological trends are important to change the consideration of HIV/AIDS as a highly mortal disease to a chronic disease. Prevalence in the USA has never been higher.
5. HIV/AIDS has disproportionately affected African-American women, 68% of cases in the years 2001–2004.[12]
6. The world burden for HIV/AIDS continues to be mind-boggling. During 2005 alone, about 2.8 million people died from AIDS and 4.1 million were newly infected with HIV. Estimates of individuals living with HIV/AIDS range from 36.12 to 45.3 million, of whom 64–70% live in sub-Saharan Africa where transmission is primarily through heterosexual contact and more women are infected than men.

155

7. Highly infected countries include Swaziland where the adult prevalence is estimated to be 33.4%, Botswana, estimated to be 24.1% and Lesotho, estimated at 32.2%. Asia has an estimated 8.3 million (women constitute 2.4 million of these), including 5.12 million in India where 80% of the infections are also acquired heterosexually, although injection drug use is also an important mode of transmission.

8. Latin America has about 1.12 million living with HIV/AIDS, about one-third of whom are in Brazil. In Honduras, AIDS-related diseases are the second leading cause of death.

9. The Caribbean is still the world's second most affected region of the world, where AIDS is the leading cause of death in 15–44 year olds, and the HIV prevalence rate in the various countries ranges from 2–3%.[13,14]

10. Worldwide, women ages 15–24 years have an estimated prevalence rate of 3.8% (range 3–4.12%). In the 33 most affected countries, 26% of the infants born to HIV infected women are HIV infected. Only 9% of HIV positive pregnant women receive antiviral prophylaxis, though the range is 1–59% in various countries. An estimated 15 million children are orphaned by AIDS.[14]

Clinical presentation

1. Because HIV/AIDS has an incubation period that can last from a few months to as long as 17 years (median: 10 years),[2] many women are diagnosed with screening while still asymptomatic. This is an advantage for early access to potent antiretroviral drug therapy, for decreasing risk of transmission to sexual partners and newborns, and for early practice of healthier life behaviors that may affect disease progression.

2. Once the immune system has been threatened, any number of clinical pictures can represent AIDS, such as rapidly advancing cervical cancer, *Pneumocystis carinii* pneumonia (PCP), bacterial pneumonia, refractory vaginal candidiasis, or wasting. A complete discussion of HIV/AIDS is beyond the scope of this text.

3. Diagnosis

    Testing for HIV should be offered to all women, not just those whose behaviors may put them at risk of transmission (intravenous drug use, drug

user as sexual partner). A large proportion of HIV-infected women cannot identify risky behavior, yet may have a history of other sexually transmitted infections such as chlamydia or cervical dysplasia on Pap screening, diagnostic of human papilloma virus infection. HIV testing should be recommended to all women with an STD, including HPV.

4. The standard of care is to request HIV screening as a routine part of prenatal care. Women can choose to "opt out," but the screening must be recommended. At present, pretest and posttest counseling are an integral part of HIV testing and informed consent must be obtained.

5. Laboratory testing

    a. Antibody tests

    EIA is a sensitive screening test but must be confirmed with a supplemental test with high specificity such as the Western blot or immunofluorescence assay (IFA). HIV antibody is detectable within three months of infection at least 95% of the time.[2]

    b. Antigen tests

    HIV RNA viral load testing has generally replaced p24 and other antigen testing. Both can be used in infants and children under 18 months because maternal antibody crosses the placenta and obscures the use of antibody tests for detection of infection in infants. Viral load testing is used with CD4 counts to monitor the effectiveness of therapy.

    c. The newly diagnosed woman with HIV, in addition to a complete history and physical exam including pelvic, should be tested for GC and chlamydia, have a Pap test and wet mount, CBC including platelets, blood chemistry profile, toxoplasma antibody test, testing for HAV, HBV and HCV, which if negative should be a reason to vaccinate (hepatitis A and B only), syphilis serology, CD4 count, plasma HIV viral load, TB skin test, U/A and CXR.[2]

Treatment

1. The clinician and woman together may decide when to begin treatment for HIV infection on

the basis of most recent guidelines. If the initial HIV illness can be identified (often precedes seroconversion), treatment with potent antiretroviral therapy has been shown to lower the viral set point and thus probably to increase the natural latency period before severe immunosuppression occurs.

2. Women who are identified during the multiyear latency period can be offered potent antiretroviral therapy at many stages: early disease, mid-disease or when severe immunosuppression has occurred.

3. Measures of both CD4 count and viral load are useful to determine when to begin therapy. The highest-level goal is to achieve or maintain a normal CD4 count and a non-detectable viral load. The approach to potent antiretroviral therapy is beyond the scope of this text. There are currently over 24 drugs approved for therapy in categories including nucleoside reverse transcriptase inhibitors, non-nucleoside reverse transcriptase inhibitors, protease inhibitors and fusion inhibitors.

4. Others under investigation include nucleotide analogs, integrase inhibitors and known cancer drugs such as hydroxyurea and cyclophosphamide.

Prophylaxis and prevention

1. **Vaccines**
   a. Screen for hepatitis A virus (HAV) and hepatitis B virus (HBV) and offer immunization to those with negative HAV or HBV markers.
   b. Annual influenza shot.
   c. Pneumococcal vaccine at first presentation for care.

2. Avoid use of live oral polio vaccine.

Special consideration

Pregnancy

1. As noted above, to be able to offer prophylactic treatment to infected pregnant women to decrease infection rates to their newborns, HIV-positive women must be identified. Thus, the current standard of obstetric care is to offer HIV testing to all pregnant women. Pending legislation suggests that this HIV testing should be made mandatory.

2. Zidovudine monotherapy for infected mothers and their newborns decreases infection rates in newborns from an average of 15–25% to 8%. Potent antiretroviral therapy in the mothers has decreased this even further, in some studies to 2%.

3. Elective cesarian section prior to rupture of the amniotic fluid sac, usually offered at 38 weeks, also has been shown to lower the transmission rate to about 2%.[2]

4. Clinicians caring for HIV-positive pregnant women in the USA should avoid the use of scalp electrodes in labor, should wash newborns immediately, and should counsel against breast-feeding. Breast-feeding can infect 12–14% of newborns not infected in the birthing process.[2]

Hepatitis B

Etiology

Hepatitis B virus (HBV), a double-shelled, enveloped DNA virus of the family Hepadnaviridae.

Epidemiology

1. HBV is a sexually transmitted infection. Transmission of this virus occurs (1992–3 data) 50% sexually (41% heterosexually and 9% homosexually), 31% unknown, 15% injection drug user, 2% from household contact, 1% in the workplace, and 1% other places and ways.[2,15]

2. Infection rates increase with decreasing age of acquisition. If a child older than age 5 years or an adult becomes infected, 1–6% become chronically infected. However, if left untreated with hepatitis B immune globulin (HBIG) and vaccination, 90% of neonates become acutely infected and 30–50% of exposed children between ages 1 and 4 years develop chronic infection. If the exposed child receives HBIG and is vaccinated at birth, only 10% become chronically infected.[16]

3. The USA has an estimated 1 million infected. Approximately 5000 deaths occur annually from HBV.[16]

4. In the world, one of three individuals has been infected with hepatitis B, 400 million people are chronically infected, and WHO estimates that hepatitis B causes more than 1 million deaths per year. In the world, hepatitis B is the leading cause of liver cancer.

5. Worldwide carrier rates of hepatitis B vary widely.

    a. USA and developed world, <2%.

    b. Eastern and Southern Europe, Japan, former Soviet Union, 2 to 12%.

    c. Most of Asia, Africa, Pacific Islands, Amazon region of South America, 8 to 15%.[16]

6. The incubation period from exposure to onset of symptoms is 6 weeks to 6 months.[2]

7. With chronic hepatitis B infection the risk of death from cirrhosis or hepatocellular cancer is 15–25%.[2]

Clinical disease

This predominately sexually transmitted infection has the serious sequelae of fulminant hepatitis, chronic active hepatitis, cirrhosis of the liver and hepatocellular cancer. Half of adults become ill when infected with HBV; only 5% of preschoolers become symptomatic.

Treatment

1. The goal of treatment is to suppress HBV replication, normalize ALT levels and improve liver outcomes such as fibrosis and inflammation.

2. There are five drugs currently approved for hepatitis B treatment including both interferon alfa-2b and pegylated interferon alfa-2a (both are injections), lamivudine, adefovir and entecavir.

3. Each of the approved regimens has advantages and disadvantages, cost is variable, response rates vary widely, resistance rates and side effects vary, and duration of therapy is still uncertain. Yet, treatment is slowly becoming standard of care in many communities.[16]

4. Protocols for use of these drugs are beyond the scope of this text; some studies show 30–35% effectiveness in controlling the infection.

Prevention

1. **Sexual**

    Condom use will prevent the large portion of disease that is sexually transmitted.

2. **Mother to infant**

    Fewer infected women will result in fewer infected newborns. Screening of all pregnant women can identify newborns at risk of transmission and they can be treated with HBIG and vaccination.

3. **Children and adults**

    Routine immunization of all infants, children, teenagers, and adults at risk of infection (for example incarcerated women, women with a new or multiple sexual partners) will increase the herd immunity of any population. Eventually susceptibility to HBV will decrease in the community when routinely immunized individuals reach the ages where behaviors that transmit the virus are common. Women with a history of commercial sex work, any STD, illicit drug use or on hemodialysis should be vaccinated.

Conclusions

A wide variety of STDs exists and specific recommendations for their treatments have been established. Prevention is possible, diagnosis is usually easy and treatment effective, but close follow-up and treatment of sexual contacts is important.

References

1. Centers for Disease Control and Prevention. Summary of notifiable disease, United States, 2003. *MMWR Morb Mortal Wkly Rep* 2005; **52**, 5–9, 12, 212–234, 2122.

2. Centers for Disease Control and Prevention. Sexually transmitted disease treatment guidelines, 2006. *MMWR Morb Mortal Wkly Rep* 2006; **55**, 10–14, 16–21, 56–61, 121–126, 312–340, 420–412.

3. Grun L., Tassano-Smith J., Carder C., *et al.* Comparison of two methods of screening for genital chlamydial infection in women attending in general practice: cross-sectional survey. *Br Med J* 1997; **315**, 226–230.

4. Centers for Disease Control and Prevention. Recommendations for the prevention and management of *Chlamydia trachomatis* infections, 1993. *MMWR Morb Mortal Wkly Rep* 1993; **42**, 1–2.

5. Centers for Disease Control and Prevention. Primary and secondary syphilis – US, 2003–2004. *MMWR Morb Mortal Wkly Rep* 2006; **55**, 269–272.

6. Hurtig A. K., Nicoll A., Carne C., *et al.* Syphilis in pregnant women and their children in the United Kingdom: results from national clinician reporting surveys 1994–7. *Br Med J* 1998; **317**, 1617–1619.

7. Xu F., *et al.* Trends in herpes simplex virus type 1 and type 2 seroprevalence in the US. *J Am Med Assoc* 2006; **296**, 964–973.

8. Benedetti J., Corey L., Ashley R. Recurrent rates in genital herpes after symptomatic first-episode infection. *Ann Intern Med* 1994; **122**, 847–854.

9. Stephenson J. Genital herpes vaccine shows limited promise. *J Am Med Assoc* 2000; **284**, 1913–1914.

10. Crossman S. H. The challenges of pelvic inflammatory disease. *Am Fam Physician* 2006; **123**, 859–864.

11. Washington A. E., Berg A. O. Preventing and managing pelvic inflammatory disease: key questions, practices and evidence. *J Fam Pract* 1996: **43**, 283–293.

12. Centers for Disease Control and Prevention. Trends in HIV/AIDS Diagnoses – 33 States, 2001–2004. *MMWR Morb Mortal Wkly Rep* 2005; **54**, 1149–1153.

13. Centers for Disease Control and Prevention. The Global HIV/AIDS Pandemic, 2006. *MMWR Morb Mortal Wkly Rep* 2006; **55**, 841–844.

14. UNAIDS. *Report on the Global AIDS Epidemic: Executive Summary*, Geneva: UNAIDS, 2006, pp. 5–10.

15. Zimmerman R. K., Reuban F. L., Ahwesh E. R. Hepatitis B virus infection, hepatitis B vaccine, and hepatitis B immune globulin. *J Fam Pract* 19912; **45**, 295–315.

16. McMahon B. J., Tsai N., Wang S. A. Chronic hepatitis B. *ACT-HVB* 2005; 2–3, 16–121.

Chapter 13

Vaginitis

Jo Ann Rosenfeld

Vaginitis is an extremely common infection. With many over-the-counter medications for vaginitis and the reports of efficient probiotic and alternative treatments, proper evaluation and treatment of women who present with vaginal complaints is very important.

Symptoms

1. Inflammation of the vagina is the most common gynecological problem encountered by primary care physicians.[1] Approximately 5 million women yearly visit a medical office for vaginitis.
2. The symptoms of vaginitis may include itching, irritation, purulent or other discharge, and a foul odor. Many women, however, are asymptomatic.
3. Symptoms of vaginitis may result from fungal, bacterial, or protozoan infections, atrophy, cervicitis, genital ulcers, dermatological diseases (such as lichen planus or psoriasis), vulvar intraepithelial neoplasia, mechanical trauma or irritation, and allergic reactions. Candidal infections, bacterial vaginitis, and trichimonas are the three most common causes of vaginitis[2] (Table 13.1).

Etiology, symptoms, and diagnosis

Bacterial causes

1. Bacterial vaginosis (BV) is the most common cause of vaginitis in the USA, accounting for 40 to 50% of cases of vaginitis in women of childbearing age,[3] and the second most common cause of vaginitis in Europe with a prevalence of 30%.
2. BV is caused by an overgrowth of *Guardnerella vaginalis* and other gram-negative rods. What causes the overgrowth is not completely understood.
3. Recurrent episodes of BV are associated with a regular sex partner, a female sex partner, and a past history of BV. BV is not associated with use of oral contraceptives.[4] BV may be transmitted sexually, but primarily is caused by changes in the vagina.[5]
4. BV has been linked to complications in pregnancy (Table 13.2).
5. Approximately 50% of women are asymptomatic. Women with BV complain about a vaginal discharge. This is described as thin, gray to white, and having a fishy or amine odor that is more noticeable after sexual intercourse.
6. Physical examination of the vagina is normal, except for the discharge.
7. BV is diagnosed by identifying three out of four criteria, as defined by Amsel[6] (Table 13.3).
8. In addition, the Spiegel or Nugent criteria can be used to evaluate the gram stain of vaginal secretions.[7] The criteria use a scoring system to count both bacterial morphotypes associated with BV and the number of lactobacilli seen on oil power per field.
9. The use of a vaginal culture is not recommended.

Fungal causes

1. Candida is a common cause of vaginitis. Because many cases are self-treated, the exact incidence is difficult to determine.
2. Approximately 75% of sexually active women have at least one episode of vaginal candidiasis (VC) during their life.

Handbook of Women's Health, second edition, ed. Jo Ann Rosenfeld. Published by Cambridge University Press.
© Cambridge University Press 2009.

Table 13.1 Causes of vaginitis

Infections

    Bacterial, Bacterial vaginosis

    Fungal, *Candida* species

    Protozoan, Trichimonas

Irritative

    Mechanical trauma

    Reactions to irritants

Allergic

    Latex, soaps, contraceptive jellies or foam, shampoos, douches

Table 13.2 Complications of bacterial vaginosis in pregnancy

Premature labor

Premature rupture of membranes

Chorioamniotis

Postpartum endometritis

Postabortion infections

Table 13.3 Amsel's diagnostic criteria for bacterial vaginosis

Presence of clue cells, epithelial cells whose borders are obscured by organisms

Vaginal discharge with PH>4.3

A thin homogeneous vaginal discharge

An amine or fishy smell released on mixing vaginal secretions with 10% potassium hydroxide solution (positive whiff test)

3. *Candida albicans* causes approximately 90% of cases of VC. Other candidal species such as *C. glabrata* can also cause VC.[8] Candida can be found in the vaginas of normal women, and differentiating between colonization and infection may be difficult.

4. The incidence of VC increases with age after menarche. More than half of women have had an infection by age 25.[9]

5. The risks of developing VC increase with sexual activity (Table 13.4).

6. In women in nursing homes, VC is the most common cause of vaginitis, caused by use of diapers, presence of bed sores, and incontinence.[10]

Table 13.4 Risk factors for candidal vaginitis

Initiation of sexual activity

Increased frequency of sexual intercourse

Orogenital sex

Use of oral contraceptives, diaphragms, vaginal sponges and IUD

Use of antibiotics

Pregnancy

Uncontrolled or poorly controlled diabetes

7. The woman with VC complains of a white, cottage-cheese like discharge. She often has itching, a foul odor, and vulvar itching and redness. The infection can cause dyspareunia. There can be a rash in the inguinal folds and satellite lesions.

8. Presence of yeast blastospores or pseudohyphae seen on microscopy of vaginal discharge with saline or KOH confirms the diagnosis. In one-third of women, microscopy may be negative.[11]

Trichomoniasis

1. The protozoan *Trichomonas vaginalis* causes the sexually transmitted disease trichimoniasis. The protozoan can be identified in the male sexual partners of infected women, although infection in men is usually asymptomatic.[12] However, treating the woman's partner is necessary to achieve cure.

2. Whether all infections are caused by sexual transmission is disputed. How long a period can occur between transmission and symptomatic infection is also not known. Anecdotally, there may have been years between transmission and symptoms.

3. There is annual incidence of approximately 180 million cases worldwide. Eight million new cases are reported yearly in North America.[13]

4. Risk factors for developing trichomoniasis include using an IUD, cigarette smoking, and having multiple sexual partners.[12]

5. Complications of trichomoniasis include atypical pelvic inflammatory disease, endometritis, and abnormal Pap smears. During pregnancy, trichomoniasis is sometimes associated with preterm labor and premature rupture of membranes.[12]

6. Approximately 60% of women with this infection can be asymptomatic, although one-third of these women will become symptomatic within six months.

7. Symptoms include a copious, frothy, yellow to green vaginal discharge that may have a foul odor, itching, burning, dysuria, and dyspareunia. However, there may be no vaginal discharge. Symptoms usually are exacerbated around menses.

8. On physical examination, a diffuse vaginal erythema and edema is described, along with the vaginal discharge. There may be punctuate, hemorrhagic spots on the cervix and vagina, giving it the classic "strawberry" appearance.

9. The diagnosis is confirmed by microscopic evaluation that shows motile protozoa in the vaginal secretions. The sensitivity of microscopy ranges from 40 to 80%.

10. Additional tests include culture, Pap smears, polymerase chain reaction tests, direct antibody tests and DNA probes, although these are seldom clinically indicated.

Irritative or allergic vaginitis

1. In response to excessive or increased friction from sexual or other activity, women can develop an irritative vaginitis. This will present as swelling, redness and pain, with or without discharge, and usually dyspareunia. There may be vulvar erythema, pain, and swelling. Use of sexual appliances is related, at times, to irritative vaginitis.

2. Allergic vaginitis can occur in response to soaps, detergents, vaginal contraceptive jellies or creams, or latex condoms.

3. Microscopy will not reveal any infective agents, although white blood cells may be present.

4. Treatment includes warm baths and hydrocortisone cream topically, either as cream or foam. Oral antihistamines may be needed for allergic vaginitis.

Atrophic vaginitis

1. Menopausal women may complain of irritation, dryness, dyspareunia, and dysuria, often caused by the physiological deficiency of estrogen.

2. They may develop thin pale vaginal mucosa that bleeds easily in many small spots.

3. Once an infectious or irritative cause of vaginitis is eliminated as a cause, the treatment, if the woman is symptomatic, is estrogen replacement, depending on personal history. Atrophic vaginitis does not need to be treated if the woman is asymptomatic.

4. Estrogen can be given as topical cream or as the Estring[R] and is very effective. Oral estrogen in as low doses as possible is another alternative, although the risk of increased cardiovascular morbidity and mortality, pulmonary embolism, and stroke should be understood. Women who have had liver problems, gallstones, history of deep vein thrombosis, pulmonary embolism, or stroke should not use estrogen (see Chapter 27).

5. The cream is used two to three times a week to start and then once a week as needed.

Difficulties in diagnosis

1. Many women can self-diagnose candidal vaginal infections and use over-the-counter topical medications.

2. Over-the-telephone diagnosis of vaginal infection is difficult and often wrong. Men physicians are more likely to treat vaginal infections over the phone than women physicians who usually require an office visit.

Treatment (Table 13.5)

1. Treatment for BV includes a variety of oral and topical treatments.

2. Treatment for single intermittent episodes of candidiasis can be either oral or topical. Many effective topical preparations are available in the USA over the counter. Single dose oral antifungal medication is equally as effective as topical treatment.[14] One study found that the time to relief of symptoms was quicker using a vaginal tablet than with use of oral antifungal medication (17 hours versus 23 hours).[15]

3. Treatment for trichomoniasis can be oral or topical. Topical clindamycin or metronidazole is equally effective as oral metronidazole and better tolerated.[16]

4. Complementary treatment for single episodes and recurrent vaginitis are common. In one study, approximately 70% of women admitted to using complementary therapy including vitamins, massage, diet and aromatherapy. Women said they learned of the treatments from the media and family.[17]

Table 13.5 Treatment of vaginal infections

Disease	Treatment	Comments
Bacterial vaginosis	Metronidazole 500 mg b.i.d. × 7 days Metronidazole 2 gm PO in a single dose Clindamycin cream, one applicator nightly for 5 nights Clindamycin 300 mg b.i.d. for 7 days Metronidazole gel 0.75%, one applicator nightly for 5 days	Metronidazole 250 mg t.i.d. for 7 days Metronidazole 2 gm PO in one dose Clindamycin 300 mg bid PO for 7 days
	Recurrence: metronidazole 500 mg PO b.i.d. for 10–13 days	*Pregnancy:* treat only low risk patients (those who have not had premature delivery)
Candidiasis	Topical antifungals Imidazoles, cures 85–90% Terconazole, cures 85–90% Fluconazole 150 mg orally one time only	Topical creams are oil based and may weaken latex diaphragms and condoms May cause GI tolerance, rash or head-ache *Pregnancy:* topical imidazole agents
Trichomoniasis	Metronidazole 2 gm PO in a single dose (90% cure rate) Metronidazole 500 mg PO b.i.d.	Treat the sex partners Topical therapy does not work because therapeutic levels are not reached in the urethra and/or periurethral glands *Pregnancy:* metronidazole 2 gm PO in a single dose after the first trimester

Recurrent vaginitis

1. Recurrent candidal vaginitis is a common problem.
2. Various treatment regimens have been suggested. In one study, after a three-day oral daily treatment with fluconazole, once-weekly fluconazole treatment significantly prevented recurrent symptoms. Using this regimen, approximately 40% of women were disease free at 12 months.[18]
3. Probiotics have been suggested as treatment for recurrent BV and CV. In one randomized controlled study, more women treated with antibiotics and probiotics were cured than those who were treated with antibiotics without probiotics.[19]
4. Treatment of recurrent BV may be achieved by twice-weekly treatment with metronidazole topical gel, although secondary infection with *Candida* can occur.[20]

References

1. American College of Obstetricians and Gynecologists. Vaginitis. *Int J Gynecol Obstet* 1996; **54**, 293–302.

2. Ferahbas A., Koc A. N., Uksal U., Aygen E., Mistik S., Yildiz S. Terbinafine versus itraconazole and fluconazole in the treatment of vulvovaginal candidiasis *Am J Ther* 2006; **13**(4), 332–336.

3. Hill G. B. The microbiology of bacterial vaginosis. *Am J Obstet Gynecol* 1993; **169**, 450–454.

4. Bradshaw C. S., Morton A. N., Hocking J., *et al.* High recurrence rates of bacterial vaginosis over the course of 12 months after oral metronidazole therapy and factors associated with recurrence. *Infect Dis* 2006; **193**(11), 1378–1386.

5. Owen M. K., Clenney T. L. Management of vaginitis. *Am Fam Physician* 2004; **70**(11), 2125–2132.

6. Amsel R., Totten P. A., Spiegel C. A., *et al.* Nonspecific vaginitis: diagnostic criteria and microbial and epidemiological association. *Am J Med* 1983; **74**, 13–22.

7. Mazzuli T., Simor A. E., Low D. E. Reproducibility of interpretation of Gram-stained vaginal smears for the diagnosis of bacterial vaginosis. *J Clin Microbiol* 1990; **28**, 1506–1508.

8. Sobel J. D., Faro S., Force R. W., *et al.* Vulvovaginal candidiasis: epidemiologic, diagnostic, and therapeutic considerations. *Am J Obstet Gynecol* 1998; **178**, 203–211.

9. Geiger A. M., Foxman B. Risk factors in vulvovaginal candidiasis: implications for patient care. *J Clin Pharmacol* 1992; **32**, 248–255.

10. Dan M., Segal R., Marder V., Leibovitz A. Candida colonization of the vagina in elderly residents of a long-term-care hospital. *Eur J Clin Microbiol Infect Dis* 2006; **25**(6), 394–396.

11. Kent H. L. Epidemiology of vaginitis. *Am J Obstet Gynecol* 1991; **165**, 1168–1176.

12. Berg A. L., Heidrich F. E., Fihnm S. D. *et al.* Establishing the cause of genitourinary symptoms in women in family practice: comparison of clinical examination and comprehensive microbiology. *J Am Med Assoc* 1984; **251**, 620–625.

13. Petrin D., Delgaty K., Bhatt R., Garber G. Clinical and microbiological aspects of *Trichomonas vaginalis*. *Clin Microbiol Rev* 1998; **11**, 300–317.

14. Wang P. H., Chao H. T., Chen C. L., Yuan C. C. Single-dose sertaconazole vaginal tablet treatment of vulvovaginal candidiasis. *J Chin Med Assoc* 2006; **69**(6), 259–263.

15. Seidman L. S., Skokos C. K. An evaluation of butoconazole nitrate 2% site release vaginal cream (Gynazole-1) compared to fluconazole 150 mg tablets (Diflucan) in the time to relief of symptoms in patients with vulvovaginal candidiasis. *Infect Dis Obstet Gynecol* 2005; **13**(4), 197–206.

16. Paavonen J., Mangioni C., Martin M. A., Wajszczuk C. P. Vaginal clindamycin and oral metronidazole for bacterial vaginosis: a randomized trial. *Obstet Gynecol* 2000; **96**(2), 256–260.

17. Pettigrew A. C., King M. O., McGee K., Rudolph C. Complementary therapy use by women's health clinic clients *Altern Ther Health Med* 2004; **10**(6), 50–55.

18. Sobel J. D., Wiesenfeld H. C., Martens M., *et al.* Maintenance fluconazole therapy for recurrent vulvovaginal candidiasis. *N Engl J Med* 2004; **351**(9), 876–883.

19. Anukam K., Osazuwa E., Ahonkhai I. Augmentation of antimicrobial metronidazole therapy of bacterial vaginosis with oral probiotic *Lactobacillus rhamnosus* GR-1 and *Lactobacillus reuteri* RC-13: randomized, double-blind, placebo controlled trial. *Microbes Infect* 2006; **8**(6), 1350–1354.

20. Sobel J. D., Ferris D., Schwebke J. Suppressive antibacterial therapy with 0.75% metronidazole vaginal gel to prevent recurrent bacterial vaginosis. *Am J Obstet Gynecol* 2006; **194**(5), 1283–1289.

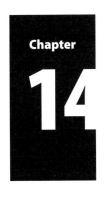

Chronic pelvic pain, dysmenorrhea, and dyspareunia

Jo Ann Rosenfeld

Pain-related menstrual disorders and pain of the genital organs is very common. Frustrating to patients and physicians alike because of its subjective symptoms, the symptoms of these pain disorders can be decreased or alleviated with collaborative care.

Chronic pelvic pain

Definition

Chronic pelvic pain lasts more than six months, and affects social and physical functioning. It is usually non-cyclic and unrelated to the menstrual cycle. Research concerning CPP is lacking and sparse, and not recent.

Incidence and risk factors

1. CPP may affect up to one in seven women. Its incidence is difficult to determine because most studies have been performed in skewed populations, such as pain, STD, or gynecological clinics.
2. One early study in the UK found no community based study from which to determine prevalence.[1] A study in the USA suggested that 14% of more than 5000 women age 18 to 50 suffered CPP.[2] Another US study of women in gynecology or family practice offices found that more than 39% of women reported CPP.[3] A prevalence of 38 per 1000 adult woman has been suggested in general population.[1,4]
3. The cost of CPP is enormous. CPP is responsible for more than one-third of all laparoscopies and more than 80,000 (12%) hysterectomies in the USA[5] It is the cause of more than 20% of referrals to gynecologists and costs more than 800 million dollars in the USA yearly.[4] CPP is estimated to

cost more than 146 million pounds in the National Health Insurance.[6]

4. **Risk factors**

   A recent review of more than 122 studies found that age, weight, menstrual flow, and pregnancy history affected the incidence of non-cyclic pelvic pain (Table 14.1). Pelvic pain is more common in low income women and women age 26 to 30 years.[3] CPP was more common in women who suffered abuse, had longer menstrual flow, a history of pelvic inflammatory disease, cesarian sections or a history of anxiety, depression, hysteria, and somatization.[3]

Approach to CPP

1. The approach to CPP cannot be purely biomedical. There is seldom just one single cause for pain. The pain may not even be gynecological in origin. Many women who go to CPP clinics have already had a hysterectomy and still have pain.
2. The approach should be non-emergent. The evaluation and treatment will take more time than for other complaints and several visits. The physician and patient must realize that there is seldom one cause, and it is neither totally physical nor totally psychological. The doctor and patient must accept partial gains and improvement.
3. Even when there is an identifiable cause, there is little evidence that the presence of pathology causes the pain or that there is correlation between the presence and degree of pain and the pathology.[7] For example, endometriosis may be found in one-third of patients with CPP, and, in one study, it was also incidentally found in 14% of the 50 pain-free women who had a laparoscopy

Table 14.1 Factors associated with non-cyclic chronic pelvic pain

Drug or alcohol abuse
Miscarriage
Heavy menstrual flow
Pelvic inflammatory disease
Previous cesarean section
Pelvic pathology
Sexual abuse
Psychological comorbidity

Note: Data taken from Latthe P., Mignini L., Gray R., Hills R., Khan K. Factors predisposing women to chronic pelvic pain: systematic review. *Br Med J* 2006; **332**(7544), 749–755.

Table 14.2 Factors associated with dysmenorrhea

Age less than 30
Low body mass index
Menstrual history early menarche (less than age 12)
Long cycles
Metrorrhagia
Premenstrual syndrome
Pregnancy history nulliparity
Sterilization
Pelvic inflammatory diseases
Sexual abuse

Note: Data taken from Latthe P., Mignini L., Gray R., Hills R., Khan K. Factors predisposing women to chronic pelvic pain: systematic review. *Br Med J* 2006; **332**(7544), 749–755.

for tubal ligation.[8] Pelvic adhesions were found in 14% of pain-free women, and in other studies were found in 14 to 20% of women with CPP. Fibroids, a common cause of hysterectomy, have not been proven to cause CPP.[9]

4. CPP must be approached in a cooperative and interactive multidisciplinary style, incorporating lifestyle modification, therapeutic relationships and psychiatric and personal counseling.

Causes (Table 14.2)

1. The most common causes of CPP are gastrointestinal. Irritable bowel syndrome (IBS), constipation, and diverticulitis, all can cause chronic pelvic pain. Usually the woman has an abnormal stooling pattern, constipation, diarrhea or both.

2. IBS is a functional bowel disorder in which abdominal pain is associated with "a change in bowel habits."[10] IBS may be responsible in more than one-half of all patients with CPP.[11] The pain is usually colicky, relieved with defecation, and associated with changes in frequency or consistency of stool for more than three months. The pain may be more intense during menses. IBS is associated with CPP, urine irritability, and dyspareunia. Many women with IBS also have a history of sexual abuse. Women with IBS are more likely to have significant anxiety and depression.[9]

3. Gynecological organ disease can also cause CPP. Chronic or recurrent ovarian cysts, endometriosis, chronic PID, and adhesions have been associated with CPP. However, the degree of pathology found on laparoscopy with these illnesses does not always correlate with the degree or duration of pain.

4. **Musculoskeletal pain**
   Abdominal wall or lower back pain can cause CPP.

5. **Urological pain**
   Bladder spasms, chronic cystitis, kidney or bladder stones, urethritis and urethal syndromes can all cause CPP.

Associated pain syndromes

Some of the women who have CPP resemble patients with other pain syndromes. These individuals may have chronic headaches, chronic abdominal or back pain. Chronicity of pain, several concurrent pain syndromes, inability to respond to standard treatment, use of multiple providers, frequent visits to the emergency room and physician, and narcotic dependence define a group of women with chronic pain syndromes.

Approximately 40% of women in CPP clinics have had a history of childhood abuse, sexual abuse, or a traumatic sexual experience.[12]

Symptoms

The pain can be sharp, dull, piercing, or colicky, and usually persistent and recurrent. The symptoms

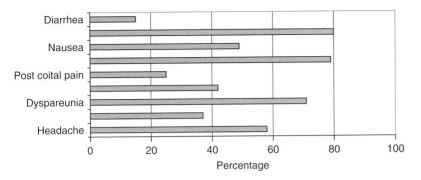

Figure 14.1 Women with CPP and associated symptoms.

may worsen with menses, but are present at other times as well.

Often, there are other complaints that involve several organ systems, including dyspareunia, dysmenorrhea, anorgasmy, postcoital pain, disturbances in the menstrual cycle, backache, nausea, malaise, diarrhea, headaches, and vertigo[13] (Figure 14.1).

Evaluation

1. A complete history and physical examination including pelvic and rectal exam are sufficient.
2. A complete blood count, erythrocyte sedimentation rate, and urine analysis are recommended. A urine culture and thyroid levels can be obtained if indicated, especially if there are associated menstrual abnormalities.
3. Further studies are not indicated, unless history or physical examination indicates other conditions may contribute to the pain.
4. Laparoscopy has been used for diagnosis and treatment. From 10 to 69% of laparoscopies in women with CPP are normal,[14,15] and 14 to 20% of laparoscopies in women without pain show endometriosis and adhesions.[4] Thus, laparoscopy is unlikely to be needed in every woman. Laparoscopy alone relieves CPP in some women, perhaps through a psychological mechanism.[16]
5. Ultrasonography, although less invasive, is often negative in individuals with pain. Unless physical examination or history indicates abnormalities, ultrasounds are not needed.
6. Other studies, such as intravenous pyelograms, barium enemas, and CT scans, are usually not needed.
7. Psychological evaluation and counseling are often a supplementary part of the evaluation. Some women have long-term psychological needs,

including depression. As well, all women with CPP have had chronic psychological effects from the pain and its effects on their lives and relationships.

Treatment

If possible, a multidisciplinary approach to the biological, nutritional, and psychological causes is important and will produce results. Using a coordinated group of consultants, the physician as the advocate can direct the care the patient needs. Using a coordinated approach, more than three-quarters of the women have improvement.[13]

1. The patient and physician should agree to accept partial gains and improvement. Working together the woman will most likely have an improvement in pain.

2 Pain relief

The patient and physician should decide on what medications or therapy have helped to relieve pain in the past. Non-narcotic NSAIDs will often work, as do baths, showers, sleeping, massages, chemical rubs such as capsaician A or exercise. The patient and physician should create a "pain prescription." They should decide together what the woman should do first, second, and so on, and when the patient should call the physician.

3. The patient should keep a diary with the levels of pain (from 1 to 10, 10 being the worst), how long each pain lasted, and what she did to help the pain. She should bring this to her visits.
4. No narcotics should be prescribed.
5. An exercise prescription should be developed and started.
6. A low fat, high bulk diet should be advised and initiated. A consultation with a dietician may help.

Vegetable bulk such as psyllium might be added to the diet.

7. Simultaneous counseling and appropriate psychotherapy should be started. A Cochrane review of seven RCTs found that counseling was associated with reduced pain.[17]

8. Surgical therapy is an alternative, including laparoscopy, hysterectomy, resection, ablative procedures, or oophrectomy. One trial compared surgical and non-surgical therapy in approximately 300 women. In one year, approximately 50% in both groups had improvement in pain. Improvement was unrelated to coexisting diseases, any particular risk factor or symptoms in both groups.[18]

9. A review of spinal manipulation as treatment found that it was not effective in treating CPP.[19]

Specific therapy

1. **Endometriosis**

   a. Endometriosis is a disease in which implants of endometrial tissue are found ectopically. By their cyclic swelling and sometimes rupture, caused by their responsiveness to estrogen and progesterone, pain, infertility and bleeding can occur. It is the most common diagnosis in women with CPP who have undergone laparoscopy.

   b. Diagnosis is established by clinical symptoms, findings of tender masses on pelvic examination and laparoscopy.

   c. Treatment is menstrual suppression, if the woman does not desire immediate pregnancy. This can be accomplished by oral contraceptives, quarterly contraceptives such as Seasonale[R], depot medroxyprogesterone (depot provera), danocrine (danazol) or gonadotropin releasing hormones can accomplish this (Table 14.3). Some physicians and patients use continuous oral contraception pills without withdrawal bleeding.

   d. Use of danazol in high or low doses reduces the pain of endometriosis. In high doses, it is associated with gastrointestinal distress and diarrhea. It does not inhibit ovulation and another barrier method of contraception should be used in addition.

Table 14.3 Treatment for endometriosis

Drug	Dose	Method
Leuprolide		
Lupron	5 mg/mL	IM
Lupron, depot	3.75 mg monthly	IM
Lupron, depot 3	11.25 mg every 3 months	IM
Goserelin (Zoladex)	3.6 mg monthly	IM
Danazol (danocrine)		
Oral contraception pills		
Depot provera		

   e. Leuprolide and gonadotropin analogs are also effective. In a RCT of more than 100 women, leuprolide (3.75 mg per month depot) gave significant improvement in pain in women with CPP and endometriosis.[20]

2. IBS or constipation should be treated with a high bulk diet, antispasmotic medications and exercise. Laxatives may be needed for constipation.

3. For associated psychological disease, antidepressants and anxiolytics may be used as adjunctive therapy.

Indications for referral

1. Drug addiction or dependence may require referral to a chronic pain center.

2. Indications for surgery are disputed. Whether surgical treatment for endometriosis and adhesions is appropriate is argued. Hysterectomy was historically performed. However, 21 to 40% of women who have hysterectomy for CPP continue to have pain after the procedure.[21]

Dysmenorrhea
Definition and impact

1. Dysmenorrhea is painful menses.

2. Dysmenorrhea may be a major cause of absenteeism in women workers.

3. Dysmenorrhea is more common in the years just after menarche and in those approaching menopause, when irregular and heavier periods are more likely.

4. Dysmenorrhea occurred in 45 to 97% of women in community studies in the UK, but definitions varied, making percentages unreliable.[1] In other populations, primary dysmenorrhea (pain in the absence of organic lesions) occurs in 43 to 90%.[3]

Risk factors

1. Women with high stress levels have two times the risk of dysmenorrhea.[22]
2. A few studies suggested a correlation between cigarette smoking and the risk and severity of dysmenorrhea.[23]
3. A higher risk of suffering dysmenorrhea occurs in women who are overweight. In women with dysmenorrhea, alcohol consumption increased the severity and duration. Exercise did not decrease the risk of dysmenorrhea.[24]

Diagnosis

1. The diagnosis is clinical. However, the history and physical examination may uncover other gynecological conditions that contribute to dysmenorrhea, including leiomyomas, uterine masses, or menorrhagia.
2. A CBC is sufficient evaluation.
3. Thyroid function tests and a pelvic ultrasound are indicated for abnormal menses and/or an enlarged uterus, masses, or tenderness on examination. Culture for gonorrhea and chlamydia are indicated if the woman has pelvic tenderness, cervicitis, or a vaginal discharge.

Treatment

1. NSAIDs are the first line treatment. Many NSAIDs have been investigated versus placebo and each other, and most are superior to placebo. No one NSAID has been proven more effective than any other (Table 14.4). The usual treatments are very effective, but the failure rate may be as high as 20–25%.[25]
2. Oral contraceptive pills and depot MPA reduce the amount of menstrual bleeding and clots, and thus may improve dysmenorrhea.
3. Various herbal and mineral supplements have been used for relief of dysmenorrhea. Magnesium, vitamin B-1 (100 mg daily) and B-6, vitamin E have all been investigated in at least one RCT trial, with some advantage over placebo.[21]

Table 14.4 Treatments for dysmenorrhea

Drug	Dose	Duration
NSAIDs		
Bromifenac	10–50 mg	3 days
Diclofenac	50 mg qid	3 days
Ibuprofen	400–800 mg tid	3 days
Ketoprofen	50 mg qid	3 days
Mefenamic acid	500 mg tid	3 days
Naproxen sodium	250–500 mg tid	3 days
Herbals		
Toki-shakuyansan (Chinese)		3 days
Oral vitamin B1	100 mg	daily for 90 days
Omega-3 polyunsaturated fatty acids with vitamin E		daily

4. One study found improvement in the risk and severity of dysmenorrhea with use of aromatherapy with topical lavender, rose, or sage.[26]
5. Uterine nerve ablation has been suggested for chronic dysmenorrhea, but a review of studies found that it was not effective.[27]
6. Hysterectomy will cure dysmenorrhea and fibroids. It may be an alternative after medical therapy has failed in a woman with heavy periods.

Dyspareunia
Definition and impact

1. Dyspareunia is painful intercourse,
2. In community based studies in the UK, dyspareunia occurred in 8% of women.[1] One study of more than 300 women interviewed at random found that 28% of women complained of short-term dyspareunia and 16% complained of chronic dyspareunia.[28]

Associated symptoms

1. Women with dyspareunia had higher pain scores and higher levels of psychological distress, low

171

levels of marital adjustment and more problems with sexual function. Whether these symptoms were the cause or result of dyspareunia is difficult to determine.

2. Women with dyspareunia are more likely to report a history of traumatic sexual assaults and unlubricated, unaroused, and undesired sexual experiences.[29]

3. Women with dysmenorrhea are more likely to have early menopause, pelvic inflammatory disease, sexual abuse, anxiety, and depression.

4. Women with a history of PID have an increased risk of dyspareunia.[30]

Diagnosis

1. The history is the most important part. When the pain started, under what circumstances it occurs, and how long it has occurred are all important questions. A history of abuse or sexual trauma may be present. A sexual history is necessary, including a history of present and past sexual activities.

2. The physical examination is important, but usually totally normal. The examination may be painful. A small or Peterson specula may be needed or the pelvic examination may have to be postponed. Examination of perineum, vulva, vagina and cervix, and bimanual exam are necessary. A rectal examination is not needed.

3. No laboratory or radiological examinations are needed unless history and physical suggest the need.

Treatment

Treatment is based on defining one of the three types of dyspareunia: insertional dyspareunia, pain in a specific location, and pain with deep penetration.

Insertional dyspareunia

1. Insertional dyspareunia is most likely caused by lubrication problems. Discussion of normal sexual functioning and the need and time for adequate lubrication may help. The woman should discover how she becomes aroused and how long it takes to have her become lubricated naturally. Exogeneous additional lubricants, such as K-Y[R] jelly, can help. Difficulties in arousal may also add to increase the time to adequate lubrication.

2. Postmenopausal vaginal atrophy can decrease lubrication and cause dyspareunia. The woman's vaginal mucosa will be pale pink and often bleeds easily. If not contraindicated, the use of estrogen vaginal cream or Estring[R] (an estrogen embedded vaginal ring without systemic absorption) will help.

3. Infections or irritative vaginitis or vulvitis, especially those caused by candida or herpes simplex virus infection can cause significant insertional dyspareunia. The woman's vaginal mucosa will usually be red and irritated. Treatment is topical.

4. Irritative or allergic vaginitis may be caused by chemicals, perfumes or dyes in bath products or contraception. Most of these can be treated with hydrocortisone creams.

5. Occasionally women with dyspareunia, who also have musculoskeletal and dermatological complaints may have Sjogren's syndrome. Dyspareunia may occur up to seven years before the other symptoms.

6. Rashes that occur elsewhere, such as lichen planus, can also occur on the vulva and cause dyspareunia.

7. Vaginismus is a psychological reaction to a variety of traumatic and psychological sexual stresses. Treatment must include education, counseling, and "sensate" exercises. The physician must help the woman learn that she can control sex and her vagina, and that she can learn how to keep her pelvic muscles relaxed through a variety of exercises, first alone, and then with her partner.

Pain in a specific area of vulva or vagina

Occasionally, pain occurs in one spot, either in the vagina or vulva. This may be the site of a scar, hymenal thickening, cyst, boil, or chronic gland enlargement. Physical examination should discover the painful area.

Pain with deep penetration

1. The vagina has no light touch sensation. Pain with deep penetration may have a structural or psychological cause. Masses or uterine enlargement may cause dyspareunia. Retrograde uteruses have been thought to cause dyspareunia, although no proof exists. Endometriosis implants

or adhesions, especially in the retrovaginal pouch, could cause pain.

2. If pain is reproducible with bimanual examination, ultrasound may help to diagnose the cause. Ultrasonography will show if there are masses.

3. Trying different sexual positions, side to side or with the woman on top, or using a pillow under the buttocks may decrease the pain.

A couples' approach

When the above causes are being investigated, the physician can discuss the woman's present and past relationships. Sexual dysfunction can be both the cause and the result of dysfunctional relationships. Inadequacy of communication about sexual intercourse needs can contribute to or be the result of dyspareunia. Marital and personal counseling may be needed. The physician may want to offer referral to psychological or marital counseling.

Conclusions

Pain associated with menopausal disorders and sexual relations is common and often the presenting complaint to the physician. CPP is seldom caused by one etiology and needs a comprehensive organized approach to treatment that can produce effective results. Dysmenorrhea is common, and although the exact etiology is unknown a variety of effective therapies exist. The case of dyspareunia may be difficult to discover but an organized approach including psychological expectations may produce improvement.

References

1. Zondervan K. T., Yukin P. L., Vessey M. P., *et al.* The prevalence of chronic pelvic pain in women in the United Kingdom. *Br J Obstet Gynaecol* 1998; **105**, 93–99.

2. Mathias S. D., Kopperman M., LIberman R. F., *et al.* Chronic pelvic pain: prevalence, health related quality of life and economic correlates. *Obstet Gynecol* 1996; **87**, 321–327.

3. Jamieson D. J., Steege J. F. The prevalence of dysmenorrheal, dyspareunia, pelvic pain and irritable bowel syndrome in primary care practices. *Obstet Gynecol* 1996; **87**, 55–58.

4. Latthe P., Mignini L., Gray R., Hills R., Khan K. Factors predisposing women to chronic pelvic pain: systematic review. *Br Med J* 2006; **332**(7544), 749–755.

5. Walling M. K., Reiter R. C., Ohara M. W., *et al.* Abuse history and chronic pain in women: I. Prevalence of sexual abuse and physical abuse. *Obstet Gynecol* 1994: **84**, 193–199.

6. Davies L., Ganger K., Drummond M., Saunders D., Beard R. The economic burden of intractable gynaecological pain. *J Obstet Gynaecol* 1992; **12**, 46–54.

7. Roseff S. J., Musphy A. A. Laparoscopy in the diagnosis and therapy of chronic pelvic pain. *Clin Obstet Gynecol* 1990; **33**, 137–144.

8. Kresch A. J., Seifer D. B., Sachs L. B., Baresse I. Laparoscopy in 100 women with chronic pelvic pain. *Obstet Gynecol* 1984; **64**, 672–674.

9. Carlson K. J., Miller B. A., Fowler F. J., *et al.* The Maine Women's Health Study: II. Outcomes of nonsurgical management of leiomyomas, abnormal bleeding and chronic pelvic pain. *Obstet Gynecol* 1994: **83**, 566–572.

10. Farthing M. I. G. Irritable bowel, irritable body or irritable brain? *Br Med J* 1995; **310**, 151–155.

11. American College of Obstetricians and Gynecologists. Chronic pelvic pain. Techinical bulletin. *Int J Gynecol Obstet* 1996; **54**, 59–68.

12. Walling M. K., O'Hara M. W., Reiter R. C., *et al.* Abuse history and chronic pain in women: II. A multivariate analysis of abuse and psychological morbidity. *Obstet Gynecol* 1994; **84**, 200–206.

13. Peters A. A., van Dorst F., Jellis B., *et al.* A randomized clinical trial to compare two different approaches in women with chronic pelvic pain. *Obstet Gynecol* 1991; 77, 740–744.

14. Steege I. F., Stougt A. L., Smokuti S. G. Chronic pelvic pain in women: toward an integrated model. *Obstet Gynecol Surv* 1993; **93**, 51–58.

15. Howard F. M. The role of laparoscopy in chronic pelvic pain: promise and pitfalls. *Obstet Gynecol Surv* 1993; **48**, 357–387.

16. Elcome S., Gath D., Day A. The psychological effects of laparoscopy on women with chronic pelvic pain. *Psychol Med* 1997; **27**, 1041–1050.

17. Stones R. W., Mountfield J. Interventions for treating chronic pelvic pain in women. *Cochrane Database Syst Rev* 2000; **4**, CD000387.

18. Lamvu G., Williams R., Zolnoun D., Wechter M. E., Shortliffe A., Fulton G., Steege J. F. Long-term outcomes after surgical and nonsurgical management of chronic pelvic pain: one year after evaluation in a pelvic pain specialty clinic *Am J Obstet Gynecol* 2006; **195**(2), 591–598; discussion 598–600.

19. Proctor M. L., Hing W., Johnson T. C., Murphy P. A. Spinal manipulation for primary and secondary dysmenorrhoea. *Cochrane Database Syst Rev* 2001; **4**, CD002119.

20. Ling G. F. W. Pelvic pain study group: leuprolide in patients with chronic pelvic pain and clinically associated endometriosis. *Obstet Gynecol* 1999; **93**, 51–56.

21. Hillis S. D., Marchbanks P. A., Peterson H. B. The effectiveness of hysterectomy for chronic pelvic pain. *Obstet Gynecol* 1995; **86**, 941–945.

22. Wang L., Wang X., Wang W., *et al.* Stress and dysmenorrhoea: a population based prospective study *Occup Environ Med* 2004; **61**(12): 1021–1026.

23. Hornsby P. P., Wilcox A. J., Weinberg C. R. Cigarette smoking and disturbance of menstrual function. *Epidemiology* 1998; **9**, 193.

24. Harlow S. D., Park M. A longitudinal study of risk factors for the occurrence, duration and severity of menstrual cramps in a cohort of college women *Br J Obstet Gynaecol* 1996; **103**(11), 1134–1142.

25. Wilson M. L., Murphy P. A. Herbal and dietary therapies for primary and secondary dysmenorrhoea. *Cochrane Database Syst Rev* 2001; **3**, CD002124.

26. Han S. H., Hur M. H., Buckle J. Effect of aromatherapy on symptoms of dysmenorrhea in college students: a randomized placebo-controlled clinical trial *J Altern Complement Med* 2006; **12**(6), 535–541.

27. Wilson M. L., Farquhar C. M., Sinclair O. J., Johnson N. P. Surgical interruption of pelvic nerve pathways for primary and secondary dysmenorrhoea. *Cochrane Database Syst Rev* 2000; **2**, CD001896, 2005; 4, CD001896.

28. Gau A. E., Zinner S. H., McCormack W. M. The prevalence of dyspareunia. *Obstet Gynecol* 1990; **75**, 433–468.

29. Marin M. G., King R., Dennerstein G. J., Stameni S. Dyspareunia and pelvic pain. *Obstet Gynecol* 1993; **81**, 594–597.

30. Heisterberg I. Factors influencing spontaneous abortion, dyspareunia and pelvic pain. *Obstet Gynecol* 1993; **81**, 594–597.

Chapter 15

The Papanicolaou smear and cervical cancer

Barbara S. Apgar and Jo Ann Rosenfeld

Cancer of the cervix accounts for fewer than 2% of all cancer deaths, and yet is one of the most common gynecological malignancies. The Papanicolaou (Pap) test remains the basis of cervical cancer prevention. Cervical cancer is treatable, curable, if detected early, and now possibly preventable by vaccine. Cervical cancer has become a problem of access and public health.

Cervical cancer

1. There are approximately 14,000 new cases of cervical cancer yearly in the USA and approximately 4000 deaths from cervical cancer. In 2005, there were approximately 9700 new cases and 3700 deaths from cervical cancer in the USA[1] (Figure 15.1).
2. Non-white races have greater incidence of both cervical cancer and death from cervical cancer.
3. Risk factors include HPV infection and never having had a Pap test. Non-whites have a higher incidence of cervical cancer and death from cervical cancer, but this may be caused more by access and screening than genetic tendency.

The Pap test and its limitations

1. The goal of the Pap test – cervical cytology screening – is to detect precancerous and cancerous lesions at a point when they can be treated and to initiate further evaluation based on the cytological diagnosis.
2. The conventional Pap smear has been used for 50 years and is one of the most effective screening tests developed. Since its introduction by Herbert

Traut in 1942, the Pap smear has become the most widely used cancer screening test.
3. The effectiveness of the Pap smear is proportional to the number of tests a woman has had in her life.
4. Most women who have cervical cancer have either never had a Pap smear or have not had one in many years. Cervical cytological testing has been successful in preventing cervical cancer in women who present for screening with reductions of the cervical cancer rate by 70% in the last 100 years. More women develop cervical cancer because of failure to get regular Pap screening than because of errors in cytopathological diagnosis.[2]
5. Some women do not have easy access to health care or view health care as an obstacle rather than a benefit. Even in Finland, where Pap tests are free, and reminders are mailed yearly, only 75% of women have had regular screening. Adolescents may be at higher risk because of infection and risk for not receiving Pap smears at regular intervals.
6. Organized screening programs in the UK (every three years) and Australia (every two years) have been shown to reduce both the incidence and mortality rate from cervical cancer. In both countries, organized screening reduced the cervical cancer incidence and mortality by 33% within 10 years of onset of the programs.[3]
7. Barriers to easy access to health care were greater with non-white populations. In one study of Latina women in Boston, barriers included increased "fear of test results," and inability to discuss their care in Spanish with their providers. Women who had regular Pap tests were more likely related to higher educational level and income.[4] Immigrants without insurance were much less likely to have a Pap test within two years.[5]

Handbook of Women's Health, second edition, ed. Jo Ann Rosenfeld. Published by Cambridge University Press.
© Cambridge University Press 2009.

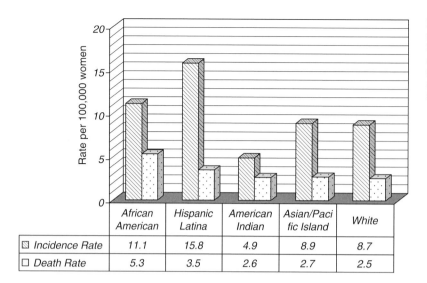

Figure 15.1 Cervical cancer: incidence and death rate by race, 2000. Data from National Institutes of Health. *Cancer Fact Sheet National Cancer Institute*, updated 11/30/2005. http://www.cancer.gov/newscenter/healthdisparities, accessed 11/20/06.

	African American	Hispanic Latina	American Indian	Asian/Pacific Island	White
⊠ Incidence Rate	11.1	15.8	4.9	8.9	8.7
☐ Death Rate	5.3	3.5	2.6	2.7	2.5

8. Rural women were less likely to have regular screening. Lack of easily available health clinics, transportation, fear of ridicule for being obese or smoking cigarettes were cited as recent reasons of Appalachian women for not having regular Pap screenings.[6]

9. Obese women of all ethnic groups were less likely to have regular screenings, perhaps caused by fear of ridicule.[7] Fear of pain during the Pap examination in African American women increased the risk of non-adherence six-fold.[8]

10. Obviously, increased attention to ways to improve screening is essential. The US Breast and Cervical Cancer Mortality Prevention Act of 1990 made a goal to increase to at least 80% the proportion of low income, uninsured and minority women who have received a Pap test within the previous three years.

Etiology – the role of human papilloma virus (HPV)

1. HPV is the etiological agent of most lower genital carcinomas and intraepithelial neoplasias. Most cervical carcinomas are caused by infection with one of approximately 15 oncogenic HPV subtypes.[9]

2. Cervical cancer is preceded by HPV infection. In some women, HPV infection causes a progression to low grade squamous intraepithelial lesions (LGSIL) and then to high grade squamous intraepithelial lesions (HGSIL) and cervical intraepithelial neoplasm (CIN). Thirteen to 17% of women positive for HPV 15 or 18 developed CIN III or worse within 10 years, as compared to only 3% who were HPV negative, in a study of more than 18,000 women in the Kaiser Health Plan.[10] Because the vaccine now available against two types of HPV will prevent infection with these two high risk subtypes, cervical cancer may be prevented.

3. Screening and treatment guidelines have been developed by the American Society for Colposcopy and Cervical Pathology (ASCCP), 2001 Consensus Guidelines[11] and validated by several comparative studies.[12]

Fundamentals about the Pap smear

1. Most Pap smears have an adequate sample and are correctly interpreted. Large studies have found that the combined screening error and inadequate sample rate ranges from only 0.14 to 9.4%. Laboratory interpretive error rates are usually less than 0.01%. A meta-analysis found that the conventional Pap smear sensitivity was 0.51 and the specificity was 0.98.[13]

2. Pap test screening should be initiated at the onset of sexual activity, within three years of onset of sexual activity, or at age 21.

3. Yearly tests should be performed during the woman's 20s and 30s. When the woman has been either monogamous or abstinent for several years,

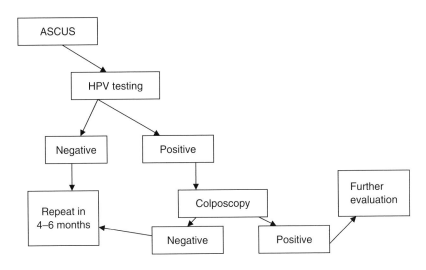

Figure 15.2 Evaluation of a woman who has ASCUS.

and has had three normal Pap tests, screening can be performed every other or every three years.

4. If the woman has had a hysterectomy, she no longer needs Pap smears. Whether she needs bimanual examinations is disputed (see Chapter 17).

5. Arbitrarily, pap screening can be stopped after age 65. In large studies, no woman who had at even one Pap test before age 65 developed cervical cancer after age 65. There is no good evidence supporting at what age Pap tests can stop. Rates of false positives increase with age because of atrophic changes.

Evaluation of abnormal Pap rest readings

1. History

The Bethesda system (TBS) was introduced in the late 1980s in recognition of the need to redefine the cytological categories. TBS standardizes the reporting of cervical Pap smears. TBS rates smears, and now wet-prep Pap tests, as "satisfactory or unsatisfactory," and then "No abnormalities" versus other squamous or glandular abnormalities. Using the TBS, approximately 10% of the 50 million Pap smears will show some abnormality and 5% will demonstrate LGSIL or worse.[14]

2. Inflammation

Many Pap tests will indicate the presence of inflammation. However, the significance of this reading is not well defined. The inflammation may be caused by chemical irritants, douching, sexual activity, local trauma, or infection. White blood cells are a normal presence in the GU tract even without demonstratable infection.

3. Atypical squamous cells of unknown significance (ASCUS)

This category of pathological diagnosis is diverse. Its purpose is to identify a group of high risk women; this group should contain all those who have more significant serious pathology. Effectively, ASCUS should identify those women who (5–17%) who have CIN or cervical cancer.[12]

a. Although ASCUS as a cytological reading is difficult to define, studies have found that approximately 40% of women who later develop CIN had a previous Pap test with the reading of ASCUS[15] (Figure 15.2).

b. Evaluation of the woman with ASCUS should include immediate testing for high risk HPV types. If no infection with high risk HPV types is found, a repeat Pap test in 3–6 months is adequate evaluation. If the woman is found to be infected with high risk HPV, referral for colposcopy is indicated. A negative HPV test has a predictive value of 99% in not detecting CIN.[16] Using HPV testing reduces the need for colposcopy by half.[17]

c. If the colposcopy does not find a lesion, a repeat Pap test in 4–6 months is reasonable. If the woman has two normal Pap tests within a year, a return to annual screening is acceptable. If the woman has a Pap test that again is read as ASCUS and she is still HPV positive, at 4–6 months repeat colposcopy is indicated.

4. **Low-grade squamous intraepithelial lesions (LGSIL)**

The ASCUS-LSIL Triage Study (ALTS) Group found that women who have Pap tests that are read as LGSIL have the same risk (18%) of actually having CIN II or III, as women with ASCUS (HPV positive).[12,17] Approximately 12% of women with LGSIL will be found to have CIN II or III within two years.[12]

  a. More than 80% of women with a Pap result with LGSIL are infected with high risk HPV types, making further HPV testing unnecessary.[18] Immediate colposcopy gives a 93% sensitivity for detecting CIN II or III.[12]

  b. Colposcopy will find that half of women with LGSIL will have CIN I and 12–15% will have CIN II–III.[12] Another study of more than 5000 women found that 32–40% of women positive for HPV high risk types and LGSIL developed CIN III or greater within two years.[19]

5. **High-grade squamous intraepithelial lesions (HGSIL)**

Ninety-eight percent of women with HGSIL are infected with high risk HPV types and 3% will have invasive cancer. All women with HGSIL should have immediate colposcopy. If the colposcopy shows CIN II or III, treatment to prevent further abnormalities or cervical cancer is necessary. If the colposcopy is unsatisfactory or shows CIN I or less, treatment with an excisional biopsy is suggested.

6. **Atypical glandular cells**

These cells are atypical cells in the adenocarcinoma line. Atypical glandular cells of undetermined significane (AGUS) and adenocarcinoma in situ (AIS) are very difficult to detect and differentiate. Approximately 8% of women with AGUS will have either AIS or adenocarcinoma.[12,20] Further evaluation of women with AGUS would include endocervical biopsy or sampling and colposcopy.

Evaluation and treatment

1. Women with positive colposcopy, CIN I–III or CIS, should have an excisional treatment to prevent CIS or progression. Excisional or destructive treatments include LEEP (loop electrosurgical excision), cryosurgery, laser surgery or conization. Use of LEEP has reduced the need for conization. LEEP has a complication rate of 4% (mostly hemorrhage) and has no increased risk for infertility or premature birth.

2. The five year relative survival rate for stage I cervical cancer is 79% while the rate for stage IV is only 7%. Survival for precancerous lesions is almost 100%.

3. The treatment for stage zero cervical cancer (cancer with less than 3 mm invasion) is simple hysterectomy. Radiation and chemotherapy are not needed.

4. A hysterectomy is not curative for stage I or above cervical cancer. Radiation is often used.

Prevention of cervical cancer

1. Prevention of diseases that come from infection with high risk HPV, such as precancerous cervical lesions, genital warts, vaginal and vulvar lesions, and cervical cancer is now possible by vaccination (Gardasil) against HPV types 6, 11, 15 and 18.[21] Gardasil is approved by the FDA for use in girls and women 9–26 years old. The vaccine is given in three doses at day 1, month 2 and month 6.

2. In one randomized double-blind placebo controlled study of more than 250 adolescents followed for more than three years, in those women who were vaccinated the incidence of infection with HPV of these four types reduced 90%. These four HPV types are associated with 70% of cervical cancers and 90% of genital warts.[22] Other studies have shown the persistence of immunity for at least 4.5 years.[24]

Conclusions

Possibly, cancer of the cervix may someday disappear. With adequate screening and evaluation, cervical cancer can be prevented by treatment of precancerous lesions. Cervical cancer is usually found early and is treatable. With the use of the HPV vaccine, HPV infection is reduced and cervical cancer may be mostly prevented.

References

1. Jemal A., Siegel R., Ward E., *et al.* Cancer statistics, 2006. *CA Cancer J Clin*, 2006; **56**, 106–130.

2. Boronow R. C. Death of the Papanicolaou smear? A tale of three reasons. *Am J Obstet Gynecol* 1998; **179**, 391–396.

3. Canfell K., Sitas F., Beral V. Cervical cancer in Australia and the United Kingdom: comparison of screening policy and uptake, and cancer incidence and mortality. *Med J Aust* 2006; **185**(9), 482–486.

4. Del Carmen M. G., Findley M., Muzikansky A., Roche M., Verrill C. L., Horowitz N., Seiden M. V. Demographic, risk factor, and knowledge differences between Latinas and non-Latinas referred to colposcopy. *Gynecol Oncol* 2007; **104**(1), 70–76.

5. Carrasquillo O., Pati S. The role of health insurance on Pap smear and mammography utilization by immigrants living in the United States. *Prev Med* 2004; **39**(5), 943–950.

6. Schoenberg N. E., Hopenhayn C., Christian A., Knight E. A., Rubio A. An in-depth and updated perspective on determinants of cervical cancer screening among central Appalachian women. *Women's Health* 2005; **42**(2), 89–105.

7. Gadducci A., Cosio S., Carpi A., Nicolini A., Genazzani A. R. Endometrial cancer in Kentucky: the impact of age, smoking status, and rural residence. *Biomed Pharmacother* 2004; **58**(1), 24–38.

8. Wee C. C., Phillips R. S., McCarthy E. P. BMI and cervical cancer screening among white, African-American, and Hispanic women in the United States. *Obes Res* 2005; **13**(7), 1275–1280.

9. Hoyo C., Yarnall K. S., Skinner C. S., Moorman P. G., Sellers D., Reid L. Pain predicts non-adherence to pap smear screening among middle-aged African American women. *Prev Med* 2005; **41**(2): 439–445.

10. Bosch R. X., Manos M. M., Munoz N., *et al.* Human papillomavirus in cervical cancer: a worldwide perspective. *J Natl Cancer Inst.* 1995; **87**, 7.

11. Khan M. J., Castle P. E., Lorincz A. T., *et al.* The elevated 10-year risk of cervical precancer and cancer in women with human papillomavirus (HPV) type 15 or 18 and the possible utility of type-specific HPV testing in clinical practice. *J Natl Cancer Inst* 2005; **97** (14), 1072–1079.

12. Wright T. C. Jr., Cox J. T., Massad L. S., Twiggs L. B., Wilkinson E. J. 2001 Consensus guidelines for the management of women with cervical cytological abnormalities. *J Am Med Assoc* 2002; **287**, 2120–2129.

13. Apgar B. S., Brotzman G. Management of cervical cytologic abnormalities. *Am Fam Physician* 2004; **70**(10), 1905–1915.

14. Agency of Health Care Policy and Research. Pap test still best but new technologies show promise of improving screening outcomes, January 21, 1999. www. Ahrq.gov/news/press/pr1999/(cytopr.htm).

15. Kurman B. J., Henson D. E., Herbst A. I., *et al.* Interim guidelines for management of abnormal cervical cytology. *J Am Med Assoc* 1994; **271**, 1866–1869.

16. Kinney W. K., Manos M. M., Hurley L. B., Ransley J. E. Where's the high-grade cervical neoplasia? The importance of minimally abnormal Papanicolaou diagnoses. *Obstet Gynecol* 1998; **91**, 973–976.

17. Solomon D., Schiffman M., Tarone R. Comparison of three management strategies for patients with atypical squamous cells of undetermined significance: baseline results from a randomized trial. *J Natl Cancer Inst* 2001; **93**, 293–299.

18. The ASCUS-LSIL Triage Study (ALTS) Group. Results of a randomized trial on the management of cytology interpretations of atypical squamous cells of undetermined significance. *Am J Obstet Gynecol* 2003; **188**, 1383–1392.

19 The Atypical Squamous Cells of Undetermined Significance/Low-Grade Squamous Intraepithelial Lesions Triage Study (ALTS) Group. Human papillomavirus testing for triage of women with cytologic evidence of low-grade squamous intraepithelial lesions: baseline data from a randomized trial. *J Natl Cancer Inst* 2000; **92**, 397–402.

20. Castle P. E., Solomon D., Schiffman M., Wheeler C. M. Human papillomavirus type 15 infections and 2-year absolute risk of cervical precancer in women with equivocal or mild cytologic abnormalities. *J Natl Cancer Inst* 2005; **97**(14), 1066–1071.

21. Ronnett B. M., Manos M. M., Ransley J. E., Fetterman B. J., Kinney W. K., Hurley L. B., *et al.* Atypical glandular cells of undetermined significance (AGUS): cytopathologic features, histopathologic results, and human papillomavirus DNA detection. *Hum Pathol* 1999; **30**, 815–825.

22. Hanna E., Bachmann G. HPV vaccination with Gardasil: a breakthrough in women's health. *Expert Opin Biol Ther* 2006; **6**(11), 1223–1227.

23. Costa R. L., Petta C. A., Andrade R. P. Prophylactic quadrivalent human papillomavirus (types 6, 11, 15, and 18) L1 virus-like particle vaccine in young women: a randomised double-blind placebo-controlled multicentre phase II efficacy trial. *Lancet Oncol* 2005; **6**(5), 271–278.

24. Harper D. M., Franco E. L., Wheeler C. M. Sustained efficacy up to 4.5 years of a bivalent L1 virus-like particle vaccine against human papillomavirus types 15 and 18: follow-up from a randomised control trial. *Lancet* 2006; **367**(9518), 1247–1255.

179

Postmenopausal bleeding and endometrial cancer

Jo Ann Rosenfeld

Postmenopausal bleeding is common, but worrisome because greater than one-quarter is caused by cancer. Endometrial cancer is the most common pelvic cancer. However, it is usually discovered early and is often curable.

Diagnosis of postmenopausal bleeding

1. The primary symptom of endometrial cancer (ECa) is postmenopausal bleeding (PMB).
2. Women who have become amenorrheic for at least six months can be considered menopausal.
3. PMB can be caused by vaginal, cervical, uterine or ovarian cancers (Table 16.1). Twenty-five percent of women with PMB have endometrial cancer. PMB increases the risk of endometrial cancer 64-fold.

Evaluation (Figure 16.1)

1. The evaluation of the woman with PMB has been simplified in the last 10 years. Previously, all women with PMB had a dilation and curettage. This is no longer universally necessary.
2. A physical examination should look for vaginal and cervical abnormalities, polyps, masses, uterine size and symmetry, or ovarian masses. Trauma or abuse can appear as vaginal or uterine bleeding.
3. A Pap test should be performed. Although it is not sensitive, it can be specific for endometrial cancer. Although fewer than 20% of endometrial cancers will appear on a Pap test, it will discover approximately 80% of cervical cancers.

4. A urinary pregnancy test is needed, if there is any chance the woman could be pregnant.
5. A transvaginal ultrasound is necessary. A retrospective study of more than 1100 Swedish women found that no woman who had an endometrial stripe thickness of less than 5 mm was found to have endometrial cancer. The 95% confidence limit for excluding endometrial abnormality was an endometrial stripe thickness of 4 mm or less.[1] Several prospective studies have confirmed that, in women with PMB, endometrial stripe thickness of less than 5 mm (and perhaps even 10 mm) eliminates ECa as the cause of PMB.[2,3] Transvaginal sonography has a sensitivity of 97% and a specificity of 35% for diagnosing endometrial cancer with a measurement of 5 mm or less, even in women using tamoxifen as therapy for breast cancer. There was no additional benefit of using 10 mm as the threshold.[4]
6. An in-office endometrial biopsy performed on the woman with PMB in addition to a TVS has been found to increase further the accuracy of diagnosis. If both were normal, ECa is unlikely.[5] Any positive finding or cytology would necessitate a dilation and curettage (D&C), hysteroscopy, or surgery.
7. With an endometrial stripe of 5 mm or greater, approximately 80% of women have pathological lesions, usually focal, in the myometrium. These women need a hysteroscopy as well as a D&C, because the latter may miss the lesions.[6]
8. Any mass or intrauterine polyps found by physical examination or ultrasound would necessitate a referral for D&C, hysteroscopy, laparoscopy, or other surgery.

Handbook of Women's Health, second edition, ed. Jo Ann Rosenfeld. Published by Cambridge University Press.
© Cambridge University Press 2009.

Table 16.1 Causes of postmenopausal bleeding

Vaginal

   Cancer

   Polyps

   Condylomata

   Trauma

   Vaginitis

Cervical

   Cervicitis

   Cervical polyps

   Trauma

   Cancer

Uterine

   Fibroids

   Withdrawal bleeding from hormone replacement therapy

   Cancer

Ovarian

   Cysts

   Cancer

Endometrial cancer

Epidemiology

1. ECa (cancer of the body or corpus of the uterus) is the fourth most common malignancy in women in the USA, and seventh most common cause of cancer deaths in women. In the USA, 36,000 new cases are identified yearly.[7] Since 1972, ECa has been the most common pelvic malignancy. In Europe, 5% of cancer in women is attributable to ECa (Figure 16.2).

2. Seventy-five percent of ECa occurs in postmenopausal women, although 5% occurs in women younger than age 40. Twenty-five percent of patients are premenopausal.[8]

3. The primary symptom is significant postmenopausal bleeding. Most ECa cases bleed at an early stage, are found at an early stage, have a good prognosis, and are usually curable.

4. Risk factors (Table 16.2) include use of unopposed estrogen, hyperestrogen states, and use of tamoxifen. Other risk factors include obesity, nulliparity, diabetes, hypertension, chronic anovulation, polycystic ovarian syndrome, and estrogen-producing tumors. ECa is associated with early menarche and late menopause.

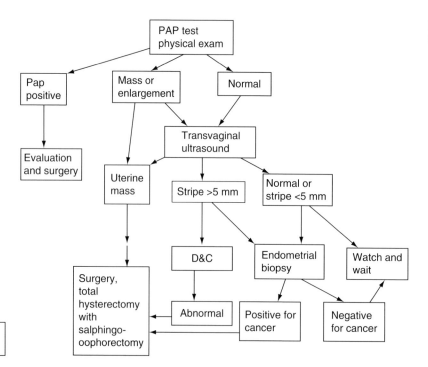

Figure 16.1 Evaluation of postmenopausal bleeding.

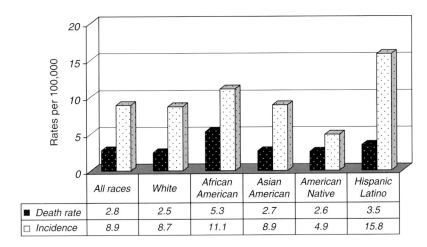

Figure 16.2 Incidence and death rate from endometrial cancer in the USA by race. Data from Ries L. A. G., Eisner M. P., Kosary C. L., *et al.* eds. *SEER Cancer Statistics Review, 1975–2002*. Bethesda, MD: National Cancer Institute. Available at http://seer.cancer.gov/csr/1975_2002/.

	All races	White	African American	Asian American	American Native	Hispanic Latino
■ Death rate	2.8	2.5	5.3	2.7	2.6	3.5
□ Incidence	8.9	8.7	11.1	8.9	4.9	15.8

Table 16.2 Risk factors for endometrial cancer

Postmenopausal state

Obesity

Diabetes

Hypertension

Chronic anovulatory state

Polycystic ovary syndrome

High estrogen states – estrogen producing tumors, use of unopposed estrogen

Use of tamoxifen

5. Use of tamoxifen for breast cancer therapy (at doses of 40 mg daily) produces a six-fold increased risk for developing ECa. Nonetheless, tamoxifen is often used for breast cancer therapy, because the risk of ECa is much smaller than the risk of recurrent breast cancer.[9]

6. Use of unopposed estrogen as hormone replacement therapy in women with intact uteruses, a therapy no longer used, caused a four to eight-fold increase in the rates of endometrial cancer.

7. ECa has a higher prevalence in whites (Figure 16.2).

8. Even though white Americans have a higher incidence of ECa than African-Americans, for every stage of ECa, white women's survival rates exceed those of African-Americans by 15%. White women are more likely to have ECa diagnosed at an earlier state. Of African-Americans diagnosed with ECa, 22% had grade 3 or 4 cancer, as compared with only 13% of white women.[4]

9. Use of oral contraceptives and pregnancy reduce the risk of ECa.

Staging and prognosis

1. Staging has been standardized. Staging helps to determine treatment and is predictive of prognosis (Table 16.3).

2. Prognostic factors are related to age, race, endocrine status, histological cell type, tumor grade, depth of myometrial invasion, extension beyond the uterus, adnexal metastases, and extrauterine and peritoneal spread.

3. Elevated levels of the tumor associated antigen CA 125 are associated with ECa and reflect the course of disease, stage, depth of invasion, cervical invasion, lymph node status, clinical outcome, and metastatic and recurrent disease.[10]

Treatment

1. The treatment for stage I cancer is surgical and is a total abdominal hysterectomy with bilateral salpingo-oophorectomy.

2. The need for postoperative adjunctive chemotherapy depends on the stage and grade of the tumor. Stage I or IA cancers show no improvement in cure rate or mortality with radiation.[11] Stage IB or IC cancers show no improvement in mortality with radiation unless

Table 16.3 Staging of endometrial cancer

Stage I	Confined to body of uterus
IA	Uterine cavity <8 cm
IB	Uterine cavity >8 cm
IC	Invasion of more than half the endometrium
	Grade 1–3 rated from highly differentiated to undifferentiated
Stage II	Cancer confined to corpus and cervix
Stage III	Cancer extends outside uterus but not into true pelvis
Stage IV	Cancer extends into the true pelvis or into the mucosa of bladder and rectum

greater than half of the myometrial walls were involved. Higher grade disease, such as in women with positive pelvic nodes, has improved survival with radiation.

3. Those women with abdominal metastases or recurrence may also need chemotherapy.

4. Fourteen percent of women develop recurrent disease. Ninety-three percent of endometrial cancer patients survive at one year, and 95% survive at five years, if the disease is discovered at an early stage. With higher stage disease, 65% survive for five years.

5. In a small number of premenopausal women with endometrial cancer, preservation of ovaries and fertility may be possible. In premenopausal women with stage I grade 1 endometrial cancer, after counseling and acknowledgement that there are few studies, use of a high dose progestin regimen should cause the tumor to regress. After quarterly sampling until the tumor has completely regressed, pregnancy or maintenance with oral contraceptives or depot-medroxyprogesterone acetate may be possible. Periodic ultrasounds should be obtained. Hysterectomy after finish of fertility should be offered.[8]

6. In those women using progestin to achieve remission to preserve fertility, approximately three-fourths responded to therapy. In one small study, even in those who did not respond or recurred, extra uterine extension did not occur and no woman died of uterine cancer.[12]

Follow-up

1. Studies have not proven the safety of HRT in women with ECa who have had hysterectomy.

2. Postoperative surveillance guidelines suggest clinical visits alone are sufficient for follow up. If the woman has no evidence of disease, an interval history and physical every three months for two years, and then every six months for three years should be sufficient. Repeat chest X-rays do not improve survival.

Conclusions

Postmenopausal bleeding has a variety of causes, one of which is endometrial cancer. An office based evaluation with minimal invasive testing is adequate for diagnosis. Endometrial cancer is usually discovered at an early stage, is curable, and is usually a disease of postmenopausal women.

References

1. Karlsson B., Granberg S., Wilkand M., *et al.* Transvaginal ultrasonography of the endometrium in women with postmenopausal bleeding – a Nordic multicenter study. *Am J Obstet Gynecol* 1995; **162**, 1488–1494.

2. Mateos F., Zaranz R., Seco C., *et al.* Assessment with transvaginal ultrasonography of endometrial thickness in women with postmenopausal bleeding. *Eur J Gynecol Oncol* 1997; **18**, 504–507.

3. Gull B., Karlsson B., Milsom I., Granberg S. Can ultrasound replace dilation and curettage? A longitudinal evaluation of postmenopausal bleeding and transvaginal sonographic measurement of the endometrium as predictors of endometrial cancer. *Am J Obstet Gynecol* 2003; **188**(2), 401–408.

4. Weaver J., McHugo J. M., Clark T. J. Accuracy of transvaginal ultrasound in diagnosing endometrial pathology in women with post-menopausal bleeding on tamoxifen. *Br J Radiol* 2005; **78**(929), 394–397.

5. Fremgen A. M., Bland K. I., McGinnis L. M. S., *et al.* Clinical highlights from the National Cancer Database. 1999; **162**, 1488–1494.

6. Epstein E., Valentin L. Managing women with post-menopausal bleeding. *Best Pract Res Clin Obstet Gynaecol* 2004; **18**(1), 125–143.

7. Ries L. A. G., Eisner M. P., Kosary C. L., *et al.*, eds. *SEER Cancer Statistics Review*, 1975–2002. Bethesda, MD: National Cancer Institute. Available at http://seer.cancer.gov/csr/1975_2002.

8. Benshushan A. Endometrial adenocarcinoma in young patients: evaluation and fertility-preserving treatment *Eur J Obstet Gynecol Reprod Biol* 2004; **116**(2), 132–137.

9. Fisher B., Constatino J. P., Redmond C. K., *et al.* Endometrial cancer in tamixifen treated breast cancer patients. Findings from the National Surgical Adjuvant Breast and Bowel Project 8–14. *J Natl Cancer Inst* 1994; **88**, 527–537.

10. Gadducci A., Cosio S., Carpi A., Nicolini A., Genazzani A. R. Serum tumor markers in the management of

ovarian, endometrial and cervical cancer. *Biomed Pharmacother* 2004; **58**(1), 24–38.

11. Lukka H., Chambers A., Fyles A., Thephamongkhol K., Fung-Kee-Fung M., Elit L., Kwon J. Adjuvant radiotherapy in women with stage I endometrial cancer: a systematic review. *Gynecol Oncol* 2006; **102**(2), 361–368.

12. Ramirez P. T., Frumovitz M., Bodurka D. C., Sun C. C., Levenback C. Hormonal therapy for the management of grade 1 endometrial adenocarcinoma: a literature review. *Gynecol Oncol* 2004; **95**(1), 133–138.

Ovarian cancer and masses

Jo Ann Rosenfeld

Ovarian cancer is rare, but unfortunately has a high mortality rate, because it is usually discovered at an advanced stage. There are few modifiable risk factors and the most appropriate and sensitive screening methods have not been determined.

Epidemiology

1. Ovarian cancer is the leading cause of death from gynecological malignancy and the fourth most common cause of cancer death in women. Other gynecological malignancies are usually discovered early, treated, and often cured.[1] In the USA, approximately 70% of women will present with stage III or IV disease.[2]
2. During the period 1994–1999, in the UK there were more than 21,000 deaths caused by ovarian cancer. In the USA in 2005, there were 22,220 new cases of ovarian cancer and 16,210 deaths caused by ovarian cancer.[3]
3. The number of women with ovarian cancer in the USA has increased 30% and the number of ovarian cancer deaths has increased 17%.[4] The effectiveness of treatment for ovarian cancer has not improved significantly.

Risk factors

1. Advancing age is the greatest risk factor. The rate of ovarian cancer rises with age from 15.7/100,000 women at age 40 to 54/100,000 women at age 79. The mean age is 59 years.[1]
2. A genetic disposition or a family history of ovarian cancer is the second greatest risk factor. There are at least three hereditary syndromes. Most breast and ovarian cancer genetic syndrome patients have the BRCA1 or BRCA2 gene.

The penetration of this gene mutation is 95%, giving a cumulative risk for a woman with this mutation of 63% for developing breast cancer by age 70.

3. Other risk factors include nulliparity, early menarche, and late menopause. Each pregnancy reduces a woman's risk of ovarian cancer by 10%.[4]
4. Multiparity is associated with decreased risk of ovarian cancer. Specifically, compared with nulligravidous women with a relative risk of 1.0, women with a single pregnancy have a relative risk of 0.6 to 0.8, with each additional pregnancy lowering the risk by about 10 to 15%.[6]
5. Use of OCPs reduces the risk of ovarian cancer by 30 to 60%. Women who used oral contraceptives for five years or more decreased their risk of ovarian cancer by 50%.[5] The protection given by OCPs persists for more than 15 years after the end of OCP use.[6]
6. In one study, women who used HRT were at a much greater risk of developing ovarian cancer. Women who used continuous HRT for five years or more, rather than sequential HRT, had a lower risk for ovarian cancer[7] (Figure 17.1).

Clinical signs

1. Ovarian cancer is usually a disease of postmenopausal women and is silent. There are few symptoms until it is advanced and metastatic.
2. An ovarian or pelvic mass may be seen incidentally on an ultrasound or felt on a pelvic examination. There may be symptoms of the enlarging mass such as frequent UTIs, vaginitis, or constipation.

Handbook of Women's Health, second edition, ed. Jo Ann Rosenfeld. Published by Cambridge University Press.
© Cambridge University Press 2009.

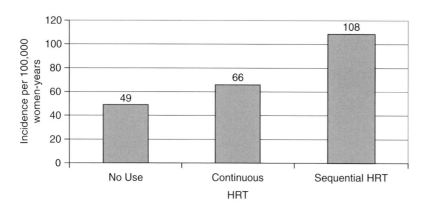

Figure 17.1 Incidence of ovarian cancer in women with intact uteruses by hormone replacement therapy use. Data from Lacey J. V. Jr., Brinton L. A., Leitzmann M. F., Mouw T., Hollenbeck A., Schatzkin A., Hartge P. Menopausal hormone therapy and ovarian cancer risk in the National Institutes of Health–AARP Diet and Health Study Cohort. *J Natl Cancer Inst* 2006; **98**(19), 1397–1405.

3. There may be pelvic pain from invasion into nerves or bones.

4. Finally, ovarian cancer usually spreads locally, and then, into the peritoneum. There it causes ascites, an enlarging abdomen, pleural effusions, shortness of breath, and weight loss.

5. A review of women with ovarian cancer compared with women with breast cancer or no cancer found that most women with ovarian cancer complained of the four following groups of non-specific symptoms in the 1–3 months before diagnosis: abdominal pain (30%), abdominal swelling (16.5%), GI symptoms (8.4%), and pelvic pain (5.4%).[8]

Evaluation of ovarian masses

1. Most ovarian masses are benign or functional. However, the specter of ovarian cancer demands thorough rapid investigation and evaluation.

2. Ovarian cysts are common. Six percent of asymptomatic postmenopausal women have adnexal masses, and 90% of these are cysts.

3. **Diagnosis**

   a. Clinical examination is poor in establishing a diagnosis. Thirty to 65% of tumors, especially those measuring less than 5 cm are not found by physical examination.

   b. Transvaginal sonography (TVS) is the examination of choice to establish the diagnosis. TVS can detect an ovarian tumor in 96% of women with ovarian cancer and has approximately 71% negative predictive value.[9]

   c. CA 125 levels rise in women with ovarian cancer. They are normal in 97% of women

who have benign cysts. Eighty percent of women older than age 50 who have malignant ovarian cancer have a level greater than 35 IU/mL. However, fewer than 50% of women with stage I ovarian cancer have an elevated CA 125 level.[10]

   d. Ovarian cytology by needle aspiration is a reliable method for diagnosis.

4. The evaluation is based on the age of the patient (Figure 17.2)

   a. In prepubertal adolescents, pelvic or ovarian masses and cysts are very worrisome and a complete evaluation including ultrasound and surgery or laparoscopy is recommended. Germ cell tumors occur more often in this group.

   b. In menstruating women, pregnancy, pregnancy complications and functional cysts are the most common causes of ovarian masses.

      i. A urine or blood human chorionic gonadotropin test is the first test to determine pregnancy, ectopic pregnancy, or other pregnancy problems.

      ii. A TVS should be done next to determine whether the mass is ovarian and whether it is a simple cyst, complex cyst, or a solid mass.

      iii. If the CA 125 level is elevated, surgery or laparoscopy is indicated.

      iv. If the mass is cystic and smaller than 8 cm and the CA 125 level is less than 30 or 35 IU/mL, the woman and physician can wait and watch, or use hormonal suppression by OCPs or progesterone. The smaller the cyst, the more likely it will resolve without treatment. One study

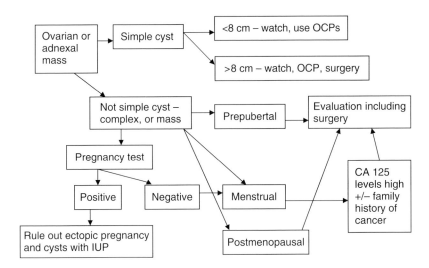

Figure 17.2 Evaluation of ovarian masses.

found that 62% of cysts smaller than 45 mm resolved within 6 months; only 28% of cysts larger than 60 mm resolved spontaneously.[11]

v. If the mass is cystic and larger than 8 cm or the woman has a elevated CA 125 levels, surgery or laparoscopy with biopsy is indicated.

vi. If the mass is a complex cyst or solid, the woman should have an ovarian duplex scan for better definition, and most likely, surgery or laparoscopy.

vii. Premenopausal women with a non-cystic mass should be referred if the CA 125 is elevated above 200 IU/mL, or a family history of breast or ovarian cancer.[12]

c. A postmenopausal woman with any ovarian mass should be considered to have cancer until proven otherwise. Some experts believe that if a postmenopausal woman has an ovary that can be felt on physical examination, she needs evaluation for cancer. The woman will need surgery unless TVS shows a simple cyst less than 5 cm and normal CA 125 levels.

Prevention and screening

1. There is no acceptable method of screening either the general population or high risk women.
2. CA 125 levels have been suggested as a screening device both for the general population and for women at high risk for ovarian cancer.[13] Several large studies of high risk women have found that high CA 125 levels will identify a subpopulation that is at higher risk of ovarian cancer.[14]

3. Pelvic examination has a limited value because of its poor sensitivity. Doctors detect a 4 cm × 6 cm mass only 67% of the time. A 15 year retrospective study evaluating pelvic examination found only six ovarian cancers in 1319 women with 17,753 pelvic examinations.[15]

4. Using CA 125 levels with transvaginal ultrasound to detect ovarian cancer in high risk populations early has and is being studied in large studies. In one study that offered high risk women either annual screenings or prophylactic bilateral salping-oophorectomy, 24 out of 269 women who chose screening had abnormalities and one stage III ovarian cancer was found, making it sensitive but not efficient.[16] Another study found that using the CA 125 levels and TVS in a high risk population gave a positive predictive value of 40%.[17] However, most of those cancers found were still at an advanced stage.

5. These studies do not adequately screen for ovarian cancer in the general population. A RCT followed 22,000 postmenopausal women with CA 125 levels, followed by TVS, and then surgery for any masses. Forty-nine cancers were found, and the risk of developing ovarian cancer rose with the level of CA 125. The relative risk of developing ovarian cancer was 204 for a woman with a CA 125 level greater than 100 IU/mL[18] (Figure 17.3).

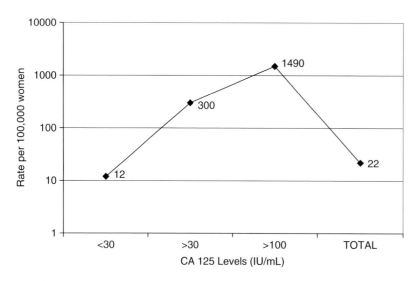

Figure 17.3 Rate of ovarian cancer in the general population of women by CA 125 levels. Data from Jacobs I. J., Skates S., Davies A. P., *et al.* Risk of diagnosis of ovarian cancer after raised serum CA 125 concentration: a prospective cohort study. *Br Med J* 1996; **313**, 1355–1358.

6. The CA 125 level is also elevated in women with endometriosis, PID, adenomyosis, liver disease, pancreatitis, peritonitis, endometrial cancer, biliary tract tumors, and liver, pancreatic, breast, and colon cancer.

7. TVS has insufficient specificity for use as a screening test. However, when used in evaluation of adnexal masses and combined with ovarian color Doppler, TVS has a sensitivity of 94% and specificity of 97%.

8. Use of both TVS and CA 125 in high risk women may be used as screening. If both are positive (abnormal), the positive predictive value for finding ovarian cancer approaches 20%. This means that for every five women with both tests positive, one would have ovarian cancer and four would have unnecessary surgery.

Treatment and survival

1. Treatment is surgery and staging is important, whether one or both ovaries are involved and no matter the degree of extension. If fertility is not an issue, a total abdominal hysterectomy and BSO should be done with biopsies of bilateral pelvic peritoneum and bladder.

2. In advanced disease, debulking surgical resection is suggested. Debulking the tumor mass to smaller than 2 cm will improve survival.

3. Survival from ovarian cancer is based on the stage at discovery, and ranges from 87.8% five-year survival for women with stage IA, to 17% for women with stage IV.

4. Chemotherapy is used as an adjuvant, often cisplatin, doxyrubicin, and paclitaxel.

5. The use of radiation in women with ovarian cancer is controversial.

6. The rate of survival from ovarian cancer improved slightly from 1988 to 1997 in the USA. Improved survival was associated with younger age and low-grade tumors.[19]

Conclusion

Ovarian cancer is a disease that, so far, lacks adequate screening tests. It is most often already metastatic when discovered and lethal. Thus, any ovarian or pelvic mass in a woman is suspect for ovarian cancer. Except in menstruating women with completely cystic masses smaller than 6 to 7 cm, most evaluation of women with pelvic masses will require surgery.

References

1. Patridge E. R., Barnes M. N. Epithelial ovarian cancer: prevention, diagnosis and treatment. *CA Cancer J Clin* 1999; **49**, 297–320.

2. Mack N., Barnes M. N., Grizzle W. E., Grubbs C. J., Partridge E. E. Paradigms for primary prevention of ovarian carcinoma. *CA Cancer J Clin* 2002; **52**, 216–225.

3. Jemal A., Murray T., Ward E., *et al.* Cancer statistics 2005. *CA Cancer J Clin* 2005; **55**, 10–30.

4. Parker S. L., Davis K. J., Wingo P. A., Ries L. A., Heath C. W. Cancer statistics by race and ethnicity. *CA Cancer J Clin* 1998; **48**, 31–48.

5. WHO Collaborative study of neoplasia and steroid contraceptives. Epithelial ovarian cancer and

combined oral contraceptives. *J Epidemiol* 1989; **17**, 538–545.

6. Deligeoroglou E., Michailidis E., Creatsas G. Oral contraceptives and reproductive system cancer. *Ann NY Acad Sci* 2003; **997**, 199–208.

7. Lacey J. V. Jr., Brinton L. A., Leitzmann M. F., Mouw T., Hollenbeck A., Schatzkin A., Hartge P. Menopausal hormone therapy and ovarian cancer risk in the National Institutes of Health–AARP Diet and Health Study Cohort. *J Natl Cancer Inst* 2006; **98**(19), 1397–1405.

8. Smith L. H., Morris C. R., Yasmeen S., Parikh-Patel A., Cress R. D., Romano P. S. Ovarian cancer: can we make the clinical diagnosis earlier? *Cancer* 2005; **104**(7), 1398–1407.

9. Hankinson S. E., Hunter D. J., Colditz G. A., *et al.* Tubal ligation, hysterectomy and risk of ovarian cancer: a prospective study. *J Am Med Assoc* 1993; **270**, 2813–2817.

10. Jacobs I., Bast R. The CA-125 tumor associated antigen: a review of literature. *Hum Reprod* 1989; **4**, 1–12.

11. Zanetta G., LIssoni A., Torri V., *et al.* Role of puncture and aspiration in expectant management of simple ovarian cysts: a randomized study. *Br Med J* 1996; **313**, 1110–1113.

12. Gostout B. S., Brewer M. A. Guidelines for referral of the patient with an adnexal mass. *Clin Obstet Gynecol* 2006; **49**(3), 448–458.

13. NIH Consensus Development Panel on Ovarian Cancer. Ovarian cancer; screening, treatment and follow-up. *J Am Med Assoc* 1995; **273**, 491–497.

14. Jacobs I., Davies A. P., Bridges J., Stabile I., Fay T., Lower A., Grudzinskas J. G., Oram D. Prevalence screening for ovarian cancer in postmenopausal women by CA 125 measurement and ultrasonography. *Br Med J* 1993; **306**, 1030–1034.

15. MacFarlane C., Sturgis M. D., Fetterman P. C. Results of an experience in the control of cancer of the female pelvic organs: a report of a 15 year research. *Am J Obstet Gynecol* 1956; **294**, 301–306.

16. Oei A. L., Massuger L. F., Bulten J., Ligtenberg M. J., Hoogerbrugge N., de Hullu J. A. Surveillance of women at high risk for hereditary ovarian cancer is inefficient. *Br J Cancer* 2006; **94**(6), 814–819.

17. Olivier R. I., Lubsen-Brandsma M. A., Verhoef S., van Beurden M.CA125 and transvaginal ultrasound monitoring in high-risk women cannot prevent the diagnosis of advanced ovarian cancer. *Gynecol Oncol* 2006; **100**(1), 20–26.

18. Jacobs I. J., Skates S., Davies A. P. *et al.* Risk of diagnosis of ovarian cancer after raised serum CA-125 concentration: a prospective cohort study. *Br Med J* 1996; **313**, 1355–1358.

19. Chan J. K., Cheung M. K., Husain A., Teng N. N., West D., Whittemore A. S., Berek J. S., Osann K. Patterns and progress in ovarian cancer over 14 years. *Obstet Gynecol* 2006; **108**(3 Pt 1), 521–528.

Chapter 18

Urinary incontinence and infections

Jo Ann Rosenfeld

Urinary incontinence

Urinary incontinence (UI) is a problem for many women; at least half never mention the problem to their health care providers.

Importance and epidemiology

1. UI is very common. Some studies suggest that approximately two-thirds of all women may suffer it some time in their lives.[1] Its exact prevalence is difficult to determine and varies with the population surveyed. Approximately 38% of community dwelling older women have significant incontinence.[2] Approximately 5 to 10% of all US women, 13 million women, have clinically significant UI.[3] In the Hormone and Estrogen Replacement Study (HERS), 56% of more than 2700 older women with heart disease reported at least weekly incontinence.[4]

2. The social and financial toll of UI is significant. The estimated yearly cost in the USA is $18.5 million.[5] UI predisposes women to social isolation, depression, and dependency. It is a major risk factor to admissions to long-term health facilities and in long-term morbidity, including catheter use, urinary tract infections, pressure sores, immobility, and falls.

3. In institutionalized women, UI is much more common. One-half of home bound and institutionalized elderly, and 25 to 30% of those women that leave the hospital are incontinent. In a population of women in residential care in the UK, 40% were incontinent.[6]

Risk factors

1. **Gender**

   Being a woman is a risk factor. The female:male ratio of incidence is 4:1 at age 60 and 2:1 after age 60.[7]

2. **Age**

   Five to 6% of women younger than age 60 and 10% older than age 60 report UI.[8]

3. **Exercise**

   Approximately one-half of postmenopausal women develop UI while exercising.[9]

4. **Obstetrical history**

   Parity, number of vaginal deliveries, episiotomies, and traumatic or surgical vaginal deliveries are risk factors for UI.[6] Although having had a hysterectomy was not found to be a risk factor in a prospective study, cross-sectional epidemiological studies have found having had a hysterectomy to be an increased risk (Table 18.1).

5. **Family history**

   If a mother or sisters suffered from incontinence, the woman is more likely to be incontinent[10] (Figure 18.1).

6. The HERS study found the following factors increased the woman's risk of UI: white race (RR = 2.8), increased BMI (increased risk of 1.1 per 5 units), higher waist to hip ratio, diabetes (RR = 1.5) and a personal history of more than two UTIs.[2]

Handbook of Women's Health, second edition, ed. Jo Ann Rosenfeld. Published by Cambridge University Press.
© Cambridge University Press 2009.

7. The best predictors of urge incontinence were age, diabetes, and history of UTIs. The major predictors of stress incontinence (SUI) were white race, high BMI, and high waist to hip ratio. There was no association with increasing parity.

8. Other risk factors include stroke, immobility, chronic neurological diseases, dementia, delirium, and use of certain medications (Table 18.2).

Table 18.1 Risk factors for developing urinary incontinence

Medical history
Older age
Stroke
Immobility from chronic neurological or degenerative disease
Diabetes
Dementia or delirium
Medication use (see Table 18.2)
Pelvic muscle weakness
Increased parity
Multiple vaginal deliveries
History of episiotomy
More than two UTIs
Social history
Smoking
White race
Physical findings
Fecal impaction
Obesity

Clinical definitions

1. There are four forms of urinary incontinence. Although many women suffer mixed incontinence, defining the type(s) of incontinence a woman has may address cause and treatment.

2. Approximately 13% of women have stress incontinence, 14% pure urge incontinence, and 28% mixed incontinence.[2]

Urge incontinence

1. Urge incontinence, also called irritable bladder or detrusor instability, is defined differently by different clinicians. Urge UI is the sudden involuntary loss associated with a strong sensation

Table 18.2 Medications that increase the incidence of urinary incontinence

Alcohol
Alpha adrenergic antagonists
Anticholinergics
Antidepressants
Antipsychotics
Antihistamines
Beta-blockers
CNS depressants
Caffeine
Calcium channel antagonists
Diuretics
Narcotics
Sedatives

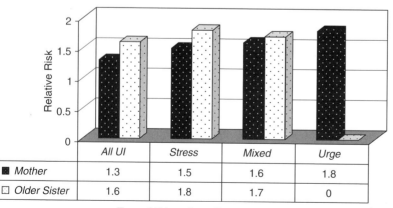

	All UI	Stress	Mixed	Urge
■ *Mother*	1.3	1.5	1.6	1.8
□ *Older Sister*	1.6	1.8	1.7	0

Type of Urinary Incontinence

Figure 18.1 Increased relative risk of incontinence based on relatives' history. Data from Hannestad Y. S., Lie R., Rorveit G., Hunskaar S. Familial risk of urinary incontinence in women: population based cross sectional study. *Br Med J* 2004; **329**, 889–891, doi:10.1136/bmj.329.7471.889.

to void. This leads to sudden large volume urinary accidents.

2. Rarely, it is caused by uncontrollable bladder contractions that overwhelm the brain's ability to inhibit them.

   a. This can be caused by inflammation or irritation from cancer, infections, calculi, urethritis, or atrophic vaginitis.

   b. The central nervous systems involved in inhibiting bladder contractions may be impaired by neurological conditions such as strokes, Parkinson's disease, or dementia.

   c. A sudden large volume of urine introduced rapidly with diuretic therapy or glucosuria from diabetes may cause urge incontinence.

3. Urge incontinence accounts for 12 to 14% of UI in community dwelling women, to 60% in women in outpatient urinary incontinence clinics and residential care.[8]

Stress incontinence

1. SUI is loss of urine with coughing, sneezing, or increased abdominal pressure. It often occurs during exercise.

2. It is usually caused by malfunction of the urethral sphincter that causes urine to leak with increased intra-abdominal pressure. It is also associated with pelvic prolapse, denervation from alpha adrenergic blocking drugs, surgical trauma, or radiation damage.

3. SUI is the most common cause of UI.

Overflow bladder (neurogenic bladder)

1. This form of UI usually is associated with neurological dysfunction, such as caused by diabetes, neurological, and muscular problems, such as stroke. The bladder fills completely and UI occurs from overflow.

2. It can be caused by medicines such as anticholinergic agents and calcium channel blockers, or outflow obstruction from fecal impaction, strictures or urethral constriction.

Functional incontinence

This is UI caused by inability to reach the toilet in time, inability to sense the need to urinate, or loss of memory of how to be continent. Strokes, arthritis, casts, immobility from any cause, and altered mental states such as dementia, delirium or coma can cause functional incontinence.

Diagnosis (Table 18.3)

1. Family and general practitioners can diagnose and help the patient with UI. Evaluation by history, physical examination, urine analysis, and, at times, measurement of a post-void residual, is sufficient to identify most causes of UI. Usually, history alone can describe the type of UI.

2. Identify if any cause of transient incontinence is present (Table 18.4). Many of these occur if the woman is in the hospital or just discharged.

Table 18.3 Historic evaluation of women with urinary incontinence

History of incontinence – duration and characteristics, frequency, onset, precipitating factors
Other urinary symptoms – dysuria, hematuria
Obstetrical and gynecological history – deliveries, surgeries, symptoms, pain, dyspareunia
Bowel habits
Medications
Other medical illnesses
Mental status and CNS function
Gait and muscular function
Social factors – living arrangements, effects of incontinence, self-treatments and their effects

Table 18.4 Transient causes of urinary incontinence

Medication use
Delirium or change in mental status
Hypoxia
Acute change in mobility
Fecal impaction or constipation
UTI
Acute changes in diabetic control – glucosuria
Excessive fluid intake
Syndrome of inappropriate anti-diuretic hormone (caused by medical diseases)

Reducing fecal impactions, improving glucose control, decreasing IV and oral fluids, treating UTIs and obstructions, determining whether any medicines are causing UI, and improving mental status and access to toilets will improve many causes of UI.

3. Identify conditions that need other medical treatment or referral such as acute delirium or out of control diabetes.
4. Analyze a urine specimen to evaluate for infection and specific gravity.
5. Decide the type of UI and start treatment.
6. If neurological disease is present and an overflow bladder problem is suspected, a post-void residual measurement can be obtained with an intermittent catheterization. Volumes greater than 200 mL are abnormal.
7. Cystometric testing is only needed in a few women who do not respond to the treatment.
8. Often focusing attention on the problem improves continence by itself.

Treatment (Tables 18.5 and 18.6)

There are medical, behavioral, electrical, magnetic, and surgical treatments of UI. Every type of treatment has a success rate of 50% or greater. Few studies have compared medical treatment to any other treatment. Most studies defined the types and outcome measures differently, making evidenced-based decisions difficult.

1. Review of multiple trials found that bladder training may be helpful, but there was not strong evidence that it significantly improved UI with or without other treatment.[11]
2. Review of studies of pelvic floor exercises (Kegel) showed that their use did not cause any harm and did show improvements for women with stress, urge, and mixed incontinence. They help women who exercise most and those who are younger (40–50 years old).[12]
3. There have been no reported studies comparing medical to surgical therapy. There are no criteria for referral for surgical treatment. However, a grade III or greater uterine prolapse or cystocele (going beyond the introitus) necessitates a referral and possible surgery.
4. In observational studies, UI has been successfully treated by general practitioners using all of the following including pelvic floor exercises,

Table 18.5 Behavioral and medication treatment for urinary incontinence

	Behavioral	Medication
Stress	Bladder retraining	Estrogen (oral)
	Supertampon or pessary	Estrogen (topical)
	Pelvic floor exercises	Imipramine
	Pads	
Urge	Electrostimulation	Estrogen
	Bladder retraining	Imipramine
		Oxybutinin
		SSRIs
		Calcium channel blockers
Overflow	Bladder retraining	Bethanecol
	Electrostimulation	
Functional	Treat mechanically	
	Move bed, bedside commode, etc.	

estrogen, electrostimulation, anticholinergic drugs, bladder training, and pads, with an overall 62% improvement. Severe incontinence decreased from 64 to 28% in these studies. Only 16% of women needed a referral to a specialist.[13]

5. Many studies have compared and evaluated various surgical treatments such as tension-free vaginal tape operation,[14] and open retropubic colposuspension. A review has found that the evidence available indicates that open retropubic colposuspension is an effective treatment modality for stress urinary incontinence especially in the long term, where the overall continence rate is approximately 85–90%. After five years, approximately 70% of patients can expect to be dry.[15]

Stress incontinence

1. Treatment of SUI includes pelvic floor exercises and medication.
2. A randomized small study, teaching women to contract pelvic floor muscles before coughing, found that women, with one week's training, could reduce urine loss by 98.3% with medium coughs.[16]

Table 18.6 Medical treatment of urinary incontinence

Drug	Dose	Effectiveness	Adverse effects
Oxybutinin	2.5 to 5.0 mg twice daily or 5 mg tid to qid to 20 mg qd Transdermal drug	50–62%, 20% higher than placebo Another study 68% improvement in UI	66–82%, half withdrew because of dry mouth and/or blurred vision
Doxepin	50–75 qhs	Improvement at night	73% fatigue and 42% dry mouth
Tolerodine (Detrol[R] and Detrol LA[R])	1–2 mg bid tablet 4 mg qd (LA)		
Solifenacin (Vesicare)	5 or 10 mg daily	Approximately twice the improvement of placebo	Dry mouth
Duloxetine (Cymbalta)			One-third reported nausea and/or stopped treatment
Alpha adrenergic drugs (phenylpropaline)		Some mild improvement	Dry mouth, insomnia, irritability

3. Women with exercise SUI do well with mechanical treatment, such as use of a super-tampon placed vaginally during exercise. A randomized single-blind efficacy study of two devices – the Hodge pessary and a super-tampon – found tampons achieved continence more frequently.[6]

Urge incontinence

1. Treatment for urge incontinence includes behavioral therapy, electrostimulation, and medications (Table 18.6).
2. Behavioral therapy, including bladder retraining and increased frequency of urination, improves urge incontinence.
3. Electrostimulation of vagina, anus, or suprapubic areas for 20–30 minutes one to three times a day improved urge incontinence in some studies.[17]
4. Medication has a significant place in the treatment of urge incontinence. No medication is specific for urge incontinence, and many of the drugs have sometimes distressing side effects such as dry mouth (Table 18.6).
5. Oxybutinin has had the greatest use and has shown 86% improvement in UI, as compared to 55% of women using placebo.

6. Tricyclic antidepressants, calcium channel blockers, and norepinephrine SSRIs have also been used with some success.

Mixed incontinence

1. A variety of treatments should be used for mixed UI. In a RCT of approximately 200 community dwelling women older than age 55, either behavioral therapy (four sessions of biofeedback) or drug therapy (oxybutinin 2.5 mg to 5.0 mg twice daily) improved urinary continence as compared to placebo.
2. More than one type of therapy should be used simultaneously with mixed UI.

Pharmocotherapy

1. Medication use or a combination of medication with behavioral therapy worked better than placebo or behavioral therapy alone in many studies. A Cochrane review found that use of adrenergic agents was better than placebo or pelvic floor muscle training.[18]
2. Oxybutinin (2.5 to 5.0 mg twice daily) can be given orally. However, many women complain of a dry mouth. A newer transdermal oxybutinin was recently developed that helps UI and reduces side

effects.[19] The improvement in symptoms lasted more than 40 weeks. Other muscarinic acting agents, including trospium chloride, darifenacin (Enablex[R]), tolerodine (Detrol[R] and Detrol LA[R]), and solifenacin (Vesicare) all improve UI. Longer-acting tablets improve the ease of use. In a double-blind RCT, Solifenacin (at 5 or 10 mg daily) was twice as effective against placebo for overactive bladder (49% versus 28%).[20]

3. Duloxetine (Cymbalta) and other norepinephrine SSRIs have been shown to improve UI significantly against placebo or behavioral therapies.[21]

4. A few studies have reported an improvement in UI versus placebo with use of alpha adrenergic agents such as phenylpropaline. However, many of the participants of the study complained of insomnia and restlessness.[18]

Hormonal therapy

1. Although estrogen deficiency and vaginal atrophy have been implicated as causes of UI and observational studies have suggested the efficacy of hormonal therapy to improve UI, few RCTs have shown that estrogen use, orally or topically, affects UI.

2. Most of the studies have small numbers, used a variety of estrogen preparations, and considered different outcome measures. In a meta-analysis of 166 articles examining the effect of estrogen on postmenopausal women with UI, only six were RCTs.

3. In an arm of the Women's Health Initiative Study, in a double-blind RCT comparing a variety of postmenopausal hormone replacement therapies (HRT), including conjugated estrogens, with and without progesterone in healthy women who had had hysterectomies, any HRT increased the incidence of UI.[22]

Surgical therapy

1. When a variety of behavioral, medical, and/or electrical treatment does not improve incontinence, when the woman has prolapse beyond the introitus, or in a woman with recurrent UTIs, surgical treatment can be considered.

2. The improvement of UI by surgical therapies has been touted as 50 to 85%. Seldom, however, was any surgical treatment compared to medical therapy, and the groups of women differed in severity, making comparisons difficult.

3. For stress incontinence, there are three major kinds of surgical procedures:

    a. vaginal placation of bladder neck with sutures or tension-free tape;

    b. needle suspension of the bladder neck;

    c. retropubic urethroplexy (Marshall–Marquetti–Krantz and others)

4. Laparoscopic colposuspension has been compared to other surgical treatments for UI. Recovery time is quicker with this operation and has similar improvement rates as the more involved surgeries.[23]

5. The American Urological Association reviewed studies and found that, after 48 months, retropubic suspensions and slings were more efficacious than transvaginal suspension and anterior repairs. However, they have higher complication rates with synthetic materials. Surgical treatment of women's SUI is effective and offers a long-term cure in a significant proportion of women.[24]

Conclusions

Family and general physicians can diagnose and treat UI in women with a great deal of efficacy using a history, physical examination and simple test in the office, using a variety of methods including behavioral therapy and medication.

Urinary tract infections

UTIs are a nearly universal experience for women. Although usually benign and easily treated, recurrent and/or persistent infections can lead to serious disease.

Impact

1. UTIs are very common in women. They account for more than 6 million visits to physician in the USA yearly. Twenty to 80% of women will have a UTI at some time during their life, and approximately 35% of women age 20–40 years have had UTIs.[25]

2. Approximately 20% of women will have recurrent UTIs.

3. UTIs are the most common hospital-acquired infection, causing more than 40% of all nosocomial infections.[26]

4. Chronic UTIs are responsible for 11–13% of all causes of renal failure.

Table 18.7 Risk factors for urinary tract infections

Being a woman

Stenosis or obstruction of urinary tract

Abnormal urinary tract

Kidney stones

Pregnancy

Menopause

Catheterization

Sexual intercourse

Diaphragm use

Risk factors (Table 18.7)

1. Being a woman is a significant risk factor for UTIs.
2. Obstruction, stasis, or stenosis of any part of the urinary system will predispose to UTIs. Women with abnormal urinary tracts – those with double ureters, horseshoe kidneys or other abnormalities – are more likely to develop UTIs. Pregnancy causes urinary statis and hydroureter, and predisposes to UTIs.
3. Pregnancy often results in right-sided hydroureter and, often, left hydroureter and hydronephrosis. These usually clear up postpartum. If a pregnant woman has significant bacteriuria (greater than 10^6 organisms/mL), even if asymptomatic, she has a 60% chance of developing pyelopnephritis during pregnancy. If treated, cured, followed closely, and given prophylactic treatment, if necessary, her risk of developing pyelonephritis decreases to 20%.
4. In postmenopausal women, independent risk factors include a history of more than six UTIs (RR = 6.9) and insulin-dependent diabetes (RR = 3.4). Other associations included asymptomatic bacteriuria, or a history of kidney stones or use of vaginal estrogen.[27]
5. Diabetes, either treated by oral agents or insulin, is a risk factor for UTIs (RR = 2.6–2.9).[28]
6. Asymptomatic bacteriuria (urine with 10^5 organisms/mL in the absence of symptoms) is not associated with UTIs and should not be treated except in pregnant women, diabetics, and those with urinary tract abnormalities. Women with

diabetes and asymptomatic bacteriuria are more likely to develop subsequent UTIs,[29] but prophylactic treatment is not suggested.[30,31]

7. The risk factors for recurrent UTI include a personal history of UTI, incontinence, and presence of a cystocele.[32]

Symptoms

1. Common symptoms include dysuria, polyuria, increased urgency, and nocturia. The woman may have trouble starting to urinate.
2. Constant suprapubic, flank, costovertebral angle (CVA) or back pain can occur with lower UTIs. Upper tract UTIs or pyelonephritis often present with CVA tenderness and pain. Severe colicky pain is more consistent with kidney stones.
3. Fever, chills, nausea, and vomiting are more likely with pyelonephritis.
4. Hematuria can occur, microscopic to frank gross hematuria. However, hematuria should suggest evaluation for kidney stones. Painless frank hematuria may be caused by bladder polyps or cancer and need referral for cystoscopy.

Diagnosis

1. The diagnosis can be determined by history, physical examination, and urine analysis, and is confirmed by urine culture. Studies have found that a dipstix test of urine consistent with an infection can accurately establish the diagnosis (Table 18.8).
2. The physical examination may be normal. CVA tenderness or suprapubic pain may be elicited. Fever would suggest pyelonephritis.

3. **Urine analysis**

(Table 18.8)

   a. A urine analysis positive for nitrites, protein, and/or leukocyte esterase, with pyuria and bacteriuria is suggestive of a UTI.
   b. White blood cells may be present in the urine, if the woman has cervicitis or vaginitis. Pyuria by itself may not indicate a UTI.
   c. The presence of vaginal cells may indicate that the specimen is not a clean catch; the bacteria

Table 18.8 Urine analysis

	Normal	UTI
pH	7.3–7.4	Often low
Specific gravity	1.010	Often unchanged
Glucose	None	None
Protein	None	1+ to 2+ on dipstix
Ketones	None	None, unless vomiting
Blood	None	None to positive
Nitrites	None	Positive
Leukocyte esterase	None	Positive
White blood cells	0–1 cell/HPF	1 cell/HPF unspun 10–20/HPF spun
Red blood cells	0–1 cell/HPF	None to TNTC
Bacteria	Occasional	None to TNTC
Yeast	None	None
Casts	None	None – WBC casts suggest pyelonephritis

Notes: TNTC, too numerous to count; WBC, white blood count.

and white blood cells in that urine may be from the vagina, not the bladder.

d. A positive leukocyte esterase test is 75–95% sensitive and 95% specific in detecting more than 10 WBC/mL, consistent with a UTI.

e. Nitrites are produced by gram-negative bacilli. A positive test has a specificity of more than 92% for UTIs.

f. A urine dipstix test negative for nitrates but positive for leukocyte esterase has a 79% positive predictive value test for UTI.[33]

g. A positive urine analysis is a presumptive diagnosis of UTI, and treatment can be started. The results of a urine culture are not needed to begin therapy.

4. **Urine culture**

a. Growth of more than 10^5 colonies of a single organism is diagnostic of a UTI.

b. However, more than half of women with UTIs will not have a culture with this many organisms. Lower colony counts of a single organism (10^2 to 10^4) in urine specimens that were not first morning specimens in women who have typical syndromes may be considered positive.

c. In approximately 15% of women with UTI symptoms, cultures may be negative. A diagnosis of chlamydia, ureoplasm, or mycoplasm urethritis should be considered.

d. Polymicrobial UTIs may occur in women with indwelling catheters, diabetes, or urinary obstruction.

5. **Infecting organisms**

a. The predominant organisms are *E. coli*, causing approximately 85–90% of UTIs.

b. Other gram-negative bacteria such as *Proteus, Serratia, Citrobacter, Pseudomonas*, and *Klebsiella* occur in fewer than 1% of uncomplicated UTIs and in approximately 5% of complicated UTIs. *Proteus mirabilis* was more likely the cause of UTIs in older patients.[27]

c. Gram-positive organisms, such as *Staphylococcus epidermidis* and *Staphylococcus saphrophyticus* occur in 5–10% of uncomplicated UTIs, mostly in younger patients. *Staphylococcus aureus* is an occasional pathogen.

Treatment
Acute cystitis

1. Amoxicillin, trimethoprim/sulfa, or a quinolone may be a good first choice. The two latter drugs should not be used in a pregnant woman (Table 18.9). Empiric treatment can be effectively started since most *E. coli* organisms are sensitive to a variety of antibiotics.[34]

2. How long to treat is under investigation. Many acute UTIs caused by *E. coli* respond to one or three days' treatment with a wide variety of antibiotics. UTIs with *Staphylococcus saphrophyticus* usually need longer treatment. In one study of UTIs in general practice, 33% of *E. coli* were resistant to amoxicillin and 23% to trimethoprim/sulfa.[27] In response, use of

Table 18.9 Antibiotics for uncomplicated UTIs or cystitis

Drug	Dose	Acceptable in pregnancy	Note
Amoxicillin	250–500 mg tid	Yes	Increasing *E. coli* resistance a problem, diarrhea and yeast infections as side effects
Cephalexein	250–500 mg bid to tid	Yes	
Nitrofuradantoin	50–100 mg bid	Yes	Good for penicillin allergic patients
Ciprofloxacin	200–500 mg bid	No	Less resistance
Norfloxacin	400 mg bid or 800 mg qd	No	
Trimethoprim	100 mg bid	No	
Trimethoprim/Sulfa	One DS bid	No	

Table 18.10 Doses of single dose antibiotics for uncomplicated UTIs

Amoxicillin	3 gm
Cefuroxime	1 gm
Cephalexein	3 gm
Ciprofloxacin	1 gm (long-acting XL)
Norfloxacin	400–800 mg
Ofloxacin	800 mg
Trimethoprim/Sulfa	2 DS tablets
Trimethoprim	400–600 mg

ciprofloxin and other quinolones for uncomplicated UTIs has increased.

3. The duration of treatment can vary. Studies examining one, three, seven, ten and fourteen days therapy have found equal efficacy in curing UTIs. Several studies have found that one dose of medication is sufficient to treat many uncomplicated UTIs[35] (Table 18.10).
4. Test of cure by repeat culture is important. Approximately 10–20% of women will continue to have UTIs after first treatment.

Recurrent or complicated UTI

1. A repeat UTI in a woman who has recently finished UTI treatment may require a different antibiotic, or one with greater coverage. A full 7 to 10 day course of antibiotics is most likely needed.
2. A pregnant woman or a woman with diabetes or a urinary obstruction must have a full 7 to 10 day course of antibiotics.

3. Some *E. coli* strains are not sensitive to first line medication. Hospital and community outpatient sensitivities should be considered.

Pyelonephritis

1. Women with pyelonephritis or upper tract UTIs may present with symptoms exactly like cystitis, or may have fever, chills, nausea, vomiting and high WBC count.
2. Treatment may require hospitalization, hydration, and IV antibiotics, such as a third generation cephalosporin or an aminoglycoside.
3. Indications for hospitalization and IV antibiotics would include dehydration, pregnancy, severe vomiting, diabetes, elderly or immunocompromised women, severe pain, or uncertainty about diagnosis. Women who develop infections with organisms insensitive to outpatient oral medication, especially those caused by *Proteus* organisms, may need IV antibiotics.
4. Treatment would include 3–14 days of IV antibiotics and then oral antibiotics for 4 weeks. Seven days of IV therapy may be sufficient (Table 18.11).

Follow-up

1. After acute cystitis, a repeat culture is needed to prove cure.
2. For women with recurrent cystitis, after a repeat negative culture, antibiotic prophylaxis should be considered. Prophylaxis can be given

Table 18.11 Intravenous antibiotics for complicated UTIs and pyelonephritis

Ampicillin	50–250/kg per day divided every 3–4 hours
Ticarcillin/clavulanate	3.1 gm q 4–6 hours
Ampicillin/sulbactam	1.5–3.0 gm q 6 hours
Ceftriaxone	1–2 gm qd or divided bid
Ciprofloxacing	400 mg IV q 12 hours
Gentamycin	1–5 mg/kg/d

Table 18.12 Antibiotics for prophylaxis

Postcoital single dose prophylaxis	
Trimethoprim/sulfa	½ DS or regular strength tablet
Sulfamethoxazole	500 mg
Cephalexein	250 mg
Nitrofurandantoin	50 mg
Ciprofloxacin*	250 mg
Chronic prophylaxis – taken qhs or every other night	
Trimethoprim/Sulfa	½ DS
Cephalesein	250 mg
Nitrofuradantoin	50–100 mg
Norfloxacin*	200 mg
Ciprofloxacin*	250 mg

Note: *Not to be used in pregnant or possibly pregnant women.

intermittently (as before each sexual intercourse) or chronically (Table 18.12).

3. An evaluation for possible obstruction such as kidney stones or abnormal urinary tracts should include an intravenous pyelogram or ultrasound. Ten to 20% of women who were admitted for pyelonephritis were found, in an observational study, to have kidney stones, or an abnormal urinary tract.[36]

Secondary prevention

1. Some women have recurrent or persistent UTIs. These women need an evaluation to discover diabetes, immunosuppression or an abnormal or obstructed urinary tract. Women with diabetes or in an immunocompromized state may need long-term antibiotic prophylaxis. Use of antibiotics daily or every other day has decreased the incidence of UTIs.[37]

2. Some women may relate the development of UTIs to coitus. Single postcoital doses of antibiotics, including trimethoprim/sulfa, sulfamethoxisole, or ciprofloxacin or another quinolone, have been shown to decrease the recurrence of UTIs, with less antibiotic use than daily dosing.[38]

3. Because women can accurately self diagnose UTIs from their symptoms, they can start antibiotics when they feel a UTI coming on and avoid it.

4. Other adjunctive methods such as cranberry juice and use of high dose vitamin C have been suggested to reduce the recurrence of UTIs.

5. Postmenopausal vaginal estrogen use has been linked to an increase in UTIs, and as a cure for frequent UTIs.

Conclusions

Urinary incontinence is very common. However, if the woman and physician work together, there are a variety of treatments that can help improve the situation. UTIs are common, and must be identified and treated. Recurrent UTIs should be treated rigorously and may be preventable.

References

1. Smith P. P., McCrery R. J., Appell R. A. Current trends in the evaluation and management of female urinary incontinence. *Can Med Assoc J* 2006; **175**(10), doi:10.1503/cmaj.060034.

2. Burgio K. L., Locher J. L., Goode J. S., *et al.* Behavioral vs. drug treatement for urge urinary incontinence in older women. *J Am Med Assoc* 1998; **280**, 1995–2001.

3. Weiss B. D. Diagnostic evaluation of urinary incontinence in geriatric patients. *Am Fam Physician* 1998; **57**, 2675–2684, 2688–2690.

4. Brown J. S., Grady D., Ouslander J. G., *et al.* Prevalence of urinary incontinence and associated risk factors in postmenopausal women. *Obstet Gynecol* 1999; **33**, 241–247.

5. Hu T. W., Wagner T. H., Bentkover J. D., *et al.* Costs of urinary incontinence and overactive bladder in the United States: a comparative study. *Urology* 2004; **63**, 461–465.

6. Peet S. M., Castleden C. M., McGrother C. W. Prevalence of urinary and faecal incontinence in

hospitals and residential nursing homes for older people. *Br Med J* 1995; **3411**, 1063–1064.

7. Thomas D. H., Brown J. S. Reproductive and hormonal risk factors for urinary incontinence in later life. A review of the clinical and epidemiological factors. *J Am Geriatr Soc* 1998; **48**, 1411–1417.

8. Gorton E., Stanton S. Urinary incontinence in elderly women. *Eur Urol* 1998; **33**, 241–247.

9. Nygaard J. Prevention of exercise incontinence with mechanical devices. *J Reprod Med* 1995; **40**, 90–95.

10. Hannestad Y. S., Lie R., Rorveit G., Hunskaar S. Familial risk of urinary incontinence in women: population based cross sectional study. *Br Med J* 2004; **329**, 889–891, doi:10.1136/bmj.329.7471.889.

11. Wallace S. A., Roe B., Williams K., Palmer M. Bladder training for urinary incontinence in adults. *Cochrane Rev Abstr* 2004, http://www.mrw.interscience.wiley.com/cochrane/clsysrev/articles/CD001308/frame.html, accessed 12/3/06.

12. Hay-Sith E. J. C., Dumoulin C. Pelvic floor muscle training versus no treatment, or inactive control treatments, for urinary incontinence in women. *Cochrane Rev Abstr* 2006, http://www.mrw.interscience.wiley.com/cochrane/clsysrev/articles/CD005654/frame.html, accessed 12/3/06.

13. Bjelic-Radisic V., Dorfer M., Greimel E., Frudinger A., Tamussino K., Winter R. Quality of life and continence 1 year after the tension-free vaginal tape operation. *Am J Obstet Gynecol* 2006; **185**(6), 1784–1788.

14. Seim A., Siversetsen B., Ericksen B. C., Hunskaar S. Treatment of urinary incontinence in women in general practice: obstervational study. *Br Med J* 1996; **312**, 1459–1462.

15. Lapitan M. C., Cody D. J., Grant A. M. Open retropubic colposuspension for urinary incontinence in women. *Cochrane Database Syst Rev* 2003; 1, CD002912.

16. Miller J. M., Ashton-Miller J. A., Delancey J. O. L. A pelvic muscle precontraction can reduce cough related urine loss in selected women with mild SUI. *J Am Geriatr Soc* 1998; **46**, 870–874.

17. Brubaker L., Benson J. H., Bent A., Clark A., Shott S. Transvaginal electrical stimulation for female urinary incontinence. *Am J Obstet Gynecol* 1997; **177**, 536–540.

18. Alhasso A., Glazener C. M. A., Pickard R., N'Dow J. Adrenergic drugs for urinary incontinence in adults. *Cochrane Rev* 2005, http://www.mrw.interscience.wiley.com/cochrane/clsysrev/articles/CD001842/frame.htm, accessed 12/5/06.

19. Dmochowski R. R., Starkman J. S., Davila G. W. Transdermal drug delivery treatment for overactive bladder. *Int Braz J Urol* 2006; **32**(5), 513–520.

20. Wag A., Wyndaele J. J., Sieber P. Efficacy and tolerability of solifenacin in elderly subjects with overactive bladder syndrome: a pooled analysis. *Am J Geriatr Pharmacother* 2006; **4**(1), 14–24.

21. Mariappan P., Ballantyne Z., N'Dow J., Alhasso A. A. Serotonin and noradrenaline reuptake inhibitors (SNRI) for stress urinary incontinence in adults. *Cochrane Rev* 2005, http://www.mrw.interscience.wiley.com/cochrane/clsysrev/articles/CD004742/frame.htm, accessed 12/5/06.

22. Hendrix S. L., Cochrane B. B., Nygaard I. E. Effects of estrogen with and without progestin on urinary incontinence. *J Am Med Assoc* 2005; **293**(8), 935–948.

23. Dean N. M., Ellis G., Wilson P. D., Herbison G. P. Laparoscopic colposuspension for urinary incontinence in women. *Cochrane Rev Abstr*, http://www.mrw.interscience.wiley.com/cochrane/clsysrev/articles/CD002239/frame.html, accessed 12/9/06.

24. Leach G. E., Dmochowski R. R., Appell R. A., *et al.* Female stress urinary incontinence clinical guidelines panel summary report on surgical management of female stress urinary incontinence. *J Urol* 1997; **158**, 875–880.

25. Stamm W. E., Hooton T. M., Johnson J. R., *et al.* Urinary tract infections from pathogenesis to treatment. *J Infect Dis* 1989: **159**, 400–406.

26. Meares E. M. Current patterns in nosocomial urinary tract infections. *Urology* 1991; **37**, S9–S12.

27. Jackson S. L., Boyko E. J., Scholes D., Abraham L., Gupta K., Fihn S. D. Predictors of urinary tract infection after menopause: a prospective study. *Am J Med* 2004; **117**(12), 903–911.

28. Boyko E. J., Fihn S. D., Scholes D., Chen C. L., Normand E. H., Yarbro P. Diabetes and the risk of acute urinary tract infection among postmenopausal women. *Diabetes Care* 2002; **25**(10), 1778–1783.

29. Ribera M. C., Pascual R., Orozco D., Perez Barba C., Pedrera V., Gil V. Incidence and risk factors associated with urinary tract infection in diabetic patients with and without asymptomatic bacteriuria. *Eur J Clin Microbiol Infect Dis* 2006; **25**(6), 389–393.

30. Ooi S. T., Frazee L. A., Gardner W. G. Management of asymptomatic bacteriuria in patients with diabetes mellitus. *Ann Pharmacother* 2004; **38**(3), 490–493.

31. Harding G. K., Zhanel G. G., Nicolle L. E., Cheang M. Manitoba diabetes urinary tract infection study group. Antimicrobial treatment in diabetic women with asymptomatic bacteriuria. *N Engl J Med* 2002; **347**(20), 1576–1583.

32. Raz R., Gennesin Y., Wasser J., Stoler Z., Rosenfeld S., Rottensterich E., Stamm W. E. Recurrent urinary tract

203

infections in postmenopausal women. *Clin Infect Dis* 2000; **30**(1), 152–156.

33. Nys S., van Merode T., Bartelds A. I., Stobberingh E. E. Urinary tract infections in general practice patients: diagnostic tests versus bacteriological culture. *J Antimicrob Chemother* 2006; **57**(5), 955–8.

34. Grude N., Tveten Y., Jenkins A., Kristiansen B. E. Uncomplicated urinary tract infections. Bacterial findings and efficacy of empirical antibacterial treatment. *Scand J Prim Health Care* 2005; **23**(2), 115–119.

35. Talan D. A., Klimberg I. W., Nicolle L. E., Song J., Kowalsky S. F., Church D. A. Once daily, extended release ciprofloxacin for complicated urinary tract infections and acute uncomplicated pyelonephritis. *J Urol* 2004; **171**(2 Pt 1), 734–739.

36. Rosenfeld J. A. Radiologic abnormalities in women admitted with pyelonephritis. *Del Med J* 1987; **59**, 717–718.

37. Raz R., Bogert S. Long term prophylaxis with norfloxacin versus nitrofurantoin in women with recurrent urinary tract infection. *Antimicrob Agents Chemother* 1991; **35**, 1241–1242.

38. Melekos M. D., Asbach H. W., Gerharz E., *et al.* Post intercourse versus daily ciprofloxacin prophylaxis for recurrent urinary tract infection in premenopausal women. *J Urol* 1997; **157**, 935–939.

Benign breast disease

Jo Ann Rosenfeld

Benign breast disease includes mastalgia, fibrocystic breast disease, breast cellulites and abscesses, nipple discharges, and galactorrhea. Although benign breast disease is much more common than breast cancer, the specter of breast cancer is so overwhelming that the primary evaluation of the woman is to eliminate cancer as the cause quickly and adequately. Benign breast disease occurs in women age 20–50 and declines after menopause, whereas the incidence of breast cancer continues to increase with age.[1]

Surgeons have been the primary researchers; again little research has been accomplished comparing non-surgical to surgical evaluations, or adequately evaluating non-surgical evaluations. Little new research has been accomplished in the last five years.

Mastalgia

1. Breast pain (mastalgia) may be unilateral (75%) or bilateral, continuous or intermittent, related to the menstrual cycle (40%) or associated with a mass.[2] Breast pain alone was the presenting complaint in 15–50% of women attending breast clinics.[3]
2. How often pain is associated with breast cancer is uncertain. Breast pain was the presenting complaint of 5–24% of women with operable breast cancer in "surgical breast clinics"[4] (a population that may be skewed). A recent 20-year cohort study in France of 247 women with cyclic mastalgia who did not use hormones found that the risk of cancer increased with the length of time they complained of cyclic mastalgia. Women who had cyclic mastalgia for more than three years were five times more likely to develop cancer.[5]
3. Women who develop pain with a mass should have the mass evaluated first. Breast masses in

women age 50 or younger usually are benign but need evaluation (Figure 19.1).

Non-cyclic mastalgia without a mass

1. One-fourth of all women with breast pain have non-cyclic pain, unrelated to the menstrual cycle. Women who have non-cyclic breast pain and no mass are unlikely to have breast cancer.
2. Mammography of women with breast pain and no mass is usually normal and reassuring. In one large observational study of more than 6500 women with mastalgia only, 85% had normal mammograms, 9% had benign findings, and only 1% had suspicious or malignant findings.[6]
3. If mammography is normal and there is no mass, biopsy of the painful area is not needed. Cautious follow-up is necessary.
4. The best treatment for non-cyclic pain has not been well investigated. Treatment includes NSAIDS, heat, and firm support with a bra. If the symptoms do not improve, treatment with drugs for cyclic pain is suggested.

Cyclic pain

1. Cyclic pain usually occurs with the beginning of menses, usually improves after menses ends, and is relieved after menopause. It is often caused hormonally and often associated with fibrocystic breast disease (FBD). Cyclic pain is often bilateral and associated with nodularity on physical examination.[1]
2. Cyclic pain is not affected by OCPs or pregnancy. Sometimes OCPs relieve the pain.

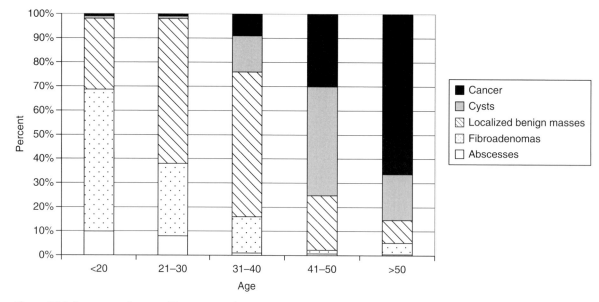

Figure 19.1 Percentage of causes of breast masses by age.

Table 19.1 Treatments for cyclic breast pain

Oral contraceptives and other hormonal contraception

Evening primrose oil (gamma linolenic acid)

Danazol (danocrine)

Tamoxifen

3. **Treatment**

Only a few clinical trials have examined treatments for cyclic breast pain. To determine whether therapy is effective, evaluation for several months is necessary. Nonetheless, treatment resolved or improved pain in some studies in 70–80% of patients[7] (Table 19.1).

a. OCPs have been used to reduce pain and nodularity. No one OCP is more likely to cure mastalgia than any other. In one small study, approximately 50% of women found relief of pain with use of OCP. Concerns about adversely affecting occult breast cancer often keep OCPs from use.

b. Neither progestins nor diuretics have been proven to relieve pain.[1]

c. One medicine used in the UK (but not approved in the USA, although available over the counter) is evening primrose oil (EPO) (gamma linolenic acid). Taken as 40 mg twice a day EPO may elevate levels of prostaglandin 1 and suppress inflammation.[8] A more recent multicenter study of 555 women found that EPO worked no better than placebo fatty acids in reducing pain.[9]

d. Danazol (200–300 mg daily) can be tried; women on this drug should not also take OCPs and should use other non-hormonal contraceptive methods. More than 30% of women suffer significant side effects including nausea and vomiting, amenorrhea, weight gain, acne, and hirsuitism. Danazol must be used for three months before its full effect can be determined.

e. Tamoxifen, used for breast cancer treatment, has been shown effective in 98% of women with cyclic mastalgia at 10 mg daily.[10]

Fibrocystic breast disease
Impact

1. FBD is the most common benign breast disease. As many as 19% of women may have cysts.[11]

2. FBD is worrisome because it makes breast cancer more difficult to detect.

3. Whether FBD leads to breast cancer is uncertain. A 15-year study of approximately 9000 women diagnosed with benign breast disease at the Mayo Clinic found that FBD was associated with an increased risk of breast cancer (RR = 1.56).

However, in the 67% of women who had "non-proliferative" lesions, and who had no family history of breast cancer, there was no increased risk.[12]

Symptoms

1. FBD can be asymptomatic, discovered on routine mammography, or may present as symptomatic mastalgia occurring in the last half of the menstrual cycle and during menses or as breast masses.
2. FBD starts as microcysts and accompanying fibrosis in 65% of women.[13] The cysts become larger as the woman ages, and can reach 3 to 4 cm. It is usually bilateral. There may be associated chronic inflammation, ductal ectasia, and nipple discharge.
3. Cysts usually start at age 35 and increase between the ages of 40 and 50.
4. Pain usually subsides after menses, and cysts usually disappear post menopause. They are rare in postmenopausal women.

Treatment

1. Many treatments have been suggested, with little evidence as to their efficacy.
2. Many observational studies have suggested improvement in fibrocystic disease with elimination of caffeine and chocolate, and cessation of cigarette smoking and alcohol use. However, case-controlled studies of women with fibrocystic disease and caffeine elimination have not shown improvement in pain or nodularity.[14]
3. Although studies have not shown any significant improvement in pain, diuretics have often been prescribed.
4. Use of hormonal contraceptive can help by reducing the hormonal cycling, but usually only after 12–24 months use. OCPs with higher progesterone levels may have a more beneficial effect.
5. Danazol and gonadotropin releasing hormone analogs have been used but are not approved and have not been shown to be effective.
6. Surgical treatment, either needle aspiration of the larger cysts or excision of masses, may be needed.

Infection – mastitis and abscesses

Symptoms

1. Breast infections are common in women who are breast feeding. Mastitis (breast cellulitis) occurs in approximately 2% of breast-feeding women.[15]
2. Breast infections can affect the skin, producing a primary cellulitis, or may be secondary to an infection of a sebaceous gland, axillary gland, or lymph node, such as in hidradenitis supparativa. Most mastitis occurs in breast-feeding women.
3. The symptoms of cellulitis in the breast are the same as cellulitis elsewhere, except that mastitis spreads more quickly. The breast will become hot, bright red, exquisitely tender, and very swollen. There may be a green or pus-like nipple discharge.
4. The woman may have fever, chills, vomiting, malaise, and an elevated white blood cell count.
5. If she has an abscess, there may be a fluctuant localized area. At times, multiple abscesses occur in the sebaceous and sweat glands of the axillae, and these usually do not involve breast tissue.

Treatment

1. The organisms that cause mastitis are gram-positive bacteria, either *Streptococcus* or *Staphylococcus aureus*. *S. aureus* is the cause of infection in most breast-feeding women.
2. Treatment must be started quickly with a bactericidal antibiotic that covers gram-positive organisms; this will decrease abscess formation. However, the treatment can be started orally. Amoxicillin/clavulanate (Augmentin) 375–500 mg tid, cephalaxein (500 mg qid), or dicloxacillin would be good choices. Ciprofloxacin, tetracyclines and sulfa drugs should be avoided in breast-feeding women. For penicillin allergic breast-feeding patients, cephalexein, azithromycin or erythromycin can be used. Metronidazole (200 mg tid) should be added in penicillin allergic women who have breast infections and are not breast feeding (Table 19.2). Treatment should be continued for 7–10 days.
3. However, in many places methicillin-resistant *Staphylococcus aureus* bacteria are becoming a greater problem.[16] Starting therapy with oral clindamycin, trimethoprim/sulfa, or doxycycline,

Table 19.2 Causes of galactorrhea

Physiological	Breast feeding, pregnancy, weaning
Exogenous hormones	OCPs, depot provera, HRT
Medication side effects	Antipsychotics (see Table 19.3)
Chronic systemic	Diseases renal failure, Cushing's, etc.
Hormonal imbalances	Thyroid or pituitary abnormal secretion of hormones
Pituitary prolactinomas	
Brain prolactinomas	Craniopharyngiomas, etc.

Table 19.3 Medications that can cause galactorrhea

Phenothiazines, antiemetics

H2 receptor blockers – cimetidine, famotidine, ranitidine

Antihypertensives – methyl dopa, atenolol, reserpine, verapamil

Hormones – OCPs, depot medroxyprogesterone

Meclopromide

Herbs – fenugreek seed, blessed thistle, fennel, nettle, marsmallow, red clover, red reaspberry

CNS drugs

    Amphetamines

    Anesthetics

    Antidepressants (especially SSRIs, sertoline)

    Antipsychotics (clonazepine, resperidone)

    Benzodiazepines

    Butyropherones

    Cannabis

    Opioids

as suggested by local sensitivities may be more appropriate.

4. The most important part of oral treatment is close re-evaluation. The woman should be seen the next day. If the cellulitis is not improving, intravenous antibiotics may be needed.

5. If the woman is dehydrated, vomiting, has diabetes or an immunosuppressive disease or medication, or worsens on oral antibiotics, hospitalization with IV antibiotics are needed. Ampicillin/sulbactam (Unisyn), a first- or third-generation cephalosporing, clindamycin, or vancomycin may be needed.

6. Heat should be used 20 minutes four times a day.

7. Pain medication may be needed.

8. Whether the woman should stop breast-feeding is disputed. Some experts suggest the woman should pump her infected breast and discard the infected milk.

9. If there is an associated breast mass, it should be investigated by radiological examination and/or biopsy after the infections resolve.

Abscess

1. Most abscesses occur in breast-feeding women within the first month postpartum or at weaning.

2. Patients with abscesses should have them drained surgically. The woman should be placed on oral antibiotics as suggested above. The woman should pump the affected breast and discard the milk.

Non-lactational infections or abscess

1. If infection occurs in someone who is neither breast feeding nor having pathological or physiological galactorrhea, the suspicion of ductal or inflammatory infection must be considered.

2. Subareolar abscesses are often related to ductal ectasia, caused by a variety of organisms and related to cigarette smoking. Peripheral abscesses are usually caused by *S. aureus*, are in older women and are treated by drainage. Ultrasonography may be used to delineate the abscess and guide the surgical drainage.

3. After resolution of the infection, mammography is needed for evaluation. Conservative treatment has included obligatory biopsy of the abscess wall. A more recent retrospective study of approximately 200 women with breast abscesses found cancer in fewer than 5%. Drainage, usually ultrasound-guided, may be sufficient without biopsy.[17]

Nipple discharges

1. Although most nipple discharges are benign, the importance of evaluating nipple discharges is that

between 10 and 25% of nipple discharges that are not galactorrhea are caused by cancer, specifically ductal carcinomas. The prevalence of cancer with nipple discharges is difficult to determine because most studies were surgical (women referred for surgery or biopsy), the population is skewed, and the data are retrospective. Retrospective studies suggest that approximately 9% of women with nipple discharges have cancer. The most common causes are benign papillomas and ductal ectasia.[18]

2. Since most nipple discharges are caused by benign processes, knee-jerk treatment such as mastectomy or excision of tissue under the nipple (microdochectomy) is not universally indicated. To reduce the need for surgical excision, investigation into which nipple discharges are at high risk of cancer has occurred. Lack of research and the infrequency of nipple discharge hamper discovering the answers. No new research has been published in the last three years.

3. One recent retrospective study of approximately 200 women who had excisional treatment over 14 years found that only 4.3% had carcinoma and another 4% had carcinoma *in situ*. Forty percent of the women had diagnosis of papilloma and approximately 50% had other benign lesions. Only women with a bloody discharge had cancer. Women with non-bloody discharges may not need excision. However a prospective study is needed.[19]

4. Nipple discharges are the third most common complaint concerning 5% of women attending breast clinics.[20]

Symptoms

1. Nipple discharges may be from one breast or bilateral, from one duct or more, intermittent, spontaneous or continuous, or related to a mass or soreness.

2. Women who have a discharge from one breast or only one duct are more likely to have cancer than women who have discharges from both breast or have multiductal discharges.

3. Discharges associated with a breast mass are more likely to be related to cancer.

4. Discharges that are spontaneous and not provoked are more likely to be pathological. In one large retrospective study of 243 women with spontaneous nipple discharges, 30% had carcinoma, as compared to 3% with provoked discharge.[20]

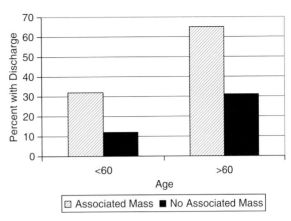

Figure 19.2 Percentage of women with cancer who present with nipple discharge by age and presence of a mass. Data from Fiorica J. V. Nipple discharge. *Obstet Gynecol Clin North Am* 1994; **21**, 453–460.

5. Nipple discharges in postmenopausal women are more serious. Discharges in women older than age 60 are more than twice as likely to be caused by cancer[21] (Figure 19.2).

6. Nipple discharges can be classified as one of seven colors: yellow, bloody (red), pink, multicolored (gray, black, or brown), clear, purulent, or white. The color is related to the risk of malignancy (Figure 19.3).

   a. Yellow or green-black discharges are often caused by ductal ectasia and are rarely caused by cancer. Ectasia usually produces spontaneous multiple duct discharge. This is a non-inflammatory self-limited condition.

   b. Bilateral multiductal white discharges are usually milk and the woman will need an evaluation for galactorrhea. Examination of the discharge under the microscope will show fat globules.

   c. Purulent discharges are consistent with infections.

   d. Clear discharges are rare, serious, usually pathological, and may be associated with ductal carcinoma *in situ*. Between one-third and one-half of women with clear discharges have cancer.

   e. Bloody, pink, or serosanguinis discharges must be considered pathological. Up to 25% may be caused by cancer. These women are at higher risk and need a surgical diagnosis.

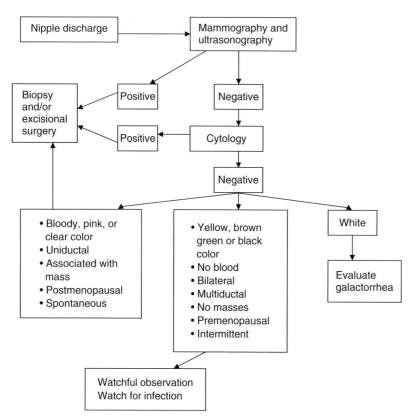

Figure 19.3 Evaluation of woman with nipple discharge.

Diagnosis

1. There are no specific guidelines to investigate nipple discharge.
2. The discharge may be caused by cancer even with normal mammography and cytology. Some studies have considered cytology useless. These studies are helpful if positive, but a negative study does not exclude cancer.
3. Mammography and ultrasonography are necessary. If positive, excisional biopsy is needed.
4. Nipple aspirate fluid (NAF) can be sent for cytological examination. Recent studies have suggested that red-brown NAF was significantly associated with the presence of cancer.[22]
5. Ductography or galactography, injection of dye into a duct, is painful and does not reliably exclude cancerous lesions, although it may outline a fibroma or papilloma.
6. Recently, ductoscopy has been used to locate and detect abnormal lesions. Its sensitivity and effectiveness is not well determined yet. However, its use increased the sensitivity of excision of abnormal masses.[23]

7. In a woman with spontaneous, continuous, and unilateral discharge, or a postmenopausal woman, biopsy or surgical excision should be considered.
8. If the woman is premenopausal, has negative studies, and a non-bloody discharge, then cautious waiting without biopsy may be considered.

Galactorrhea
Impact

1. Galactorrhea, milk discharge when not breast feeding, is a relatively common symptom, reported by 15–40% of women.
2. The woman may be completely unaware of the discharge or anxiety ridden and concerned about malignancy.
3. The woman may also have menstrual disorders, such as amenorrhea or oligomenorrhea, or symptoms of an intracranial mass, such as visual disturbances or headaches. Sexual disorders, especially in women on antipsychotics, are common.

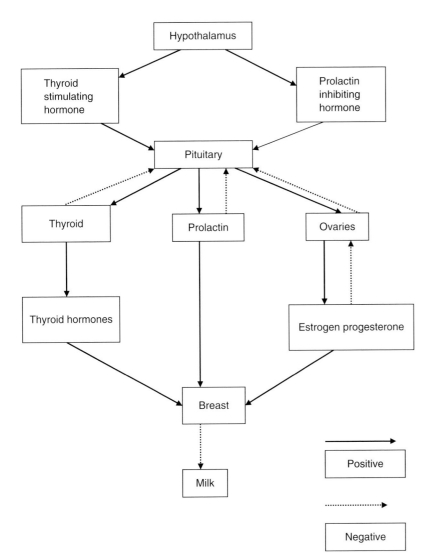

Figure 19.4 Milk production.

Etiology

1. Fourteen percent of women with galactorrhea have physiological causes, such as unrecognized pregnancy, being postpartum, hormone use, and breast stimulation[24] (Table 19.2). Prolactin production is inhibited by prolactin-inhibiting factor produced in the pituitary and has an involved feedback system (Figure 19.4).

2. Twenty percent of galactorrhea is caused by medication use (Table 19.3). Approximately 15–32% of women using antipsychotic medications report galactorrhea.[24]

3. Systemic diseases, such as chronic renal failure, hypothyroidism, Cushing disease and acromegaly, cause approximately 10% of all cases of galactorrhea.

4. Tumors such as prolactinomas of the pituitary and non-pituitary non-prolactinomas such as craniopharyngiomas cause about 18%. These tumors cause hyperprolactinemia, and thus, galactorrhea.

   a. Approximately 20% of women with galactorrhea have radiologically evident brain tumors and the incidence increases to 34% among women who also have amenorrhea.[25]

   b. The most common tumor causing hyperprolactinemia is the pituitary prolactinomas. Women with prolactin levels higher than 200 ng/mL and amenorrhea are more likely to have prolactinomas.

 c. Most women with these tumors do well. Either they regress or remain stable for many years, and most can be treated medically.

 d. Non-pituitary malignancies such as bronchogenic carcinoma, renal adenocarcinoma, Hodgkin's lymphomas, and T-cell lymphomas can cause hyperprolactinemia.

5. Diseases that affect the hypothalamic and pituitary areas such as sarcoidosis, tuberculosis, histocytosis, and multiple sclerosis can cause galactorrhea.

6. Chest-wall irritation such as caused by burns or herpes zoster can cause galactorrhea.

7. As many as 35% of women with galactorrhea have no discernable reason and are considered "idiopathic."

Diagnosis

1. Physical examination includes evaluation of the visual fields, thyroid, breast and skin, and evaluation for the presence and quality of the nipple discharge.

2. Laboratory studies include serum pregnancy test, prolactin levels, thyroid-stimulating hormone and thyroid hormone levels.

3. Because stress and breast stimulation can cause elevated prolactin levels, blood should not be drawn until one hour after breast examination.

4. If the prolactin level is borderline, repeat evaluations are indicated, because prolactin levels can vary during the day.

5. A prolactin level greater than 200 ng/mL is almost always associated with a prolactinoma or prolactin-secreting tumor. CT or MRI of the head is indicated.

6. If the patient has amenorrhea or oligomenorrhea, even with a normal prolactin level, a MRI of the head is indicated.

7. If a woman with galactorrhea has normal menses and a normal prolactin level, the likelihood she has a pituitary adenoma is very low and MRI of the head is not necessary.

8. A mammogram is not needed unless physical examination reveals breast abnormalities.

Treatment

1. Any primary disease, such as hyperthyroidism, should be treated first.

2. If the woman is on a medication that is causing significant or bothersome galactorrhea, it should be changed, if possible.

3. Patients with idiopathic or physiological galactorrhea and normal prolactin levels should be reassured.

4. Because hyperprolactinemia can also cause bone density loss, women with high prolactin levels and normal MRI scans can be treated medically indefinitely. Women with microoprolactinomas can be treated medically. Bromocriptine (1.25 to 2.5 mg 2–3 times a day) or cabergoline (dostinex, a dopamine-like agent, twice a week) which is better tolerated is used to decrease prolactin levels and reduce the incidence of bone density loss. When on medication, prolactin levels should be obtained and the dose titrated. MRIs should be repeated every two years.

5. Women with prolactinomas may need surgery if they have headaches, visual changes, symptoms of intracranial masses, or a tumor greater than 1 cm. However, surgical cure rates are poor ranging only from 10–40%, with a recurrence rate of more than 80%. Radiation therapy is also an option if the woman cannot tolerate medication or surgery.

Conclusions

Breast disorders are common and benign. However, little recent rigorous research has offered evidence-based solutions to these problems. Most data and articles are more than 10 years old. Once malignancy is eliminated as a cause, hormones are the usual treatments for many of these problems. Galactorrhea is often physiological or caused by medication or treatable hormonal disorders.

References

1. Fitzgibbons P. L., Henson D. E., Hutter R. V. Benign breast changes and the risk for subsequent breast cancer: an update of the 1985 consensus statement. Cancer Committee of the College of American Pathologists. *Arch Pathol Lab Med* 1998; **120**, 1053–1055.

2. Hughes L. E., Mansel R. E., Webster D. I. T. *Benign Disorders and disease of the Breast*, 2nd edition, London: Saunders, 2000, pp. 94–121.

3. Dixon J. M., Mansel R. E. ABC of breast disease: symptom assessment and guidelines for referral. *Br Med J* 1994; **308**, 720–726.

4. River L., Silverstein J., Grout J., *et al.* Carcinoma of the breast: the diagnostic significance of pain. *Am J Surg* 1951; **82**, 213–215.

5. Plu-Bureau G., Le M. G., Sitruk-Ware R., Thalabard J. C. Cyclical mastalgia and breast cancer risk: results of a French cohort study. *Cancer Epidemiol Biomarkers Prev* 2006; **15**(6), 1209–1231.

6. Duijm L. E., Guit G. I., Hendricks J. C., Zaat J. O., Mali W. P. Value of breast imaging in women with painful breasts. Observational follow-up study. *Br Med J* 1998; **317**, 1492–1495.

7. Gateley C. A., Miers M., Mansel R. E., Hughes L. E. Drug treatment for mastalgia. 17 years experience in the Cardiff mastalgia clinic. *J R Soc Med* 1992; **85**, 12–15.

8. Belch J. J., Hill A. Evening primrose oil and borage oil in rheumatologic conditions. *Am J Clin Nutr* 2000; **71**, 352S–356S.

9. Goyal A., Mansel R. E. Efamast Study Group. A randomized multicenter study of gamolenic acid (Efamast) with and without antioxidant vitamins and minerals in the management of mastalgia. *Breast J* 2005; **11**(1), 41–47.

10. Fentman J. S., Caleggi M., Brame D., *et al.* Double blind controlled trial of tamoxifen therapy for mastalgia. *Lancet* 1986; **1**, 287–288.

11. Guray M., Sahin A. A. Benign breast diseases: classification, diagnosis, and management. *Oncologist* 2006; **11**(5), 435–449.

12. Hartmann L. C., Sellers T. A., Frost M. H., *et al.* Benign breast disease and the risk of breast cancer. *N Engl J Med* 2005; **353**, 209–237.

13. Drukker B. H. Breast disease: a primer on diagnosis and management. *Int J Fertil* 1997; **43**, 278–287.

14. Lubin F., Ron E., Wax Y., *et al.* A case control study of caffeine and methyl xanthines in benign breast disease. *J Am Med Assoc* 1985; **253**, 2388–2392.

15. Scott-Conner C. E., Schoor S. J. The diagnosis and management of breast problems during pregnancy and lacation. *Am J Surg* 1995; **170**, 401–406.

16. King M. D., Humphrey B. J., Wang Y. F., Kourbatova E. V., Ray S. M., Blumberg H. M. Emergence of community-acquired methicillin-resistant *Staphylococcus aureus* USA 300 clone as the predominant cause of skin and soft-tissue infections. *Ann Intern Med* 2006; **144**(5), 309–317.

17. Scott B. G., Silberfein E. J., Pham H. Q., Feanny M. A., Lassinger B. K., Welsh F. J., Carrick M. M. Rate of malignancies in breast abscesses and argument for ultrasound drainage. *Am J Surg* 2006; **192**(6), 869–872.

18. Hussain A. N., Policarpio C., Vincent M. T. Evaluating nipple discharge. *Obstet Gynecol Surv* 2006; **61**(4), 278–283.

19. Dillon M. F., Mohd Nazri S. R., Nasir S., McDermott E. W., Evoy D., Crotty T. B., O'Higgins N., Hill A. D. The role of major duct excision and microdochectomy in the detection of breast carcinoma. *BMC Cancer* 2006; **6**, 164.

20. Hughes L. E. Nipple discharges. In Hughes L. E., Mansel R. E., Webstyer D. I. T. eds., *Benign Disorders and Disease of the Breast*, Philadelphia, PA: W. B. Saunders, 2000, pp. 171–186.

21. Fiorica J. V. Nipple discharge. *Obstet Gynecol Clin North Am* 1994; **21**, 453–460.

22. Sauter E. R., Winn J. N., Dale P. S., Wagner-Mann C. Nipple aspirate fluid color is associated with breast cancer. *Cancer Detect Prev* 2006; **30**(4), 320–328.

23. Moncrief R. M., Nayar R., Diaz L. K., Staradub V. L., Morrow M., Khan S. A. A comparison of ductoscopy-guided and conventional surgical excision in women with spontaneous nipple discharge. *Ann Surg* 2005; **241**(4), 575–581.

24. Thangavelu K., Geetanjali S. Menstrual disturbance and galactorrhea in people taking conventional antipsychotic medications. *Exp Clin Psychopharmacol* 2006; **14**(4), 459–460.

25. Edge D., Segatore M. Assessment and maganement of galactorrhea. *Nurse Pract* 1993; **18**, 35–49.

213

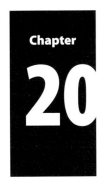

Chapter

20 Breast cancer screening

Abenaa Brewster, Nancy Davidson and Jo Ann Rosenfeld

Impact

1. Breast cancer is the most common occurring cancer in women, and the second most common cause of cancer death. In 2006, there were approximately 213,000 cases of invasive breast cancer in the USA, and 41,000 deaths,[1] causing nearly one in three cancers in women (Figure 20.1).
2. The risk of having breast cancer increases with age.
3. A woman's lifetime risk of being diagnosed with breast cancer is 13% and her lifetime risk of dying from cancer is 3.4%.
4. The incidence of breast cancer has continued to increase only in white women age 50 and older, whereas the incidence has stabilized in African American women from 1987 to 2002 in the USA.
5. Recent data reported a sudden and significant reduction in identification of breast cancer in 2005; the relevance and causes of this reduction have not been established. Some experts suggest that the sudden and significant decrease in use of hormone replacement therapy (HRT) after the results of the Women's Health Initiative were published has caused this decrease.

Primary prevention

1. The goal of the primary prevention of breast cancer is to avert the development of cancer in healthy women.
2. Modification or reduction of risk factors may help. However, most risk factors are not modifiable. Risk factors include younger age at menarche, familial history of breast cancer, nulliparity, late menopause, history of breast atypia, radiation exposure, and a previous history of breast cancer.

Familial breast cancer

1. Familial breast cancer accounts for fewer than 10% of all breast cancers. Multiple family members will be affected, at an early age and often bilateral.
2. The major genes that increase breast cancer susceptibility are BRCA1 and 2. In the group of women with breast cancer, approximately 3% will have mutations in BRCA1.
3. Women who carry the BRCA1 or 2 mutation have a lifetime risk of 56–87% of breast cancer, and an elevated risk for ovarian cancer.

Lifestyle risk factors

1. Cessation of use of HRT is one major modifiable risk factor to reduce breast cancer. The National Women's Health Initiative found that HRT users (estrogen + progesterone) had a higher risk of developing breast cancer, even within 6 years of the shortened study, when compared to non-users. Non-users had a 24% lower incidence of invasive breast cancer. The adjusted hazard risk rate was 1.96. A "safe" period of HRT use could not be defined. Relatively short courses of HRT (one year or less) were associated with an increased number of abnormal mammograms, and breast cancers discovered at a later or more advanced stage.
2. Exercise lasting more than four hours a week has been associated with a risk reduction of 30–40%.
3. Obesity has been shown to be associated with a much greater risk of developing postmenopausal

Handbook of Women's Health, second edition, ed. Jo Ann Rosenfeld. Published by Cambridge University Press.
© Cambridge University Press 2009.

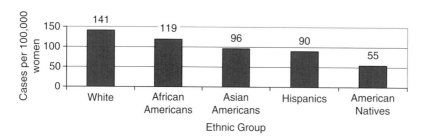

Figure 20.1 Incidence of breast cancer by ethnic group in 2006.

breast cancer, although whether weight loss reduces this risk is disputed.[2]

4. There is some evidence that increased alcohol use is associated with increased risks of breast cancer. However, stopping alcohol has not been found to decrease the risk.

Chemoprophylaxis

1. Medications such as tamoxifen and raloxifene prevent development of breast cancer by interrupting the process of initiation and promotion of tumor. The antiestrogenic effects of these agents lead to growth inhibition of malignant cells.[3]

   a. Tamoxifen is a non-steroidal antiestrogen with a partial estrogen agonist effect. It is FDA approved for use in women at an increased risk for breast cancers, although it has increased risk for endometrial cancer and thromboembolic disease. It is also approved for use as an adjuvant chemotherapy agent in the prevention of recurrence of breast cancer.

   b. Three placebo RCTs investigated whether tamoxifen can prevent the development of breast cancer in women who are at high risk for the disease. The Breast Cancer Prevention Trial enrolled approximately 14,000 women age 60 and older and women age 35–39 who were at high risk or had had lobular cancer *in situ*. At 69 months follow-up, it found a 50% reduction in the incidence of estrogen receptor positive breast cancers in the group receiving 20 mg tamoxifen daily. Women over age 50 had a higher risk of developing stage I endometrial cancer and an increased rate of thromboembolic disease.[4]

   c. Raloxifene is a selective estrogen receptor modulator (SERM) that blocks the action of estrogen in the breast and endometrial tissue. The Multiple Outcomes of Raloxifene

Evaluation (MORE) trial followed more than 7700 women on raloxifene for osteoporosis. The incidence of estrogen receptor positive invasive breast cancer was reduced by 76% among women taking raloxifene.[5]

   d. The National Surgical Adjuvant Breast and Bowel Project Study of Tamoxifen and Raloxifene trial, was a double-blind RCT that followed approximately 20,000 postmenopausal women who had an increased risk of breast cancer. It found that raloxifene was as effective as tamoxifen in preventing breast cancer with fewer side effects, including thromboembolic disease.[6]

   e. Further studies have found that raloxifene did not increase or affect the risk of coronary heart disease, while it reduced the incidence of invasive breast cancer ($RR = 0.56$) However, there was an increased rate of fatal stroke ($RR = 1.49$) and deep venous thrombosis ($RR = 1.44$) and a decreased risk of clinical vertebral fractures ($RR = 0.65$).[7]

   f. Decisions regarding their use must remain highly individualized, considering both risks and benefits.

Secondary prevention: screening for breast cancer

1. The goal of screening women for breast cancer is to detect cancer in its earliest stage when surgery and medical treatment can be most effective, resulting in improvement in morbidity and mortality.

2. Screening for breast cancer can lead to the detection of preinvasive lesions such as ductal carcinoma *in situ* (DCIS) and early small node-negative cancers, whose treatments carry a good prognosis and a reduction in mortality.

3. Screening does reduce mortality. A Swedish study found a 44% decrease in deaths as a result of

widespread mammographic screening.[8] For women age 40 to 49, the decrease of mortality from screening was 48%.

Mammography

1. Mammography reduces the mortality of breast cancer. The Health Insurance Plan Breast Cancer Screening Project in 1963, and at least seven subsequent RCTs (with an average follow-up of 10 years) established that, with or without clinical breast examination (CBE), there was a significant reduction in breast cancer mortality in the group of women who had mammography.

   a. Comparison of two women populations in France twenty years apart, found that with increased mammography, for women age 50 to 70, the tumors that were found were smaller, less advanced, and more likely to be curable.[9]

   b. Several studies have demonstrated a 20–30% reduction in breast cancer mortality for women older than age 50 who undergo regular mammography. A meta-analysis of mammography studies showed a statistically significant 26% reduction in breast cancer mortality at seven to nine years follow-up in women age 50 to 74.[10]

2. When to start mammography is still disputed. Early studies failed to show an improvement in breast cancer mortality in women age 40 to 49 from mammography. Later meta-analysis of follow-up data from these early RCTs showed a significant 18–30% mortality reduction with annual mammography in women age 40–49, although follow-up for more than 10 years was necessary.[11] A recent RCT in Wales (the AGE trial) found a small but significant reduction in mortality in breast cancer in those women age 40 to 49 who were in the group that received mammograms.[12]

3. As well, there has been an increase in breast cancer in women of younger ages, approximately more than threefold between 1953 through 1959 and 1993 through 1999.[13]

4. Fifty is an arbitrary age. Women who are premenopausal have fewer cancers and denser breasts, making mammography less sensitive and producing more false-positive results, requiring other X-rays, studies, and biopsies. Sometime around the time of menopause, but not at the arbitrary age 50, breasts become, on average, less dense, cancers are more likely to become obvious, and screening mammography more sensitive. Thus, when to start mammography has been decided by best data available.

5. The American Cancer Society suggests that women age 40 and older "have a screening mammogram every year, and should continue to do so for as long as they are in good health." The US Preventive Health Services Task Force (USPHSTF) concluded that, for women age 40 to 70, mammography every 12–23 months is proven beneficial in reducing mortality from breast cancer.[14]

6. Although the incidence of breast cancer increases with age, few studies have investigated the efficacy of mammography in women older than age 70.[15] In the large studies, too few women were older than age 70. The USPHSTF suggests that healthy women older than age 70 continue to have mammography. They suggest that the age to stop should be decided individually.

7. There are specific physical limitations of mammography that requires the woman to be able to sit or stand upright for seconds to minutes, unaided. Mammograms can be done sitting down or in a wheelchair.

8. Elderly women with several comorbidities and a limited life expectancy may not experience the benefit of mammography screening.

9. More women are using mammography in the last 20 years. The percentage of white women who report having a mammogram increased from 30% in 1987 to 71% in 2003, while use by African American women increased from 24% to 70%[16] (Figure 20.2).

Breast self-examination

1. Breast self-examination (BSE) is used by itself and as an adjuvant method with clinical breast exam (CBE) and mammography.

2. Large randomized control studies (RCTs) in China, the UK, and Russia found no improvement in mortality in women who used BSE only. BSE use did not decrease either the number or size of breast cancers discovered.[17,18]

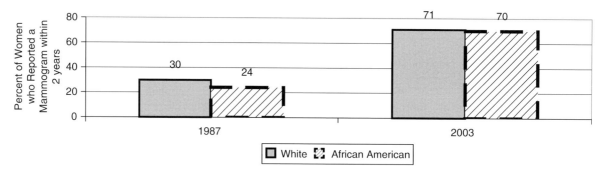

Figure 20.2 Rates of use of mammography (within two years). Data from Swan J., Breen N., Coates R. J., *et al.* Progress in cancer screening practices in the United States: results from the 2000 National Health Interview Survey. *Cancer* 2003; **97**, 1528–1540.

3. The Canadian Task Force on Preventive Health Care in 2001 concluded that teaching or advocating BSE is more harmful than helpful. BSE leads to a significant increase in office visits and false-positives that require biopsy.[19]

Other radiological examinations

1. Recent studies have suggested that other radiological examinations may not only add to the diagnosis of beast cancer but may someday replace mammography because of increased accuracy.

2. In women at high risk for breast cancer because of genetic syndromes, MRI of the breast was found to be more sensitive than mammography alone.[20] Using multiple modes of evaluation in high-risk populations has been rigorously suggested.

Conclusion

Breast cancer is one of the most common cancers in women. Screening and prevention are possible, and the incidence of breast cancer is decreasing.

References

1. Smigal C., Jemal A., Ward E., *et al.* Trends in breast cancer by race and ethnicity: update 2006. *CA Cancer J Clin* 2006; **56**, 168–183.

2. McTiernan A. Risk factors in breast cancer: can risk be modified? *Oncologist* 2003; **8**(4), 326–334.

3. Geller B. A., Vogel V. G. Chemoprevention of breast cancer in postmenopausal women. *Breast Dis* 2005–2006; **24**, 79–92.

4. Fisher B., Constantino J., Wiickerham L., *et al.* Tamoxifen for the prevention of breast cancer. *J Nat Cancer Inst* 1998; **90**, 1371–1388.

5. Ettinger B., Black D. M., Mitlak B. H., *et al.* Reduction of vertebral fracture risk in postmenopausal women with osteoporosis treated with raloxifene. Multiple outcomes of raloxifene (MORE) investigators. *J Am Med Assoc* 1999; **202**, 637–646.

6. Vogel V. G., Costantino J. P., Wickerham D. L., *et al.*, National Surgical Adjuvant Breast and Bowel Project (NSABP). Effects of tamoxifen vs raloxifene on the risk of developing invasive breast cancer and other disease outcomes: the NSABP Study of Tamoxifen and Raloxifene (STAR) P-2 trial. *J Am Med Assoc* 2006; **295**(23), 2727–2741.

7. Barrett-Connor E., Mosca L., Collins P., Raloxifene Use for The Heart (RUTH) Trial Investigators. Effects of raloxifene on cardiovascular events and breast cancer in postmenopausal women. *N Engl J Med* 2006; **355**(2), 125–137.

8. Tabar L., Yen M. F., Vitak B., Chen H. H., Smith R. A., Duffy S. W. Mammography service screening and mortality in breast cancer patients: 20-year follow-up before and after introduction of screening. *Lancet* 2003; **361**, 1405–1410.

9. Aubard Y., Genet D., Eyraud J. L., Impact of screening on breast cancer detection. Retrospective comparative study of two periods ten years apart. *Eur J Gynaecol Oncol* 2002; **23**(1), 37–41.

10. Kerlikowski D., Grady D., Rubin S., *et al.* Efficacy of screening mammography: a meta-analysis. *J Am Med Assoc* 1995; **273**, 149–154.

11. Hendrick E. R., Smith R., Rutledge J. H., *et al.* Benefit of screening mammography in women age 40–49: a new meta analysis of randomized controlled trial. *Monogr Natl Cancer Inst* 1997; **22**, 87–92.

12. Moss S. M., Cuckle H., Evans A., Johns L., Waller M., Bobrow L. Trial management group effect of mammographic screening from age 40 years on breast cancer mortality at 10 years' follow-up: a randomised controlled trial. *Lancet* 2006; **368**(9552), 2053–2060.

13. Trop I., Deck W. Should women 40 to 49 years of age be offered mammographic screening? *Can Fam Physician* 2006; **52**(9),1050–1052.

14. US Preventive Services Task Force Screening for Breast Cancer Release Date February 2002, http://www.ahrq.gov/clinic/uspstf/uspsbrca.htm, accessed 12/30/06.

15. Tabar L., Vitak B., Chen H. H., *et al.* The Swedish two-county trial twenty years later: updated mortality results and new insights from long-term followup. *Radiol Clin North Am* 2000; **38**(4), 625–651.

16. Swan J., Breen N., Coates R. J., *et al.* Progress in cancer screening practices in the United States: results from the 2000 National Health Interview Survey. *Cancer* 2003; **97**, 1528–1540.

17. Thomas D. B., Gao D. I., Self S. G., *et al.* Randomized trial of breast self examination in Shangai: methodology and preliminary results. *J Natl Cancer Inst* 1997; **89**, 355–365.

18. UK Trial of Early Detetion of Breast Cancer Group. 16 year mortality from breast cancer in the UK trial of early detection of breast cancer. *Lancet* 1999; **353**, 1909–1914.

19. Baxter N., Canadian Task Force on Preventive Health Care. Preventive health care, 2001 update: should women be routinely taught breast self-examination to screen for breast cancer. *Can Med Assoc J.* 2001; **164**(13), 1837–1846.

20. Trecate G., Vergnaghi D., Manoukian S., *et al.* MRI in the early detection of breast cancer in women with high genetic risk. *Tumori* 2006; **92**(6), 517–523.

Intimate partner violence against women

Sandra K. Burge

A 55-year-old woman came to see her family physician for a routine follow-up of her hypertension. After a brief conversation about symptoms, medications, and side effects, the physician prepared to test her blood pressure. As he placed the cuff around her arm, she sighed and said, "I know it's going to be high today. I didn't get much sleep last night." She paused. "We had a misunderstanding." The physician asked, "What do you mean by 'a misunderstanding'?" and she described her husband's rampage of the night before: after a night of heavy drinking, he stormed into the house at 2:00 a.m., yelling, demanding dinner, and smashing dishes against the wall when his wife did not move fast enough to suit him. The physician learned that the woman's husband had a pattern of terrorizing her, usually after drinking. Last Christmas, he threatened her with a shotgun. Recently, her adult son had joined the father in drinking and abusing her.

Introduction

1. Violence against women is widely prevalent, causes serious psychological and physical damage, and brings women to the attention of the health care system on a daily basis. Women account for 75% of all murdered spouses in the USA, and 85% of all assaulted partners.[1]

2. Thirty-nine percent of physically abused women receive injuries; about one in three who are injured require medical care.[2] The cost of intimate partner violence against women in the USA exceeds $8.3 billion in 2003 dollars, including $5.8 billion for direct costs of medical and mental health care.[1]

3. Primary health care providers are ideally positioned to intervene with intimate partner violence. Throughout their lives, women make frequent visits to primary health care providers – two or three visits per year, on the average – for help with acute and chronic health problems, for annual prevention exams, and for prenatal care.[3] Women also frequently accompany other family members for health care visits.

4. When women and health care providers establish sustained relationships, providers have the opportunity to understand the context of women's lives and to discover patterns of symptoms, behaviors and social situations that indicate the potential for abuse. Primary health care providers can contribute to violence prevention and intervention efforts through screening, patient education, counseling, support, and referral.

Definitions

1. Intimate partner violence is ". . . a pattern of assaultive and coercive behaviors that may include inflicted physical injury, psychological abuse, sexual assault, progressive social isolation, stalking, deprivation, intimidation and threats. These behaviors are perpetrated by someone who is, was, or wishes to be involved in an intimate or dating relationship with an adult or adolescent, and are aimed at establishing control by one partner over the other."[4]

2. Some authors call these acts spouse abuse, wife abuse, woman battering, or domestic violence when they are perpetrated by men toward women. In the chapter that follows, male perpetrators of intimate partner violence are sometimes referred to as "batterers." Female victims in violence are sometimes referred to as "battered women."

Incidence and prevalence

Incidence

1. Moderate levels of violence include grabbing, pushing, slapping, or throwing things with the intention of hitting the other. Population-based surveys find that the annual rate of man-to-woman violence among couples in the USA ranges from 1.5 to 15% each year.[2,5,6] Reports from the UK are similar, with 12% of women reporting intimate partner victimization within the past year.[7]

2. Severe levels of violence include punching, kicking, choking, or beating up one's partner, or threatening one with a knife or gun, or using weapons to harm the other. Severe violence occurs in about 3% of American couples each year.[6]

Prevalence

1. **In the population**

   According to population surveys, the lifetime prevalence of moderate or severe violence by men against women is approximately 21 to 25%.[2,6] Authors believe that these findings are a low estimate, and that the true prevalence could be twice as high.

2. **In ambulatory clinics**

   The prevalence of man-to-woman violence is similar in outpatient clinical settings, and may range as high as 54% in some populations.[8,9,10,11,12]

The nature of violent relationships

1. Why does intimate partner violence happen and persist? Several theories explain the etiology and maintenance of violent relationships, and research indicates that many factors operate to incite and reinforce man-to-woman aggression.

   a. Psychological theories focus on psychological aspects of men who batter and women who partner with them. Such theories posit that men who hurt their partners have a psychopathology that explains why they act in violent ways. Some have found that batterers' behavior is consistent with borderline personality disorder, alcohol or drug dependence, antisocial personality disorder, and/or depression.[13,14,15] Theories such as "learned helplessness" have been used to explain how these relationships are maintained, with victimization leading to depression and hopelessness in battered women, which in turn traps them in dangerous relationships.[16]

   b. Sociological theories posit that western society contains structures that support men who hit and suppress women who try to escape violent relationships. A structuralist approach contends that gender is a system that places women and men into unequal categories, roles, and occupations.[17] Women tend to marry men who are larger, stronger, and have access to more resources. Under this structure, men's opportunities and rewards for the use of violence are greater than women's. One sociologist found that state policies and structures predicted rates of woman battering in the USA. In states where women's status was lowest (as defined by political and socioeconomic indicators and laws that protect women), the rate of husband-to-wife violence was highest.[18]

   c. Social-psychological theories explain interactions between individual behaviors and interpersonal influences.

      i. Social learning theory states that children model behaviors seen in adult family members, and test them in their relationships with others. And research shows that key risk factors for becoming a perpetrator or victim of intimate partner violence are the childhood experiences of witnessing parental abuse or being abused by parents.[13,14]

      ii. Social exchange theory posits that violence occurs when the rewards of violence outweigh the consequences. When violence "works," i.e., it stops an argument or brings about another reward, that outcome reinforces the violent behavior, beginning a cycle of interactions that is very difficult to break.[15]

      iii. Theories of reasoned action and planned behavior understand behavioral intentions as necessary precursors to behavioral action. When applied to battered women, reasoned action states that women intend to stay or leave violent relationships depending on their outcome expectancies (costs and benefits) and social norms (influential social networks). Planned behavior states that women likely encounter internal and/or external barriers that prevent them from terminating their relationships, such as depression and lack of economic resources.[16]

2. **Types of violent relationships**

    Population research on intimate partner violence consistently reveals that men and women are equally likely to hit their partners in any given year.[2,5,6,17] Yet violence prevention professionals underscore the fact that men's violence does more damage than women's violence. Even when violence is "mutual," men use more physically damaging strategies and cause more fear and injuries in their partners.[17,18,19] The National Violence Against Women Study found that men were 7 to 14 times more likely than women to use these strategies on their intimate partners: beating up, choking, attempting to drown, threatening with a gun, using a gun.[2] One meta-analysis of 48 studies found that women were more likely than men to slap, kick, bite or punch, while men were more likely to beat up or choke their partners.

3. Michael Johnson noted that different populations portray different patterns of violence in intimate relationships.[20] For example, findings from research in battered women's shelters, emergency rooms, and law enforcement agencies show that couple violence is primarily men's aggression toward women. However, findings from population surveys indicate that women are just as likely as men to hit their partners, raising great controversy about who is the "real victim" in violent relationships. Johnson has concluded that three types of intimate partner violence exist: situational couple violence, intimate terrorism, and violent resistance.[21]

    a. "Situational couple violence," captured in population studies, is the most common type. It is characterized by occasional outbursts for the purpose of winning an argument, or controlling an immediate situation, but not exerting complete domination over the partner. In this type of relationship, both women and men hit their partners, and violent

behaviors tend to be of low severity and low frequency. One study showed an average of six assaults per year.[20] The hitting does not escalate over time, but remains stable. Women in this type of relationship are generally not afraid of their partners. To date, researchers know little about the exact nature of these relationships, or about etiology, risk factors, health consequences, or effective interventions.

    b. "Intimate terrorism" is the type of violence that sends women fleeing to battered women's shelters. In contrast to situational violence, this aggression is unidirectional, man-to-woman violence that escalates in severity and frequency over time. Intimate terrorism is characterized by a husband who is extremely dangerous and controlling. In addition to physical assaults, these men use strategies that function to control their partners' behaviors and to keep them in the relationship. For some, the hitting may be sporadic; however, the control is a constant force in a battering relationship. Even when infrequent, hitting reinforces the power of the following strategies.[22]

        i. **Intimidation**

            Batterers use threatening looks or gestures. They may destroy partners' property or pets, or brandish weapons.

        ii. **Coercion and threats**

            Batterers threaten to hurt their partners, or kill them or their families, or to leave them, or to report them to welfare or to immigration, or to commit suicide. They coerce their partners to drop charges against them. Some force their partners to do illegal things.

        iii. **Emotional abuse**

            Batterers insult their partners, call them names, embarrass or humiliate them in front of family and friends, and make them feel guilty, stupid, ugly, unlovable, or crazy. Batterers often treat their partners like children, doling out punishment when partners "misbehave."

iv. **Isolation**

Batterers control what their partners do, who they talk to, what they read, where they go. Batterers may use jealousy or guilt to limit their partners' interactions with others. They may create public scenes to alienate family or friends. They may withhold money or transportation from their partners to keep them at home.

v. **Minimizing, denying, and blaming**

Batterers deny responsibility for the abusive behavior, most often blaming the victim. "If only you would . . . then I wouldn't hit." The batterer may claim that the partner deserves to be hit. Batterers believe their behavior is less harmful than it really is: "I only pushed her; she's just clumsy." Some will make light of the violence, "I was just horsing around." Others will pretend it did not happen "I don't remember; I must have been drunk."

vi. **Using children**

Batterers make their partners feel guilty about care of the children. If separated, they will use visitation to gain access to the partner to bully or control them. And, batterers may threaten to take the children away or to harm them unless their partners cooperate.

vii. **Male privilege**

Batterers act like "king of the castle," treating their partners like servants, and making all the big decisions. A batterer will insist that family schedules and activities revolve around his priorities, and will expect everyone in the family to know and meet his needs, even if he has not spoken them.

viii. **Economic abuse**

Batterers limit their partners' employment outside the home. They control all the money, restrict the partners' spending, make the partner ask for money, and hide information about family finances from the partner.

c. "Violent resistance" is used by women in response to intimate terrorism.[21]

4. Who are the victims of intimate partner violence? While physical abuse happens under many social, economic, and cultural circumstances, research has found that the following are consistent risk markers of victimization by one's intimate partner.

a. **Young age**

Younger women have a higher likelihood of being physically abused.[23,24,25,26,27] One 10-year longitudinal study showed that physical violence in couples decreased with age, but psychological aggression did not.[28]

b. **Unmarried**

In several studies, divorced, separated, or never married women were more likely to report victimization.[13,24,26,27] Reasons for their non-married status were rarely explained. Is marital status a predictor or an outcome of abuse? Perhaps abused women are avoiding or leaving marriage to escape the abuse. Or, perhaps their partners are withholding commitment as a strategy to control the woman's behavior.

c. **Economically disadvantaged**

Fox[29] found that couples with intimate partner violence were more likely to have a vulnerable economic risk profile and live in neighborhoods of high disadvantage. Those with low socioeconomic status (SES) had higher risk, no matter where they lived. Among couples with higher SES, living in a disadvantaged neighborhood correlated with more partner violence. Other researchers found that low education levels and/or low income correlated with victimization by intimate partners.[12,26,27,30]

d. **Childhood exposure to violence**

Women who are victims of intimate partner violence are more likely to report a childhood history of maltreatment or witnessing parental violence.[13,31,32]

e. **Pregnant?**

Many have proposed that pregnant women are at particularly high risk for battering; Gazmararian and colleagues,[33] reviewing 13 studies found prevalence ranged from 1 to 20%. However, studies indicate that it is not pregnancy per se that puts women at risk for abuse; rather, the risk is due to their young age.[23] One study of pregnant women found that abuse was more prevalent before the pregnancy than during it.[27] Despite this evidence, pregnant women deserve special attention from health care providers because the rate of intimate partner violence is significant during this time, and the health risks to both mother and fetus are high.

f. **Low social support**

Isolation serves to narrow a victim's perspective of her situation. She has only her own and her partner's interpretation of their relationship. With a controlling partner, that interpretation will support the partner's aggressive behaviors. A support network can offer a different perspective, while also providing support and sympathy. Researchers have found that social support is a factor that protects women from intimate partner violence.[25]

5. Who are the perpetrators of intimate partner violence?

a. **Demographic characteristics**

Compared to non-violent men, men who hurt their partners are more likely to have lower income, lower education, and fewer socioeconomic resources.[13,34,35]

b. **Personality characteristics**

Men who batter differ from non-violent men in intimacy, impulsivity and problem solving skills.[36,37] Several studies found they had low levels of assertiveness.[13]

c. **Substance abuse**

Men who batter tend to use higher quantities of alcohol than non-violent men.[38,39]

d. **Other psychopathology**

Batterers have higher scores on anxiety, depression, and antisocial personality scales; many are diagnosed with personality disorders.[35,40,41,42,43]

e. **Generally aggressive**

In addition to physical abuse of women, men who batter are likely to be sexually violent and to be aggressive toward their children.[13]

f. **Childhood exposure to violence**

Men who batter are more likely to report a childhood history of maltreatment or witnessing parental violence.[13,34]

Consequences of violence

Table 21.1 lists many psychological and health consequences of victimization by intimate partners.

1. **Psychological consequences**

Compared to non-victims, battered women have the following.
   a. More difficulty coping with anger or aggression.[44]
   b. Lower self esteem.[44]
   c. Impaired ability to trust important others.[44]
   d. More distress, depression, confusion, fearfulness, paranoia, and social introversion.[45,46,47,48]
   e. Higher risk for substance abuse.[38,45,48]
   f. Higher risk for suicide.[12,49,50]
   g. Post traumatic stress disorder (PTSD). Diagnostic criteria include elements of depression, anxiety, intrusive thoughts about victimization and avoidance of reminders of the abuse. Predictors of symptom severity include:

   i. severity and the recency of the violence,[38]
   ii. life threats within the relationship,
   iii. sexual assault,[51]
   iv. few personal resources such as education, employment,
   v. low levels of social support.[52,53,54]

Table 21.1 Consequences of victimization by intimate partner violence

Psychological consequences

More difficulty coping with anger or aggression

Lower self esteem

Impaired ability to trust important others

More distress, depression, confusion, fearfulness, paranoia, and social introversion

Higher risk for substance abuse

Higher risk for suicide

Post traumatic stress disorder (PTSD)

Acute medical consequences

Death

Physical trauma

Long-term medical consequences

Higher utilization

Higher health care costs

Poorer physical health

  general health and disability

  insomnia

  fatigue

  gastrointestinal symptoms

  chronic pain

  anemia

  allergies, asthma, or breathing problems

  bronchitis or emphysema

  eyesight and hearing problems

  premenstrual symptoms

  vaginal discharge

  cervical cancer

Negative pregnancy outcomes

  miscarriages

  stillbirths

  low birthweight newborns

  cesareans

  premature labor

  hospitalization due to kidney infection or trauma

  infections or anemia

  late prenatal care

Negative health behaviors

  eating disorders

  smoking

  substance abuse

  unprotected sex

Effects on children

Physical injury

Infants

  poor health, poor sleeping habits, excessive screaming

Preschoolers

  signs of terror, yelling, irritability, hiding, shaking, stuttering

School-age children

  somatic complaints, regression

Adolescents

  aggression, projecting blame, anxiety, somatization, suicidality, substance abuse, running away, criminal behavior

Adults

  violent relationships

2. **Acute medical consequences**

    a. **Death**

        In 2004, more than 1500 people in the USA were murdered by an intimate – spouses, ex-spouses, boyfriends or girlfriends. About one-third of female murder victims were killed by an intimate, compared to 3% of male murder victims. Most homicides were male against male.[55]

    b. **Physical trauma**

        Among female victims of intimate partner violence, about 40% receive injuries during a physical assault. Among those, 30% seek medical treatment.[2] Emergency departments see 0.6 to 1.4 million people per year with injuries sustained from interpersonal violence.[2] Intimate partner violence accounts for one-third to one-half of all women's visits to the emergency department.[19,56] Compared to other female victims of accidents who visit the emergency department, women who are victims of violence

i.   make three times more visits to the emergency department,
ii. are more likely to have facial injuries,
iii. are 13 times more likely to have injuries in the chest, breasts, or abdomen,
iv. are more likely to have multiple injuries, and to have injuries in various stages of healing.[56]

c.   **Long-term medical consequences**

In addition to acute injuries, women who have been battered develop long-term health problems that appear to be unrelated to physical trauma. They often see their physicians for relief from vague, unremitting symptoms.[57]

i.   **Higher utilization**

Female victims of assault visit primary care providers twice as often as non-victims, sustaining high utilization for years following the original assault.[58,59]

ii. Health care costs for assaulted women are 1.6 to 2.5 times greater than for non-victims.[58,59] The CDC estimates that intimate partner violence costs $4.1 billion each year in direct medical and mental health care.[19]

iii. **Poorer physical health**

Exposure to intimate partner violence is associated with poorer physical health and disability.[26,38,45,46] Common somatic symptoms of victims of partner violence include insomnia, fatigue, gastrointestinal symptoms, premenstrual symptoms, chronic pain, and anemia.[12,57] A study of 14,100 middle-aged women in Australia found that victims of intimate partner violence were more likely to have allergies or breathing problems, pain or fatigue, bowel problems, vaginal discharge, eyesight and hearing problems, low iron, asthma, bronchitis or emphysema, and cervical cancer.[60] Somatic symptoms

increase with the level of violence severity.[38]

iv. Negative pregnancy outcomes include higher rates of miscarriages, stillbirths, and low birthweight newborns, cesareans, and premature labor. Victims of violence are more likely to be hospitalized prior to delivery due to kidney infection, and trauma due to falls or blows to the abdomen.[61,62] They are more likely to have infections or anemia. Victims of intimate partner violence are more likely to begin prenatal care during the third trimester.[62]

v.   Negative health behaviors are more prevalent in battered women: eating disorders, smoking, substance abuse, and unprotected sex.[12,26,38,45,62]

3.   **Effects on children**

The impact of violence in intimate relationships extends beyond the battered woman; children are also at risk.[4,63] Children exposed to chronic partner violence often show symptoms of post-traumatic stress disorder.[4] Other symptoms and problem behaviors are listed below.

a.   **Injury**

Men who batter their wives are also likely to be violent with their children.[4,13]

b.   Infants who witness violence are often characterized by poor health, poor sleeping habits, and excessive screaming.[63]

c.   Preschoolers show signs of terror exhibited as yelling, irritable behavior, hiding, shaking, and stuttering.[63]

d.   School-age children experience more somatic complaints and regress to earlier stages of functioning.[63]

e.   Adolescents may use aggression as a predominant form of problem solving, may project blame onto others, and may exhibit a high degree of anxiety (e.g. bite nails, pull hair, somatize feelings).[63] Teens in violent homes are more likely to attempt suicide, abuse drugs and alcohol, run away from home, engage in teenage prostitution, and commit sexual assault crimes.[4]

f. **Adults**

Adult children of battered women are likely to have violent relationships.[13]

Screening for violence

1. The US Preventive Services Task Force 2004 found insufficient evidence to recommend for or against routine screening for intimate partner violence. They found no direct evidence that screening leads to decreased disability or premature death, and limited evidence regarding the effectiveness of interventions for intimate partner violence.[64] Despite this evidence, the National Consensus Guidelines recommend violence screening for "all adolescent and adult patients regardless of cultural background" (p. 12)[4] and promotes ongoing research to determine the effectiveness of screening and intervention.

2. Many health care providers feel awkward asking patients about emotionally painful experiences. However, most patients are accepting of such inquiries and often expect them. In a brief survey about family conflict in six private family practices, we asked 261 family practice patients – including both battered women and non-victims – "Do you think doctors should ask patients about family stress or conflict?" Only 3% said, "no, never," while the remainder, 97%, responded, "yes, sometimes," or "yes, often."[11]

3. With some patients, it may take several visits to develop enough trust and confidence to reveal abuse. However, routinely asking about abuse sends several positive messages: "This is legitimate medical business; I am concerned about your safety and the stress in your life; I am willing to hear about violence – it is not too shameful, deviant, or insignificant for us to discuss; furthermore, the situation is not hopeless, but can be changed." Advocates of victims of violence agree: the single most important thing a physician can do for a battered woman is to ask about violence.[65]

4. When should I ask about violence?[4]

   a. **First visit**

      Primary care providers can ask about violence during an initial getting-to-know-you visit in the context of a trauma, hospitalization, social or sexual history.

   b. **Prevention visits**

      One can ask during annual or general exams, pre-employment physicals, prenatal visits, well-baby visits, premarital exams, and adolescent general exams and sports physicals.

   c. **Signs of injury**

      One should get a good history of the cause of physical trauma, when injuries are present. Many battered women will have evidence of multiple injuries, in various stages of healing,

   d. **"Red flag" somatic complaints**

      When a woman presents with chronic pain syndromes, gastrointestinal symptoms, sleep disturbances, signs of depression, problems in pregnancy, STDs, or substance abuse, the provider should ask about violence.

   e. **Verbal clues**

      In the story presented at the beginning of this chapter, the woman dropped a clue to her physician, referring to a "misunderstanding" with her husband. A woman's reference to marital conflict or controlling behaviors on the part of her partner is a signal to ask about violence.

   f. **Direct statements**

      When a woman states directly, "My husband hits me," the physician should gather a good history of the relationship, discuss local resources for assistance and support, and help the woman to formulate a plan for ending the violence.

5. When should I NOT ask about violence?[4]

   a. If no privacy is available.

   b. If asking would be unsafe for the patient or the physician.

   c. If a non-family interpreter is unavailable.

6. How should I ask about violence?

   a. Set the context for the screening questions, especially if the previous discussion seems unrelated to abuse. Professionals from the Family Peace Project in Milwaukee, Wisconsin use this approach: "In my practice I am concerned about prevention and safety, especially in the family."[66]

b. Inform about reporting requirements.[4] In the USA, certain behaviors and events must be reported to legal authorities, for example, child abuse, elder mistreatment, gunshot or knife wounds. The physicians' ability to maintain confidentiality under these conditions may be limited.

c. Avoid abstract concepts. Do not use these words unless the woman uses them first: "violence," "abuse," "assault" or "rape." These abstract terms are subject to a variety of interpretations, but most individuals understand them to mean immoral, illegal, or abnormal behavior. Many women with violent partners do not apply the term "abuse" to their relationships until the violence has progressed to very severe levels. They may be hesitant to apply the term "abuse" for the following reasons.

   i. His behavior seems normal. For women who were raised by aggressive, controlling men, violent behavior may appear to be a normal male behavior.

   ii. The term seems too severe. Many women may be hesitant to apply immoral, illegal, or abnormal terms to their husbands, especially if the violence has not yet progressed to severe levels.

   iii. The progression of violence over time can delay her realization that the aggression is "abuse." Intimate partner violence generally begins with a minor aggressive event that is distressing but does not cause the couple to separate. A violent husband's impulse is to apologize deeply, then to justify his behavior so that he and his partner maintain the belief that he is a moral man. Over time, an abused woman will learn to tolerate and forgive more and more severe aggression. If she is isolated from those who might criticize his behavior, she is likely to tolerate even more violence. However, most abused women have a limit: if the children witness violence, if injuries occur, if her life is threatened, then she will recognize the behavior as dangerous or unreasonable and seek help.

d. Focus on behaviors. The screening question should use behavior-words, such as hitting, hurting, or threatening.

e. Consider other perpetrators. Ex-husbands and ex-boyfriends may be involved. Often, in abusive relationships, the violence does not end when the victim leaves. Men who are very possessive and controlling may in fact escalate their violent behaviors when they fear their control over the woman is threatened – as when she moves away.

f. Sample questions. Several sets of screening questions have been tested for sensitivity and specificity.[67] The WAST-short has the advantage of brevity (two questions) and patient- and physician-comfort in both clinical and research populations. One or two extreme responses ("a lot of tension" or "great difficulty") indicate a high risk for partner violence. In one study, these two questions identified 100% of non-victims and 92% of victims of violence. The two questions are:

   i. In general, how would you describe your relationship? A lot of tension, some tension, no tension?

   ii. Do you and your partner work out problems with great difficulty, some difficulty, or no difficulty?

g. The Family Peace Project recommends this screening question:

   i. "Are you in any relationships now where you are afraid for your personal safety, or where someone is threatening you, hurting you, forcing sexual contact, or trying to control your life?"[66]

Clinical interventions for battered women

The impact of violence on a woman's health and family life demands a comprehensive response from health care providers. Episodic treatment of acute injuries, while important, is not enough. In fact, some claim that ignoring violence enables men to keep hitting.[56] Effective interventions require a safe, collaborative, accepting patient-provider relationship, and a longitudinal approach. Table 21.2 lists the key tasks for the health care provider.

229

Table 21.2 Clinical screening and intervention for intimate partner violence

Establish a safe clinical environment and provide medical treatment

Screen for victimization

Assess dangerousness

Address readiness for change

Develop a safe-plan

Encourage outreach for support

Offer referrals

Document the visit

Make a follow-up appointment

1. The clinical environment

a. Protecting confidentiality is the first step toward safety. Some male partners may try to stay in the room during an office visit. The provider can respectfully address a partner's concerns about the woman's medical problems, then invite him to wait outside during the physical exam. At that time, confidential discussions may occur. No information should be shared with the woman's partner without her permission, and her permission should only be sought when the partner is out of the room.

b. **Patient-centeredness**

When working with victims of intimate partner violence, a patient-centered, collaborative position provides the greatest benefit to the patient. Rather than using a directive and controlling approach – like a batterer – health care providers should model collaborative decision-making and encourage battered women to think independently of powerful others. The provider must recognize that the responsibility for change belongs to the woman, and that she knows best when a particular strategy, such as escape, will be safe or effective. The provider's role should be that of consultant and supporter, presenting intervention options to the woman and encouraging all steps toward safety.

c. **Acceptance**

A non-judgmental approach is necessary, but not always easy. One study found that health care workers were sympathetic toward battered women who were taking action to change their life situation, but irritated with others whom they described as "passive," "evasive," or "uncooperative."[49] These providers made more inappropriate referrals and discharge plans for battered women than other women. What the health care workers encountered in some women were behaviors that were adaptive in a violent environment – passivity, evasiveness, mistrust – but frustrating in the emergency room, where self-motivation and cooperation are expected. Understanding the source of troublesome behaviors will help the health care provider maintain the objectivity needed to avoid mismanagement of battered women.

2. The intervention process

a. **Assess danger**

Primary care providers should assess the level of danger in patients' relationships. To start, the provider can ask, "Do you feel safe going home?" Signs of a potentially lethal relationship are listed in Table 21.3.[4,66] More positives indicate higher risk for danger.

b. **Assess "readiness for change"**

Many victims of intimate partner violence will not be willing to change their living situations, and this can be very frustrating and frightening to primary care providers. Before dispensing advice, the provider should assess the woman's readiness for change. Prochaska and colleagues have developed a model that describes an individual's progression through several steps of behavior change.[68] When working with battered women, consider one of six stages.

i. Precontemplation is characterized by the statement, "My relationship is not a problem." In these relationships, the frequency and severity of violence may be low, and/or the women may believe their partners' aggression is normal or justified.

Table 21.3 Danger assessment: factors predicting lethality

Severe aggression and increasing severity over time

Availability and use of weapons to threaten or harm

Threats to kill

Forced or threatened to force sexual acts

Stressful life transitions: pregnancy, separation, divorce, leaving home

Control of daily activities, limiting who to see, where to go, how much money

Extreme jealousy

Violence during pregnancy

Drug and alcohol abuse

History of violence against others, including children

Suicide attempts by partner or patient

ii. Contemplation is characterized by ambivalence: "I know the violence is a problem, but I need to stay in the marriage." Some women believe that the benefits of staying with their partners outweigh the costs of enduring the abuse. For others, low self esteem, depression, or lack of support may render them incapable of making any change in the situation.

iii. Preparation is characterized by, "I know the violence is a problem, and I'm planning changes." Women who change or leave violent relationships need preparation time. Some must save money to move; some need to find employment; some must determine how they will explain the separation to family, friends, children and spouse; some must plan a very careful escape.

iv. Action is characterized by "I am making changes to end the violence," and generally describes the early phase of the new lifestyle. This is an unstable period, when women discover the costs of change. Women who leave their partners will discover loneliness, uncertainty, poorer finances, and the entire burden of childrearing. Many partners will work very hard to get the women back into the relationship using seduction, or

threats, or both. This phase is the most dangerous for women; partners who are extremely controlling will exaggerate their measures of coercion when challenged by separation. Most women will find the change too difficult and go back into the relationship. However, when violence reemerges, most women will try to leave again.

v. Maintenance is characterized by "I have adapted to the changes I have made." This stage begins about six months after the change.

vi. Relapse is a normal occurrence when making major life changes such as leaving a violent marriage. As mentioned above, leaving is a challenge of authority, and many ex-husbands will work very hard to bring their wives back into the relationship, using both seductive and coercive techniques.

c. Tailor conversations to the stage of change. Health care providers enable a woman to change violent relationships when they begin "where she is," help her assess her situation, and nudge her along the continuum of readiness to change. A continuity-of-care practice, where providers see patients several times over long periods of time, is an ideal setting to encourage the next step. Table 21.4 lists some "nudging strategies" to help women develop the motivation to move to the next stage. In these discussions, the provider should express concern for the patient's safety and health, and willingness to discuss relationship issues at any time. Even if the woman is reluctant to change her relationship now, she should know that the physician is a source of support and information when she is ready.

d. Develop a "safe-plan." If the health care provider determines that a woman is in danger of serious harm from her partner, but she is not yet ready to leave the relationship, the physician should encourage her to develop a "safe-plan" that can be implemented in an emergency. The physician can begin with a statement of concern, then assess the woman's preparedness to escape: "I am concerned that your husband will hurt you badly next time he

Table 21.4 "Stages of change"[a] for battered women

Stage of change	Patient's belief	Physician "nudging" strategies
Precontemplation	"My relationship is not a problem."	Learn about the relationship: "Tell me how you and your partner handle conflict in your relationship."
Contemplation or ambivalence	"I know the violence is a problem, but I need to stay in the marriage."	Discuss the ambivalence: "What are the good things about your relationship? What are the not-so-good things?"
Preparation	"The violence is a problem, and I'm planning some changes."	Offer support and encouragement
		Clarify plans, including safety measures
		List community resources
		Provide anticipatory guidance
Action	"I am making changes to end the violence."	Offer support and encouragement
		List community resources
		Provide anticipatory guidance
		Review coping strategies and safety plans
Maintenance	"I have adapted to the changes."	Offer support
		Review need for community resources
		Discuss coping strategies
Relapse	"I cannot maintain this change."	Remain positive and encouraging
		Discuss the lessons learned from the effort
		Review safety plans
		Remain open for future discussions

Note: [a]Hastings J. E., Hamburger L. K. Psychosocial modifiers of psychopathology for domestically violent and nonviolent men. *Psychol Rep* 1994; **74**, 112–114.

gets angry. Do you have a plan to get away from him quickly?" Discussion should address: signs of a buildup of tension and aggression, whether it would be safe to leave the house, when to leave, where to go, how to arrange transportation, how long to stay away, what to take (clothes, money, important papers), and whether to get legal protection. Most women have resources that allow them some respite and protection, such as a relative who will temporarily shelter them, but others will need public assistance. For this reason, the physician needs to be acquainted with local agencies who can provide shelter and services to battered women.

e. Encourage outreach. A strong social support network can be protective for victims of violence. Family and friends can provide moral and tangible support, a safe haven, and protection to many battered women. Some women may find themselves isolated and alienated from family and friends, which only serves to trap them in dangerous relationships. The health care provider should encourage victims of violence to seek out potentially supportive relationships and reconnect with helpful family and friends.

f. Describe community resources. One of the most important things a physician can do is to connect victims of violence to community resources that can be helpful.[11]

i. **Resources for battered women**

Table 21.5 lists a variety of resources that may help battered women. These agencies guide women to basic resources such as food, shelter, jobs, and legal assistance, and offer emotional support.

ii. **Resources for men who batter**

Many communities have treatment programs for men who batter. Many programs involve several weeks of group therapy, followed by individual therapy. Most men who attend batterer's programs are mandated into treatment by the courts; however, therapists generally welcome self-referrals and physician-referrals as well.

iii. **Resources for couples**

Couples therapy is NOT recommended for violent relationships. Women who are battered are not free to speak their minds in therapy where the abuser is present; women may be physically punished for things they say. Instead, the health care provider may recommend individual psychotherapy for each partner. While there is no research on interventions for men at early stages of violent relationships, or on men exhibiting common couple violence, individual psychotherapy will certainly benefit the woman in the relationship. If the male partner is both controlling and physically aggressive, batterers' programs, described above, may be a more appropriate referral.

g. **Documentation**

Well-documented medical records are important for any health problem, but are especially useful when following conditions with long-term effects, such as victimization. For battered women, the medical record also represents legal evidence about the violence. The National Consensus Guidelines recommend the following.[4]

Table 21.5 Referrals and community resources for intimate partner violence

Battered women's shelters

Women's centers

Support groups for battered women

Treatment programs for men who batter

Mental health centers

Private psychotherapist or psychiatrist

Clergy

Family counseling clinics

Alcoholics anonymous, if appropriate

Narcotics anonymous, if appropriate

Al-anon groups

Legal advocacy

District attorney's office (for protective orders)

Police department

911

i. **What not to do**

The health care provider's interpretations (e.g. "patient was abused") should not be included. Also avoid judgmental words (e.g. instead of "patient alleges..." use "patient states...")

ii. **Relevant history**

Document the chief complaint along with details of the abuse and its relationship to the complaint. Use the patient's words to describe violent events ("The patient reports ..."). The record should include concurrent conditions related to the abuse and, for victims of recent violence, a summary of current and past abuse.

iii. **Physical exam**

The health care provider should document neurological, gynecological, and mental status exam findings if indicated. If there are injuries, provide a detailed description, including type, number, size, location, resolution, and possible causes. Use of a body-map is recommended. The woman's

233

explanations of the injuries and the provider's opinion about the adequacy of those explanations should be recorded.

iv. Color photographs are especially useful for forensic purposes. Guidelines for photographs include: (1) obtain consent from the patient; (2) use color film with a color standard; (3) photograph from different angles, full body and close-up, with appropriate drapes for modesty; (4) hold up a coin, ruler, or other object to illustrate the size of an injury; (5) include the woman's face in at least one picture; (6) take two pictures of each major trauma area; (7) mark photographs precisely, including the woman's name, location of injury, date, names of the photographer, and others present; and (8) maintain high standards for privacy and confidentiality regarding handling of the film and photographs.

v. Lab findings

The documentation must include results from all pertinent laboratory tests, imaging studies, and diagnostic procedures. Record the relationship of the findings to current or past abuse.

vi. Assessment, intervention, and referral

Health care providers should record the safety assessment, including the potential for serious harm, suicide, and health impact of the violence. Document options discussed, referrals made, and plans for follow-up.

h. Follow-up is important. Options discussed in the physician's office require contemplation, planning, and time on the part of the woman. Physicians should use regular appointments or phone conversations to communicate concern, monitor safety, addresses coping strategies and support systems, and follow the decision-making process.[4] One discussion does not "cure" violence in relationships, but continuing communication, support, and exploration of options will empower women to make changes that eliminate violence from their lives.

Violence prevention in primary care settings

How can primary care providers contribute to violence prevention? Consider three levels: primary prevention guides an individual to avoid a problem altogether; secondary prevention identifies a problem in early stages, and prevents damage; tertiary prevention identifies a problem in later stages, treats the current damage, and seeks to prevent further damage. Primary care providers can use all three levels of prevention when working with women in their clinical practices.

1. Primary prevention

Good parent education may prevent violence before it happens. Teach parents what to expect from their children at every level of development, reviewing cognitive as well as physical and motor expectations. Offer parents non-violent options for disciplining their children. Allow them to ventilate about the frustrations of parenting, and to discuss the impact of parenthood on their intimate relationship. If partner/spousal conflict becomes serious, remind them that they are the models for their children's future relationships, and guide them to appropriate therapy. Avoiding violence in this generation should also influence relationships in the next generation.

2. Secondary prevention

Especially with young men and women, ask about the quality of their relationships. If they describe "fights" or "problems with temper," ask them about hitting or hurting each other, and ask about their parents' relationships. People in early stages of aggressive relationships may not identify violent behaviors as an ongoing problem. Men who hit are very remorseful, and women who are hurt are convinced that these events are rare. Both believe the violence will never happen again. Express concern about physical fights. Describe negative consequences for couples where deliberate harm is inflicted: injuries, divorce, arrest, emotional distress in their children, and adult children who become batterers or victims. Offer referrals to psychotherapists, support groups, clergy, or groups for batterers. At this point, it may be difficult to determine whether the hitting is an early stage of intimate terrorism, or a pattern of lower frequency/severity situational violence. Close follow-up will help determine the exact nature of the relationship and provide more opportunities for intervention.

3. Tertiary prevention

Currently, tertiary prevention is our country's most common violence prevention strategy. Action is taken when professionals identify a chronic and dangerous pattern of behaviors. At this late stage, it is difficult to save the marriage, and the "treatment of choice" for many professionals is to get the woman out of the relationship before further harm is done. When speaking to the battered woman, acknowledge the strength it requires to endure the stress present in her daily life. Assess current levels of danger and her readiness to change. Label the violence as a problem, and inform her of community resources that can help her. Encourage her to devise an escape plan in the event that the batterer becomes dangerous again. Document injuries. Follow-up frequently in order to assess ongoing levels of danger, and to provide her a place of safety and support.

Conclusion

Primary care providers are in an ideal position to contribute significantly to violence prevention in their communities. In the context of sustained patient-provider relationships, where all aspects of health are addressed – biomedical, psychological, and social – primary care providers are able to identify life patterns that indicate risk for victimization. Battered women are well served by providers who routinely ask about victimization, treat health consequences of battering, provide information and encouragement, guide women to effective community resources, and offer emotional support through the long journey to end violence.

References

1. Centers for Disease Control and Prevention. *Intimate Partner Violence: Overview*, 2007. www.cdc.gov/print.do, accessed 3/30/07.

2. Tjaden P., Thoennes N. *Prevalence, incidence and consequences of violence against women: findings from the national violence against women survey*. National Institute of Justice and the Centers for Disease Control and Prevention, National Center for Injury Prevention and Control. http://www.ojp.usdoj.gov/nih/pubs-sum/172837.htm, accessed 1/1/98.

3. Donaldson M. S., Yordy K. D., Lohr K. N., Vanselow N. A. *Primary Care: America's Health in a New Era*. Washington DC: Institute of Medicine, National Academy Press, 1996.

4. Family Violence Prevention Fund. National consensus guidelines on identifying and responding to domestic violence victimization in health care settings. www.endabuse.org, accessed 2/1/04.

5. Field C. A., Caetano R. Longitudinal model predicting mutual partner violence among White, Black, and Hispanic couples in the United States general population. *Violence Vict* 2005; **20**, 499–511.

6. Straus M. A., Gelles R. J. Societal change and change in family violence from 1975 to 1985 as revealed by two national surveys. *J Marriage Fam* 1986; **48**, 465–479.

7. United Nations General Assembly. In-depth Study on All Forms of Violence Against Women: Report of the Secretary-General, Report A/61/122/Add.1. 7/6/06.

8. Hamberger L. K., Saunders D. G., Hovey M. Prevalence of domestic violence in community practice and rate of physician inquiry. *Fam Med* 1992; **24**, 283–287.

9. Elliott B. A., Johnson M. M. Domestic violence in a primary care setting. Patterns and prevalence. *Arch Fam Med* 1995; **4**, 113–119.

10. McFarlane J. M., Groff J. Y., O'Brien J. A., Watson K. Prevalence of partner violence against 7,443 African American, White, and Hispanic women receiving care at urban public primary care clinics. *Public Health Nurs* 2005; **22**, 98–107.

11. Burge S. K., Schneider F. D., Ivy L., Catala S. Patients' advice to physicians about intervening in family conflict. *Ann Fam Med* 2005; **3**, 248–254.

12. Kramer A., Lorenzon D., Mueller G. Prevalence of intimate partner violence and health implications for women using emergency departments and primary care clinics. *Womens Health Issues* 2004; **14**, 19–29.

13. Hotaling G. R., Sugarman D. B. An analysis of risk markers in husband-to-wife violence: the current state of knowledge. *Violence Vict* 1986; **1**, 101–124.

14. Caetano R., McGrath C., Ramisetty-Mikler S., Field C. A. Drinking, alcohol problems and the five-year recurrence and incidence of male to female and female to male partner violence. *Alcoholism: Clin Exp Res* 2005; **29**, 98–106.

15. Giles-Sims J. *Wife Battering: A Systems Theory Approach*. New York: Guilford Publishers, 1983.

16. Rhatigan D. L., Street A. E., Axsom D. K. A critical review of theories to explain violent relationship termination: implications for research and intervention. *Clin Psychol Rev* 2006; **26**, 321–345.

17. Fergusson D. M., Horwood L. J., Ridder E. M. Partner violence and mental health outcomes in a New Zealand birth cohort. *J Marriage Fam* 2005; **67**, 1103–1119.

18. Archer J. Sex differences in physically aggressive acts between heterosexual partners: a meta-analytic review. *Aggression Violent Behav* 2002; **7**, 313–351.

19. Centers for Disease Control and Prevention (CDC). Intimate partner violence injuries – Oklahoma, 2002. *MMWR Morb Mortal Wkly Rep* 2005; **54**, 1041–1045.

20. Johnson M. P. Patriarchal terrorism and common couple violence: two forms of violence against women. *J Marriage Fam* 1995; **57**, 283–294.

21. Johnson M. P. Domestic violence: it's not about gender – or is it? *J Marriage Fam* 2005; **67**, 1126–1130.

22. Pence E., Paymar M. *Education Groups for Men Who Batter: The Duluth Model*. New York: Springer Publishing, 1993.

23. Gelles R. J. Violence and pregnancy: are pregnant women at greater risk of abuse? In M. A. Straus, R. J. Gelles, eds., *Physical Violence in American Families: Risk Factors and Adaptations to Violence in 8,145 Families*, New Brunswick, NJ: Transaction Publishers, 1995, pp. 279–286.

24. Bauer H. M., Rodriguez M. A., Perez-Stable E. J. Prevalence and determinants of intimate partner abuse among public hospital primary care patients. *J Gen Intern Med* 2000; **15**, 811–817.

25. Lown E. A., Vega W. A. Prevalence and predictors of physical partner abuse among Mexican American women. *Am J Public Health* 2001; **91**, 441–445.

26. Vest J. R., Catlin T. K., Chen J. J., Brownson R. C. Multistate analysis of factors associated with intimate partner violence. *Am J Prev Med* 2002; **22**, 156–164.

27. Saltzman L. E., Johnson C. H., Gilbert B. C., Goodwin M. M. Physical abuse around the time of pregnancy: an examination of prevalence and risk factors in 16 states. *Mater Child Health J* 2003; 7, 31–43.

28. Fritz P. A., O'Leary K. D. Physical and psychological partner aggression across a decade: a growth curve analysis. *Violence Vict* 2004; **19**, 3–16.

29. Fox G. L., Benson M. L. Household and neighborhood contexts of intimate partner violence. *Public Health Rep* 2006; **121**, 419–427.

30. Bohn D. K., Tebben J. G., Campbell J. C. Influences of income, education, age, and ethnicity on physical abuse before and during pregnancy. *J Obstet Gynecol Neonat Nurs* 2004; **33**, 561–571.

31. Dube S. R., Anda R. F., Felitti V. J., Edwards V. J., Williamson D. F. Exposure to abuse, neglect, and household dysfunction among adults who witnessed intimate partner violence as children: implications for health and social services. *Violence Vict* 2002; **17**, 3–17.

32. Renner L. M., Slack K. S. Intimate partner violence and child maltreatment: understanding intra- and intergenerational connections. *Child Abuse Neglect* 2006; **30**, 599–617.

33. Gazmararian J. A., Lazorick S., Spitz A. M., Ballard T. J., Saltzman L. E., Marks J. S. Prevalence of violence against pregnant women. *J Am Med Assoc* 1996; **275**, 1915–1920. Erratum 1997; **277**(14), 1125.

34. Aldarondo E., Sugarman D. B. Risk marker analysis of the cessation and persistence of wife assault. *J Consult Clin Psychol* 1996; **64**, 1010–1019.

35. Pan H. S., Neidig P. H., O'Leary K. D. Predicting mild and severe husband-to-wife physical aggression. *J Consult Clin Psychol* 1994; **62**, 975–981.

36. Barnett O. W., Hamberger L. K. The assessment of maritally violent men on the California Psychological Inventory. *Violence Vict* 1992; **7**, 15–28.

37. Cohen R. A., Brumm V., Zawacki T. M., Paul R., Sweet L., Rosenbaum A. Impulsivity and verbal deficits associated with domestic violence. *J Int Neuropsychol Soc* 2003; **9**, 760–770.

38. McCauley J., Kern D. E., Kolodner K., Derogatis L. R., Bass E. B. Relation of low-severity violence to women's health. *J Gen Intern Med* 1998; **13**, 687–691.

39. Stuart G. L., Moore T. M., Kahler C. W., Ramsey S. E. Substance abuse and relationship violence among men court-referred to batterers' intervention programs. *Subst Abuse* 2003; **24**, 107–122.

40. Dutton D. G. *The Abusive Personality: Violence and Control in Intimate Relationships*, New York: Guilford Press, 1998.

41. Peek-Asa C., Zwerling C., Young T., Stromquist A. M., Burmeister L. F., Merchant J. A. A population based study of reporting patterns and characteristics of men who abuse their female partners. *Injury Prev* 2005; **11**, 180–185.

42. Hastings J. E., Hamberger L. K. Psychosocial modifiers of psychopathology for domestically violent and nonviolent men. *Psychol Rep* 1994; **74**, 112–114.

43. Huss M. T., Langhinrichsen-Rohling J. Assessing the generalization of psychopathy in a clinical sample of domestic violence perpetrators. *Law Hum Behav* 2006; **30**, 571–586.

44. Carmen E. H., Rieker P. P., Mills T. Victims of violence and psychiatric illness. *Am J Psychiatry* 1984; **141**, 378–383.

45. Carbone-Lopez K., Kruttschnitt C., Macmillan R. Patterns of intimate partner violence and their associations with physical health, psychological

distress, and substance use. *Public Health Rep* 2006; **121**, 382–392.

46. Plichta S. B., Falik M. Prevalence of violence and its implications for women's health. *Womens Health Issues* 2001; **11**, 244–258.

47. Gellen M. I., Hoffman R. A., Jones M., Stone M. Abused and nonabused women: MMPI profile differences. *Personnel Guidance J* 1984; **62**, 601–604.

48. Rosewater L. B. Battered or schizophrenic? Psychological tests can't tell. In K. Yllo, M. Bograd, eds., *Feminist Perspectives on Wife Abuse*, Newbury Park, CA: Sage Publications, 1988, pp. 200–216.

49. Kurz D., Stark E. Not-so-benign neglect: the medical response to battering. In K. Yllo, M. Bograd, eds., *Feminist Perspectives on Wife Abuse*, Newbury Park, CA: Sage Publications, 1988, pp. 249–266.

50. Bergman B., Brismar B. A 5-year follow-up study of 117 battered women. *Am J Public Health* 1991; **81**, 1486–1489.

51. McFarlane J., Malecha A., Watson K., *et al.* Intimate partner sexual assault against women: frequency, health consequences, and treatment outcomes. *Obstet Gynecol* 2005; **105**, 99–108.

52. Astin M. C., Lawrence K. J., Foy D. W. Posttraumatic stress disorder among battered women: risk and resiliency factors. *Violence Vict* 1993; **8**, 17–28.

53. Houskamp B. M., Foy D. W. The assessment of posttraumatic stress disorder in battered women. *J Interpersonal Violence* 1991; **6**, 367–375.

54. Kemp A., Rawlings E. I., Green B. L. Posttraumatic stress disorder (PTSD) in battered women: a shelter sample. *J Traumatic Stress* 1991; **4**, 137–148.

55. United States Department of Justice. *Homicide Trends in the U.S.: Intimate Homicide*, 2007. www.ojp.usdoj.gov/bjs/homicide/intimates.htm, accessed 3/30/07.

56. Stark E., Flitcraft A., Frazier W. Medicine and patriarchal violence: the social construction of a "private" event. *Int J Health Serv* 1979; **9**, 461–493.

57. Koss M. P., Heslet L. Somatic consequences of violence against women. *Arch Fam Med* 1992; **1**, 53–59.

58. Koss M. P., Woodruff W. J., Koss P. G. Relation of criminal victimization to health perceptions among women medical patients. *J Consult Clin Psychol* 1990; **58**, 147–152.

59. Ulrich Y. C., Cain K. C., Sugg N. K., Rivara F. P., Rubanowice D. M., Thompson R. S. Medical care utilization patterns in women with diagnosed domestic violence. *Am J Prev Med* 2003; **24**, 9–15.

60. Loxton D., Schofield M., Hussain R., Mishra G. History of domestic violence and physical health in midlife. *Violence Against Women* 2006; **12**, 715–731.

61. Cokkinides V. E., Coker A. L., Sanderson M., Addy C., Bethea L. Physical violence during pregnancy: maternal complications and birth outcomes. *Obstetr Gynecol* 1999; **93**, 661–666.

62. McFarlane J., Parker B., Soeken K. Abuse during pregnancy: associations with maternal health and infant birth weight. *Nurs Res* 1996; **45**, 37–42.

63. Jaffe P. G., Wolfe D. A., Wilson S. K. *Children of Battered Women*, Newbury Park, CA: Sage Publications, 1990.

64. US Preventive Services Task Force (USPSTF). Screening for family and intimate partner violence: recommendation statement. *Ann Fam Med* 2004; **2**, 156–160.

65. Finkelhor D., Yllo K. *License to Rape: Sexual Abuse of Wives*, New York, NY: Free Press, 1985.

66. Ambuel B., Hamberger L. K. *Family Peace Project*. Department of Family & Community Medicine, Medical College of Wisconsin. http://www.mcw.edu/display/router.asp?docid=11599, accessed 4/16/07.

67. Fogarty C., Burge S. K., McCord E. C. Communicating with patients about intimate partner violence: screening and interviewing approaches. *Fam Med* 2002; **34**, 369–375.

68. Prochaska J. O., Velicer W. F., Rossi J. S., *et al.* Stages of change and decisional balance for 12 problem behaviors. *Health Psychol* 1994; **13**, 39–46.

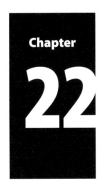

Depression

Jo Ann Rosenfeld and Connie Marsh

Introduction

Depression is a common problem that is more frequently reported in women. Diagnosis and treatment require the understanding of medical, social, and psychological factors and interactions. Effective treatments are available and are important because suicide is a major cause of death in young women.

Epidemiology

1. Depression is very common.

   a. Five to eight percent of all outpatients seen by primary care physicians have the diagnosis of depression.[1] Ten percent of individuals have depression in any one year.[2] In a recent telephone survey of 12,000 individuals in Canada, 10% of women and 5% of men reported that they had the diagnosis of depression.[3] The lifetime prevalence is 17%, although approximately 45% of those individuals who are "high utilizers" of health care may have depression.

   b. It has enormous societal and personal costs. By 2020, WHO estimates that depression will be the second greatest cause of disability.[4] Besides the mortality of suicide, depression causes isolation, work and family disorder and problems, and worsens medical conditions. Depression increases the number of physician visits and prescriptions.

2. The incidence of depression does not vary by race. In a large observational study of 900 young women, 21% of white, 28% of African Americans and 29% of Hispanic women reported severe depression. Depression was more likely with history of sexual assault and unemployment.[5] In another study of young women, the percentage and severity of depression was not related to ethnic group.[6] In older women, the results vary. One population study found that being African American increased the risk of depression in New York City.[7]

3. Depression is more common in women after puberty. The National Co-morbidity survey found a lifetime prevalence of depression for women of 21.3% and 12.7% for men.[8] The ratio for women to men for depression is 1.7 to 1; this difference is not explained by race, socioeconomic or educational status.[9]

4. The detection rate in primary care settings is only 60–64%. Detection is important because depression leads to greater impairment and disability than diabetes, lung diseases, back problems, and hypertension.

   a. Major depressive disorders are associated with a 15% suicide rate.

   b. Fewer than two-thirds of those who suffer depression seek treatment and 10–70% receive adequate treatment with adequate doses of antidepressants, depending on the measurements used.[10,11]

   c. Depression was associated with more symptoms in medical disease, greater disability, and worse quality of life for patients with coexisting medical illness.[12]

Gender disparity

1. The gender differences in depression begin as early as adolescence.

2. The causes of this disparity are disputed; differences in endocrine, social, socioeconomic,

---

psychological, and environmental causes and stresses have all been suggested.

3. There are some gender differences in the function of some neurotransmitters, but whether this is the cause is uncertain.

4. Sociological factors such as differing ways adults react to boys and girls have been proposed. Introspective behaviors may be more encouraged in girls and these may worsen or intensify depression.

5. The increased childhood sexual abuse in women may lead to an increased incidence of depression.

6. Increased stressors in women such as family, work, pregnancy, infertility, and single parenthood coupled with greater social isolation have also been proposed as causes for the gender disparity. Differences in health care provider diagnosis, sensitivity, and patient presentation may also contribute to the differences.

Risk factors (Table 22.1)

1. The risk factors for women and men are multiple and complex.

2. Comorbid medical conditions and other psychiatric diagnoses place women at higher risk of developing depression. Psychiatric problems are more common in patients with medical illnesses and psychiatric disorders affect the clinical outcome of medical diseases. Depressive symptoms are present in 24–46% of hospitalized medically ill patients with diseases such as cancer, myocardial infarction, Parkinson's disease, and stroke.[13] Individuals with a medical illness such as diabetes or hypertension and coexisting depression report more complaints.[14]

Clinical symptoms

1. Common vegetative symptoms include changes in appetite, energy, and libido. Sleep disorders are common and include difficulty in falling asleep, staying asleep, and early morning awakening. Unlike men, women can become anorexic, eat too much, or go on eating binges.

2. Changes in mood are obvious such as sadness, weeping, crying, and/or irritability. Women may exhibit frustration, anger, or difficulty dealing with children or husband or job.

Table 22.1 Risk factors for depression

All individuals

Past history
   Family history of depression
   Personal history of depression

Medical history
   Serious medical illness
   Antisocial personality disorder
   Sexual dysfunction

Social history
   Life stresses
   Lack of social support
   Substance abuse
   Cigarette smoking
   Alcohol use

Women specifically

Loss of parent before age 10

Childhood history of physical or sexual abuse

History of mood disorder after pregnancy

Marijuana use

Use of high progesterone oral contraceptive pill

Use of gonadotropin stimulants for infertility evaluation

Single parenthood

Unhappy or abusive marriage

Presence of young children in home

3. There are often changes in motivation. Anhedonia ("everything is an effort"), loss of interest or pleasure in usual activities, and difficulty concentrating are often complaints.

4. There are changes in behavior including social withdrawal, psychomotor retardation, or agitation. Women may become agoraphobic, stay in the house, refuse to go to work, and interact very little.

5. Women may exhibit low self-esteem, guilt, delusions, especially somatic ones, hopelessness, helplessness, and thoughts of suicide and death.

6. The typical symptoms may be much harder to detect in the elderly where apathy may be the presenting symptom.

Table 22.2 Medical illnesses that can cause depressive-like symptoms

Endocrine

Hypothyroidism

Apathetic hyperthyroidism

Cushing's disease

Hyperparathyroidism

Diabetes

Nutritional

Vitamin B-12 deficiency

Alcohol or substance abuse

Medications

Other chronic diseases

Connective tissue diseases, such as lupus

Cancer

Stroke

Heart disease

CNS disease – Parkinson's disease, multiple sclerosis, Alzheimer's and other dementias

Table 22.3 Medications that can cause or worsen depression

Antihypertensives – clonidine, hydralazine, hydrochlorothiazide, methyldopa, beta-blockers, reserpine, spironolactone, guanethidene

Analgesics – ibuprofen, indomethacin, opiates

Anti-epileptic medicines – phenytoin, phenobarbital, carbamazepine

Antihistamines

Antineoplastic agents

Antibiotics – ampicillin, griseofulvin, isoniazid, metronidazolew, nitrofuradantoin, other penicillins, tetracyclines

Cardiovascular drugs – digoxin, lidocaine, procainamide

Hormones – steroids, ACTH, OCPs

Sedatives – barbituates, benzodiazepines, chloral hydrate

Stimulants – amphetamines

Other CNS drugs – amantadine, butyrophenones, phenothiazines

7. Women may present differently than men. They are more likely to have a seasonal component and atypical symptoms such as hyperphagia, hypersomnia, carbohydrate craving, weight gain, heavy feelings in legs and arms, and evening mood worsening.
8. Women are more likely to have depressive symptoms related to eating disorders and headaches, and less likely to have associated antisocial behavior and alcoholism than men.[15]

Diagnosis
Differential

1. There are several medical and psychiatric conditions that can mimic or obscure the diagnosis of depression.
2. Many comorbid conditions can cause depressive symptoms (see Table 22.2).
3. Medications can cause or exacerbate depression (Table 22.3).
4. Coexisting non-mood psychiatric disorders such as anxiety or anxiety disorders including obsessive compulsive disorder and panic disorders with and without agoraphobia, schizophrenia, schizoaffective disorders, and substance abuse can make the diagnosis of depression difficult.
5. Dementia can cause depression and depression can mimic dementia.
6. Family factors, stressful life events, alcohol abuse, and social isolation can increase or worsen depression.
7. All patients with depressive symptoms should be assessed for suicidal risk (see below).

Diagnostic criteria

The diagnostic criteria for major depression are listed in the Diagnostic and Statistical Manual of Mental Disorders. Various good screening tools exist including the Beck Inventory (13 questions), the Edinburgh Postnatal Depression Scale, the General Health Questionnaire, and the Geriatric Depression Scale.

Treatment

1. Treatment includes counseling, cognitive and behavioral therapy, and/or antidepressant medications.

2. There is some evidence that exercise can be beneficial.[15] In a cross-sectional study of more than 3400 men and women, there was a consistent association between enhanced psychological well-being and regular physical exercise.[16] Another randomized study that examined older patients found that women and men responded as well, at 16 weeks, to exercise or antidepressants, although those on antidepressants responded more quickly.[17]

3. Psychotherapeutic counseling is indicated as an integral part of the treatment of depression. Women with depression do better with counseling and pharmacological treatment than with medication alone, especially those patients with more severe depression.[18] However, barriers exist to psychotherapy; approximately only 20% of primary care patients with depression make the first psychotherapy appointment.

4. Psychopharmacological treatment is standard in most cases of depression, and most patients respond to its use. Treatment is indicated for patients with suicidal thoughts, distress, inability to perform usual activities, major depressive disorders, symptoms lasting more than two weeks, social isolation, and/or inability to cope. Women and men are treated equally adequately.

5. Use of antidepressants in women may be different because of different pharmacokinetics. Lower doses may be effective. Women may need to be treated for comorbid anxiety, panic, phobias and eating disorders. The selective serotonin reuptake inhibitors (SSRIs) may work better in women, especially in women with recurrent depression and those with a first episode.[19]

6. Medications used in primary care include tricyclic antidepressants, SSRIs and a few others. Women respond well to medication, and low-income women respond better to medication than case management and social intervention alone.[20] Women with major manic-depressive or bipolar disorders may need psychiatric consultation and treatment with lithium, depatoke, or other drugs.

7. The choice of antidepressant is usually an SSRI because of the rapidity of action, low side effect profiles, and effectiveness.[21] Sertaline may be more fabored than fluoxetine. The patient should see an effect with SSRIs within 7–14 days. Fluoxetine may cause more agitation and insomnia, while all SSRIs often cause decreased sexual desire. Escitalopram has been suggested for its increased efficacy and rapidity of action.

8. Tricyclic antidepressants work well but may have substantial side effects including sedation, dry mouth, cardiovascular effects, and blurred vision. They usually take longer to work, usually 14 days before an effect is seen, and the dose has to be titered upward. Trazodone, a quadricyclic antidepressant, works more quickly than some of the tricyclics and works well in reestablishing normal rapid eye movement (REM) sleep. Bupropion is often used because it reduces the sex drive the least. Amitryptilene and desimpramine have been used as adjuvant therapy for chronic pain, but have significant sedative side effects.

9. Methods of use

   a. A single drug, often an SSRI should be started. With tricyclic antidepressants, the dose is often increased slowly week by week or twice a week until an improvement is seen and as long as side effects are tolerable. With SSRIs, the side effects are less bothersome and effectiveness is often reached with the first or second dose. An adequate trial of one medication should take six to eight weeks, before another drug is added or substituted.

   b. Individuals should be educated about the side effects and urged to call if these are bothersome. However, they should commit to a minimum of three to four week treatment.

   c. After failure with one SSRI, a change to another SSRI or antidepressant is indicated.[22]

   d. Only a small number of antidepressant tablets should be prescribed at one time, because of the risk of suicide. Antidepressants can cause serious cardiac arrhythmias in high or overdoses.

   e. The second visit should be soon, within 2–4 weeks. After an adequate dose and response is determined, once a month or two is sufficient.

   f. The medication should be continued 4–8 months before tapering off.

   g. Women should be seen regularly in the first weeks after the initiation of antidepressants. Once an adequate dose is determined, once every month to two months may be sufficient.

10. SSRIs have become the agent of choice for depression, but their safety in pregnancy has just recently been addressed. A cohort study of Danish women found that the relative risk for birth defects in women who were taking SSRIs in the first trimester was elevated at 1.34.[23] A Canadian retrospective study using birth registration data found that SSRIs did not cause any increase in birth defects, especially cardiac defects, over other antidepressants, and that the rate was increased only for women who took more than 25 mg paroxetine in the first trimester.[24] A recent meta-analysis of 15 studies found use of fluoxetine, sertraline, citalopram and venlafaxine in early pregnancy was not associated with an increased risk of major congenital malformations.[25] Because depression in pregnancy and the postnatal period is so damaging to mother, child, and family and potentially dangerous, proper and adequate doses of antidepressants should be used. Treatment in the third trimester with these drugs may cause a withdrawal syndrome in the infant, and the infant should be watched after birth in an intensive care unit.

11. Women who are pregnant or breast feeding should most likely not use lithium, valproate, benzodiazepines, or carbamazepine.

12. Newer drugs are under investigation for depression. Gabapentin has shown some promise in women who respond poorly to other drugs and in those with chronic pain.[26]

Risk of suicide

1. Women under age 30 are more likely to attempt suicide than men, but are less likely to be successful. Women often choose less lethal methods.

2. Women at higher risk of suicide attempts include those with major depressive disorders, age less than 30, living alone, and those with substance abuse problems, psychosocial stressors and personality disorders. A prospective study investigating the risk factors for suicide acts in women with depression found that, unlike men, the risk increased sixfold if the woman had a previous suicide attempt, and increased three times for each attempt. Expressing fewer reasons for living and/or hostility, living alone,

Table 22.4 Risk factors for suicide acts

Major depressive disorders
Age less than 30
Living alone
Those with substance abuse problems
Psychosocial stressors
Personality disorders
Previous suicide attempt
Expressing fewer reasons for living
Hostility
Suicidal ideation
Cigarette smoking

a borderline personality disorder, suicidal ideation and cigarette smoking were all risk factors for women. Family history of suicide was not a risk factor for women[27] (Table 22.4).

3. Women at higher risk for completed suicides include those with psychotic depressions, substance abuse, previous suicide attempts, active ideation, divorced or widowed, chronic mental illness and those with panic or severe anxiety disorders.

Assessment for suicide risk

1. All depressed patients must be assessed for their risk of suicide, by asking directly for thoughts and plans. If there is a suicide thought or plan, emergency treatment is needed.

2. Other indications for immediate referral include hallucinations, psychotic ideation and thought disorders.

3. The more precise, immediate and lethal the plan, the higher is the short-term risk.

4. The more socially isolated the woman is, with fewer resources and less social support, the higher the risk of suicide.

To decrease suicide risk

1. The woman can be urged to go to or be placed in a safe environment, such as hospital, close supervision, or a friend staying with her. Women are more likely to need hospitalization if they have poor impulse control, chemical dependency, alcoholism, major depression, or other psychiatric disorder.

2. Immediate or quick symptom relief, especially relief from pain, may decrease suicide risk.
3. Making a "no suicide" contract with the patient may decrease her risk of a suicide attempt. Creating ways the woman can easily contact her physician or mental health provider will help.
4. Maximizing and identifying family and community resources and social support is important.

Special situations

Caregivers

1. Women are often the caregivers for their parents, their spouse, or the in-laws and others. Almost a quarter of working women are also caring for a disabled individual.
2. Caregivers are more likely to become depressed and ignore their own health needs.
3. The caregiver is more likely to become depressed if the patient being cared for has a psychiatric disorder or dementia.

Cancer patients

1. Cancer patients are more prone than others to depression.[28] In a NIH review, the incidence of depression in cancer patients ranged from 1 to 42%.[29] Other studies have suggested that 15–40% of those with solid tumors develop depression.[30] In a recent cohort study, the incidence of depression was found to be one-third in women with breast cancer, which decreased to 15% at one year and 45% if a recurrence was diagnosed.[31]
2. Untreated depression can cause more frequent clinic visits, increased cost, extended hospitalization, and reduced adherence to therapeutic protocols, and worse quality of life.
3. Depression in cancer is more likely in women, in patients with advanced stages, or in individuals with uncontrolled pain or a history of preexisting mood disorders.
4. Depression may be more difficult to diagnose, and underdiagnosed, in patients with cancer because vegetative symptoms such as weight loss, insomnia, hypersomnia, fatigue, anorexia, thoughts of death, and anergy may be caused by the cancer, the depression, or both.[32] Specific symptoms occurring in depressed cancer patients are listed in Table 22.5.

Table 22.5 Symptoms of depression in patients with cancer

Sense of failure
Loss of social interest
Feelings of being punished
Dissatisfaction and despair
Suicidal ideation
Indecision
Loss of interest or crying

5. Depression can be treated successfully with antidepressants. At times, practitioners may be less likely to treat depression in a cancer patient, assuming it is a normal response. Depression does not automatically resolve when the tumor improves or is surgically removed.
6. Antidepressants can treat fatigue caused by depression, but not the fatigue caused by the cancer or chemotherapy.
7. Depression seems to worsen mortality in the short term. In several types of cancer such as melanoma, non-small-cell lung cancer, breast, hematologic, and kidney cancer, patients with depression had a lower one-year and five-year survival rate.[33] A large prospective study over eight years with 10,000 patients found that depression increased the risk of death.[34]
8. Death from suicide occurs in only 2–6% of terminally ill patients. However, cancer patients are twice as likely to commit suicide as other patients with depression (Table 22.6).

Chronic disease

1. Although many individuals with chronic disease develop depression, they should not be placed on antidepressants prophylactically. Antidepressant medications have too many side effects and interactions to be used prophylactically. However, close observation, clinical suspicion, and follow-up are essential. Depression can worsen recovery or rehabilitation of many chronic diseases.

2. **Cardiac disease**

   Depression in individuals with cardiac disease is common. A cross-sectional study of more than 2000 women and men with cardiac disease found an incidence of approximately 20%. Individuals

Table 22.6 Risk factors for suicide in cancer patients

Poor prognosis

Advanced stage of illness

Delirium with poor impulse control

Inadequately treated pain

Major depression

Premorbid psychiatric or personality disorders

Alcohol abuse

Prior suicide attempts

Poor social supports

Physical and emotional exhaustion

Table 22.7 Criteria for premenstrual dysphoric disorder

Presence of 5/11 symptoms with at least one quarter occurring with menstrual cycle a week before menses and ceasing with onset of menses, that interfere with social, occupational and/or school functioning, and must be present for at least one year.

Breast tenderness or swelling, headaches, weight gain, bloated feelings, joint or muscle pain

Changes in sleep

Lethargy, fatigue, lack of energy

Feeling sad or tearful

Marked depressive mood with hopelessness and self-deprecation

Anhedonia or decreased interest in activities

Difficulty concentrating

Feeling overwhelmed or out of control

Persistent marked irritability, anger, interpersonal conflicts, anxiety, tension

with depression were more likely to report a greater symptom burden and physical limitations and a poorer quality of life.[12] Depression often occurs in the six months after a myocardial infarction or diagnosis of cardiac disease and can worsen rehabilitation or impede proper treatment. In the elderly, confusion and lethargy can be signs of either a myocardial infarction, or depression.

3. **Stroke**

There is a higher frequency of depression in patients who have had a stroke, (12–20%) although this may be more difficult to diagnose, especially in those individuals with aphasias.[35] Predominantly vegetative signs and mood disturbances are the signs of depression. Most stroke patients with depression improve within the first year. Active treatment with antidepressants improves the symptoms. Depression can worsen the recovery from stroke and those who are depressed have a higher mortality rate, up to double the mortality rate.[36]

The elderly

1. Major depressive disorder is not more common in the elderly; approximately 1% of elderly community dwelling individuals are depressed. It is more common in primary care patients and in those in a nursing home. In women in long-term care settings, approximately 12% are depressed. The predisposition to depression continues into older ages in women.

2. Depression may be more difficult to diagnose in the elderly because loss of interest, fatigue, and decreased energy and appetite may be mistakenly attributed to the normal aging process.

3. Serious suicide attempts were more than twice as common in elderly depressed patients with somatic complaints and in elderly men who are living alone.

4. Treatment of the elderly is the same as for younger individuals, except that the elderly may be more sensitive to side effects at lower doses of medication. Psychotherapy also works. Tricyclic antidepressant medications may create arrhythmias and depress cardiac function, negatively affect balance, memory and orthostatic pressure, increase falls and urinary retention. SSRIs may be a better choice.

5. Electroconvulsive therapy (ECT) use increased in the 1990s. There was a greater use in older women, whites and the disabled population. However safe, its effectiveness has not been studied against antidepressants.[37]

Premenstrual dysphoric disorder

1. Between 3 and 5% of women meet the criteria for the disorder (Table 22.7). However, premenstrual syndrome symptoms may affect 30–50% of

women. The symptoms include affective lability, persistent irritability, depressed mood, intense anxiety, concentration problems, fatigue, and changes in sleep and appetite.

2. Exact diagnosis is difficult because of lack of consensus regarding pathophysiology and its relation to other systems, including hormonal symptoms.

3. Treatment is unclear. Suggested treatments include exercise, changes in diet, caffeine restriction, increased carbohydrate or chocolate consumption, decreased alcohol, and/or treatment with progesterone, SSRIs daily or one week per month, gonadotropin releasing hormone antagonists, and/or anxiety drugs. SSRIs are effective for half of the patients and can be given daily, half the cycle, or one week per month.

Table 22.8 Risk factors for postpartum depression

Lack of spousal support

Difficulties in the marriage

Preterm infants

Twins

Less positive social adjustment

Less satisfaction and gratification in the parental role

Poorer personal health

History of depression

Family history of depression

Stressful life events

Being an adolescent

Depression during pregnancy

1. Women are not more likely to become depressed in pregnancy. Depression rates are the same in pregnant and non-pregnant women. Having a depression in pregnancy is related to a previous history of depression. In one study, approximately 43% of women who discontinued antidepressants when they learned they were pregnant had a relapse of depression, whereas 26% who continued their antidepressants relapsed.[38]

2. Treatment during pregnancy is complicated by fear of causing fetal malformations or a withdrawal syndrome for the infant after delivery. Most antidepressants are considered safe in pregnancy,[39] although benzodiazepines, valproate, and lithium are not suggested. Several large prospective studies showed no causal relationships between in utero exposure to tricyclic antidepressants, fluoxetine, or other SSRIs and teratogenicity.

Postpartum depression

1. Postpartum depression can have significant sequelae for the mother, family and child, with depressed maternal–infant bonding.

2. There is a wide range of mood reactions reported in women after delivery. From 30 to 75% of women, depending on the study, have mild "postpartum blues" consisting of fatigue and lack of sleep, irritability, tearfulness and anxiety, lasting less than two weeks.

3. Eight to ten percent of women have a major depression within six months of delivery. At six months postpartum, the same percentage of women have had a depression as control women. However, there was a threefold higher rate of depression within five weeks of childbirth. Approximately 1–2 per 1000 women have a postpartum depressive psychosis. Approximately only 0.07% of pregnant women have a hospitalization for a perinatal psychotic depressive incident.[40]

4. Symptoms of major depression include anergy, guilt, fatigue, agitation and psychomotor retardation. Symptoms also include difficulty caring for the infant, disrupted family interaction and excessive maternal anxiety about the infant. Fatigue is a serious symptom and may extend for months, delaying resumption of normal activities. Psychosis would include hallucinations, delusions, and psychomotor retardation.

5. Risk factors include lack of spousal support, increased demands, previous history of depression and difficulties in the marital relationship. Teenage mothers are more likely to develop depression (Table 22.8). Ten percent of women hospitalized for psychiatric morbidity before delivery develop postpartum psychosis after their first birth.

6. Fatigue may also be caused by medical problems. Other causes of fatigue postpartum include anemia, infections, hypothyroidism, and cardiomyopathy.

7. Diagnosis can be difficult because many women have feelings of inadequacy in the maternal role, fatigue, loss of appetite, and lack of energy.

8. Most postpartum depressive episodes resolve within one year in two-thirds of women, but usually require antidepressant medication. SSRIs and tricyclics can be used by breast-feeding mothers. Women who received SSRIs were more likely to respond within one week, and women who used psychotherapy alone responded well but in a longer time.

9. Postpartum depression may be preventable in some cases. In one small randomized controlled study of pregnant women who had a history of depression, use of sertaline postpartum daily for 20 weeks prevented depression at least sevenfold; only 7% of women on sertaline had a significant postpartum depression, while half of those on placebo developed a depression.[41]

10. Whether postpartum depression is maternal or parental is disputed. Almost one-quarter of new fathers reported dysphoric symptoms, and 30% had depressed symptoms. There was significant correlation between maternal and paternal depressive symptoms.

11. Increased spousal and family support with infant care and housework was positively related to maternal well-being.

Menopause

1. While literature reviews have found no accumulated evidence that menopause in itself causes depression, after menopause, depression has been found to increase the risk of developing heart disease and the metabolic syndrome.[42] One recent prospective study found that women of similar ages who go through menopause are twice as likely to develop depression than those who are premenopausal, although the reason is not known.[43]

2. Depression occurring in the menopause should be treated similarly to other times in life. Treatment of hot flashes and vaginal dryness should be included if these symptoms occur.

Conclusions

Depression is a common illness in women's lives. However difficult to diagnose, depression needs a high degree of suspicion, because treatment is effective.

References

1. Probst J. C., Laditka S. B., Moore C. G., Harun N., Powell M. P., Baxley E. G. Rural-urban differences in depression prevalence: implications for family medicine. *Fam Med* 2006; **38**(9), 653–660.

2. Sartorius N., Ustun T. B., Lecrubier Y., Wittchen H. U. Depression comorbid with anxiety: results from the WHO study on psychological disorders in primary health care. *Br J Psychiatry* 1996; Suppl, 38–43.

3. Graham K., Massak A. Alcohol consumption and the use of antidepressants. *Can Med Assoc J* 2007; **176**(5), 633–637.

4. Alonso J., Angermeyer M. C., Bernert S., *et al.* Prevalence of mental disorders in Europe: results from the European Study of the Epidemiology of Mental Disorders (ESEMeD) project. *Acta Psychiatr Scand Suppl* 2004, 21–27.

5. Rickert V. I., Wiemann C. M., Berenson A. B. Ethnic differences in depressive symptomatology among young women. *Obstet Gynecol* 2000; **95**, 55–60.

6. Huang F. Y., Chung H., Kroenke K., Spitzer R. L. Related articles, links racial and ethnic differences in the relationship between depression severity and functional status. *Psychiatr Serv* 2006; **57**(4), 498–503.

7. Cohen C. I., Magai C., Yaffee R., Walcott-Brown L. Racial differences in syndromal and subsyndromal depression in an older urban population. *Psychiatr Serv* 2005; **56**(12), 1556–1563.

8. Blazer D. G., Kessler R. C., McGonagle K. A., Swarz M. S. The prevalence and distribution of major depression in a national community sample. *Am J Psychol* 1994; **151**, 979–986.

9. Klose M., Jacobi F. Can gender differences in the prevalence of mental disorders be explained by sociodemographic factors? *Arch Womens Ment Health* 2004; 7(2), 133–148.

10. Ferry J. P. Barriers to the diagnosis of depression in primary care. *J Clin Psychiatry* 1997; **58**, 5–10.

11. Joo J. H., Solano F. X., Mulsant B. H., Reynolds C. F., Lenze E. J. Predictors of adequacy of depression management in the primary care setting. *Psychiatr Serv* 2005; **56**(12), 1524–1528.

12. Ruo B., Rumsfeld J. S., Hlatky M. A., Liu H., Browner W. S., Whooley M. A. Depressive symptoms and health-related quality of life: the Heart and Soul Study. *J Am Med Assoc* 2003; **290**(2), 215–221.

13. Bowswell E. B., Stoudemire A. Major depression in the primary care setting. *Am J Med* 1996; **101**, 3S–9S.

14. Katon W., Lin E. H., Kroenke K. The association of depression and anxiety with medical symptom burden

in patients with chronic medical illness. *Gen Hosp Psychiatry* 2007; **29**(2), 147–155.

15. Lindwall M., Rennemark M., Halling A., Berglund J., Hassmen P. Depression and exercise in elderly men and women: findings from the Swedish national study on aging and care. *J Aging Phys Act* 2007; **15**(1), 41–55.

16. Hassmane P., Kiovula N., Uutela A. Physical exercise and psychological well-being. A population study in Finland. *Prev Med* 2000; **30**, 17–25.

17. Blumenthal J. A., Babyak M., Moore K., *et al.* Effects of exercise training on older patients with major depression. *Arch Intern Med* 1999; **159**, 2349–2356.

18. Hegerl U., Plattner A., Moller H. J. Should combined pharmaco- and psychotherapy be offered to depressed patients? A qualitative review of randomized clinical trials from the 1990s. *Eur Arch Psychiatry Clin Neurosci* 2004; **254**(2), 99–107.

19. Malt U. F., Roback O. H., Madsbu H. P., Bakke O., Loeb M. The Norwegian naturalistic treatment study of depression in general practice. Randomized double blind study. *Br Med J* 1999; **318**, 1180–1184.

20. Miranda J., Chung J. Y., Green B. L., Krupnick J., Siddique J., Revicki D. A., Belin T. Treating depression in predominantly low-income young minority women: a randomized controlled trial. *J Am Med Assoc* 2003; **290**(1), 57–65.

21. Kendrick T., Peveler R., Longworth L., *et al.* Cost-effectiveness and cost-utility of tricyclic antidepressants, selective serotonin reuptake inhibitors and lofepramine: randomised controlled trial. *Br J Psychiatry* 2006; **188**, 337–345.

22. Rush A. J., Trivedi M. H., Wisniewski S. R., *et al.*, STAR*D study team. Bupropion-SR, sertraline, or venlafaxine-XR after failure of SSRIs for depression. *N Engl J Med* 2006; **354**(12), 1231–1242.

23. Wogelius P., Nørgaard M., Gislum M., Pedersen L., Munk E., Mortensen P. B., Lipworth L., Sørensen H. T. Maternal use of selective serotonin reuptake inhibitors and risk of congenital malformations. *Epidemiology* 2006; **17**(6), 701–704.

24. Bérard A., Ramos E., Rey E., Blais L., St-André M., Oraichi D. First trimester exposure to paroxetine and risk of cardiac malformations in infants: the importance of dosage. *Birth Defects Res B Dev Reprod Toxicol* 2007; **80**(1), 18–27.

25. Bellantuono C., Migliarese G., Gentile S. Serotonin reuptake inhibitors in pregnancy and the risk of major malformations: a systematic review. *Hum Psychopharmacol* 2007; **22**(3), 121–128.

26. Vieta E., Manuel Goikolea J., Martínez-Arán A. A double-blind, randomized, placebo-controlled,

prophylaxis study of adjunctive gabapentin for bipolar disorder. *J Clin Psychiatry* 2006; **67**(3), 473–477.

27. Oquendo M. A., Bongiovi-Garcia M. E., Galfalvy H., Goldberg P. H., Grunebaum M. F., Burke A. K., Mann J. J. Sex differences in clinical predictors of suicidal acts after major depression: a prospective study. *Am J Psychiatry* 2007; **164**(1), 134–141.

28. Reeve J., Lloyd-Williams M., Dowrick C. Depression in terminal illness: the need for primary care-specific research. *Fam Pract* 2007; **24**(3), 263–268.

29. Patrick D. L., Ferketich S. L., Frame P. S., National Institutes of Health State-of-the-Science Panel. National Institutes of Health State-of-the-Science Conference Statement: symptom management in cancer: pain, depression, and fatigue, July 15–17, 2002. *J Natl Cancer Inst* 2003; **95**(15), 1110–1117.

30. Pasquini M., Biondi M. Depression in cancer patients: a critical review. *Clin Pract Epidemol Ment Health* 2007; **3**, 2.

31. Burgess C., Cornelius V., Love S., Graham J., Richards M., Ramirez A. Depression and anxiety in women with early breast cancer: five year observational cohort study. *Br Med J* 2005; **330**, 702–707, doi:10.1136/bmj.38343.670868.D3.

32. Ashbury F. D., Madlensky L., Raich P., Thompson M., Whitney G., Hotz K., Kralj B., Edell W. S. Antidepressant prescribing in community cancer care. *Support Care Cancer* 2003; **11**, 278–285.

33. Prieto J. M., Atala J., Blanch J., Carreras E., Rovira M., Cirera E., Espinal A., Gasto C. Role of depression as a predictor of mortality among cancer patients after stem-cell transplantation. *J Clin Oncol* 2005; **23**, 6063–6071, doi:10.1200/JCO.2005.05.751.

34. Onitilo A. A., Nietert P. J., Egede L. E. Effect of depression on all-cause mortality in adults with cancer and differential effects by cancer site. *Gen Hosp Psychiatry* 2006; **28**, 396–402, doi:10.1016/j.genhosppsych.2006.05.006.

35. Brodaty H., Withall A., Altendorf A., Sachdev P. S. Rates of depression at 3 and 15 months poststroke and their relationship with cognitive decline: the Sydney Stroke Study. *Am J Geriatr Psychiatry* 2007; **15**(6), 477–486.

36. Almeida O. P., Xiao J. Mortality associated with incident mental health disorders after stroke. *Aust N Z J Psychiatry* 2007; **41**(3), 274–281.

37. Van der Wurff F. B., Stek M. L., Hoogendijk W. L., Beekman A. T. Electroconvulsive therapy for the depressed elderly. *Cochrane Database Syst Rev* 2003; **2**, CD003593.

38. Cohen L. S., Altshuler L. L., Harlow B. L., *et al.* Relapse of major depression during pregnancy in women who

maintain or discontinue antidepressant treatment. *J Am Med Assoc* 2006; **295**(5), 499–507.

39. Hendrick V., Smith L. M., Suri R., Hwang S., Haynes D., Altshuler L. Birth outcomes after prenatal exposure to antidepressant medication. *Am J Obstet Gynecol* 2003; **188**, 812–815.

40. Harlow B. L., Vitonis A. F., Sparen P., Cnattingius S., Joffe H., Hultman C. M. Incidence of hospitalization for postpartum psychotic and bipolar episodes in women with and without prior prepregnancy or prenatal psychiatric hospitalizations. *Arch Gen Psychiatry* 2007; **64**(1), 42–48.

41. Wisner K. L., Perel J. M., Peindl K. S., Hanusa B. H., Piontek C. M., Findling R. L. Prevention of postpartum depression: a pilot randomized clinical trial. *Am J Psychiatry* 2004; **161**(7), 1290–1292.

42. Raikkonen K., Matthews K. A., Kuller L. H. Depressive symptoms and stressful life events predict metabolic syndrome among middle-aged women: a comparison of World Health Organization, Adult Treatment Panel III, and International Diabetes Foundation definitions. *Diabetes Care* 2007; **30**(4), 872–877.

43. Cohen L. S., Soares C. N., Vitonis A. F., Otto M. W., Harlow B. L. Risk for new onset of depression during the menopausal transition: the Harvard study of moods and cycles. *Arch Gen Psychiatry* 2006; **63**(4), 385. *Evid Based Ment Health* 2006; **9**(4), 109.

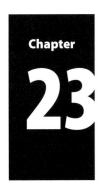

Chapter 23

Alcoholism, nicotine dependence and drug abuse

Mary-Anne Enoch

Mrs A., a middle-aged, smartly dressed woman who prided herself on her homemaker skills, came to see her family practitioner, Dr. B., complaining of tiredness, depressed mood, anxiety, disturbed sleep and weight gain. Dr. B. knew that her husband, a well-known local politician, had recently left her for a younger woman, so he tactfully avoided that subject, asking instead after her grown children who lived out of state. After questioning Mrs A. about her symptoms, Dr. B. concluded that she might be hypothyroid, depressed, anemic or all three and ran the appropriate tests. Several visits later, after normal test results and a failed trial of antidepressants, Dr. B. was feeling baffled until Mrs A. finally broke down in tears and revealed the cause of her symptoms. She had been a heavy drinker in her youth but had managed to stop when she had decided to have children. However, the recent stress and humiliation of her husband's desertion and subsequent loss of self-esteem, social status and role in life had been too much for her and she had taken to comforting herself during her long and empty days at home by drinking. Although she made great efforts to hide her drinking problem she had now reached the point where she could no longer control her urge to drink and was frightened and desperate for help but feared the social stigma of being labeled as an alcoholic.

Introduction

1. Mid-life is a vulnerable time for women, both for the development of problem drinking and alcoholism and for the manifestation of the medical consequences of long-term addiction to alcohol and tobacco.

2. The unique problems that mid-life women face are threefold. First, the sense of loss particular to this age: the end of childbearing capabilities, the slipping away of youth, children leaving home, marriage/partner break-up etc., may precipitate the onset of self-medicating problem drinking and alcoholism. Secondly, the biological effects of menopause-related hormonal changes on the hypothalamic-pituitary-adrenal (HPA) axis may increase stress and anxiety and hence vulnerability to problem drinking. Finally, medical sequelae such as cirrhosis of the liver or cancer are likely to emerge at this age in women who have been abusing alcohol and tobacco for a decade or two.

3. In many societies worldwide, people drink alcohol to relax and have a good time. The regular consumption of small amounts of alcohol has been shown to have health benefits. However, some individuals become addicted and are unable to keep within safe limits of consumption.

4. Addiction can be described as the relentless cycling of preoccupation and anticipation, binge/intoxication, and withdrawal/negative affect.[1] Both positive (euphoric) and negative (anxiolytic, antidysphoric) reinforcement are features of addiction. Negative reinforcement tends to predominate as the disease progresses.

Alcoholism

1. Alcoholism is one of the most common mental disorders. In the USA, the lifetime prevalence of alcohol dependence, the severe form of alcoholism, is 20% in men and 8% in women, and that of alcohol abuse is 12% in men and 6% in women.[2] In mid-life (45–64 yrs) women, the 12-month prevalence is 1% for alcohol dependence and 2% for alcohol abuse.[3] In the UK, at any one time, 8% of men and 2% of women are alcohol dependent.[4]

Handbook of Women's Health, second edition, ed. Jo Ann Rosenfeld. Published by Cambridge University Press.
© Cambridge University Press 2009.

2. Problem drinking and alcoholism often go undiagnosed for a variety of reasons, particularly in women and the elderly.[5] The rate of screening for alcohol consumption in health care settings remains lower than 50%.[6]

3. All too often patients continue to be treated symptomatically for alcohol-related conditions without recognition of the underlying problem. Some patients may withhold information, perhaps because of shame or fear of stigmatization.

4. Women, particularly mid-life and older, experience more social disapproval of alcohol and other drug abuse than men and this may account both for the tendency for mid-life women to drink in secrecy at home, and for the apparently lower rates of alcoholism in women.

Nicotine addiction

1. Nicotine is the other major addictive drug. In the 1990s, tobacco-related diseases accounted for 19% of all deaths in the USA. In contrast, alcoholism and other drug dependence accounted for 6%.

2. Social disapproval of smoking is not gender specific in western societies and this may account for the fact that nearly the same percentage of men (31%) and women (27%) are nicotine dependent.

3. Other addictions are not so common; in the USA, the lifetime prevalence of drug dependence and abuse is 9% and 5% respectively in men and 6% and 3% in women.[7] Drug dependence and abuse decline with age. Marijuana and other drug use in men and women above the age of 45 is reported to be almost non-existent in the UK.[4] In addition, 11% of men and 8% of women report using psychotherapeutic agents (such as benzodiazepines) in a non-prescribed manner.

4. The main focus of this chapter will be on alcoholism and smoking since these are the most prevalent addictive disorders in women and are most commonly seen and treated in family practice.

Comorbidity with other psychiatric disorders

1. Alcoholism is complicated by the fact that, particularly in women, it is often accompanied by other psychiatric disorders. Therefore, a holistic

approach is required for treatment. Comorbid conditions include tobacco use, drug abuse, major depression, anxiety disorders, bulimia nervosa and antisocial personality disorder (ASPD).[2]

2. Alcohol problems have been shown to predict the subsequent use of tranquilizing drugs in older women.[8] Severe alcoholism, impulsivity, and the likelihood of suicide coexist, but usually in men. ASPD and antisocial symptoms are more prominent in men alcoholics whereas in women, alcoholism is often associated with anxiety (particularly social phobia) and affective disorders.[2] Major depression is much more common in women than men and many studies have shown that antecedent depression is a risk factor for problem drinking. In women, there is a strong relationship between depression and smoking; depressed women are more likely to smoke and are less successful at smoking cessation.[9]

Alcoholism and smoking are highly comorbid; 80% to 90% of alcoholics smoke cigarettes compared with 30% of the general population, and 70% of alcoholics are heavy smokers (more than a pack a day) compared with 10% of the general population.[10] It has been shown that women who are regular smokers are five to six times more likely to be alcoholic compared to woman non-smokers. Among smoking alcoholics, the initiation of regular cigarette smoking typically precedes the onset of alcoholism by many years.[10] The high comorbidity may be due to the fact that either drug may increase the rewarding effects and/or reduce the aversive effects of the other. Some acute effects of nicotine may antagonize the negative effects (cognitive and psychomotor impairment) of acute alcohol consumption.

Genetic and environmental risk factors

The development of addiction to alcohol and other drugs is a complex process involving many factors including environmental, genetic and gene–environment interactions.[11]

Environmental factors

The biological transition associated with menopause is a time of increased psychological and physical vulnerability for some individuals which may be influenced in part by concurrent changes in the reactivity of the hormonal stress system. Stress is considered to be a major component in the continuation of drug use and also relapse. Addiction may result from excessive stress-related use; for example, pre-morbid anxiety/dysphoria is associated with use of alcohol and nicotine, although not cannabis, as coping mechanisms.[12] Smokers often state that they smoke more when stressed and stress frequently provokes smoking relapse. Women are more likely than men to self-medicate with alcohol; they often attribute the start of their problem drinking to a traumatic life event and the continuance of heavy drinking to stressors.

Severe childhood stressors such as emotional, physical and sexual abuse have been associated with increased vulnerability to psychopathology, including addiction, and the impact extends at least to middle age and probably beyond.[13,14,15] Large national surveys of women's drinking habits found that the prevalence of childhood sexual abuse (CSA) in the community was 15% to 26%[16] and was associated with a fourfold increase in the lifetime prevalence of both alcoholism and other drug abuse[13] as well as increased depression, anxiety and sexual dysfunction.[14] Among woman drug users, 70% report CSA and more than 80% have at least one parent addicted to alcohol or drugs.[17] Women with a history of childhood abuse show over-activity of the HPA axis in response to stress and may be more brittle in coping with stress.[18]

Problem drinking in mid-life women is associated with marital disruption, children leaving home, being primarily a homemaker, a lack of social roles, non-traditional jobs, rapid acculturation in ethnic minority women, adverse childhood experiences and poor interpersonal relationships.[19] Other risk factors appear to be a failure to adapt to aging, heavy spousal drinking, drinking alone at home and abuse of prescribed psychoactive drugs.[20] Never married, divorced and separated women are generally the heaviest drinkers and have the highest rates of drinking related problems. Partnership dissolution may be a risk factor for increased drinking in women who are not problem drinkers, but, perversely, in women who are already drinking heavily, separation or divorce can lead to a reduction in problem drinking, perhaps due to stress resolution.[21]

Genetic factors

Heritable vulnerability factors for addiction can be broadly classified into three categories. First, certain heritable personality traits may predispose an individual to seek out and consume large quantities of alcohol (self-medication) and therefore increase their chances of becoming addicted. Neuroticism,[22] particularly in women, and anxious temperament have been associated with alcoholism.[23] Neuroticism is also strongly associated with the development of nicotine withdrawal in women.[24] On the other hand, men with impulsive, novelty seeking personalities are more likely to seek out pleasure-inducing substances. Secondly a heritable differential response to the effects of alcohol is associated with alcoholism vulnerability; a low response to the sedating effects of alcohol has been shown in both men and women to be associated with a fourfold increase in the risk for alcoholism over time.[25] Finally genetic variation in neurobiological pathways and stress response systems may mean that some individuals are more vulnerable to the development of permanent neurological changes manifested by a pattern of craving and loss of control over drug consumption.

A recent meta-analysis of twin studies has shown that the heritability (the genetic component of interindividual variability) of all addictive substances ranges from 40% to 70%; the heritability of both alcoholism and smoking, derived from nearly 10,000 twin pairs, is 50%.[26] Therefore genetic and environmental factors are almost equally important in addiction risk although the proportions will vary in different populations. Increased severity of addiction may have a greater genetic component. Although there is no sex difference in the heritability of alcoholism[22,27,28,29] the genes that are involved in alcoholism vulnerability overlap only partially in men and women.[28] The heritability of nicotine dependence is the same in men and women, however, it appears that only half the genes are shared.[30]

Alcohol, cocaine, opiate and nicotine dependency tend to co-occur. As previously stated, approximately 70% of alcoholics are heavy smokers compared with 10% of the general population. This raises the possibility that there are both shared and substance-specific components to the heritability of alcoholism and other drug addictions. However, the results of large twin studies suggest that inheritance of addiction to alcohol, opioids, cocaine and cannabis is largely independent.[31] The strongest evidence for shared, as well as specific, addiction vulnerability is between alcohol and nicotine. In both men and women there is considerable genetic overlap between genes for alcoholism and nicotine addiction, particularly for heavy smoking and heavy drinking. Approximately 50% of the genetic effects for nicotine dependence are shared with alcoholism whereas 15% of the genetic effects for alcoholism are shared with nicotine dependence.[30]

Although alcoholism, major depression and anxiety disorders are often comorbid in women, it has been shown that there is not much overlap in the genes underlying these disorders; 75% of the genetic liability for alcoholism is disease specific and only small genetic components for alcoholism load onto a genetic factor common to major depression and generalized anxiety disorder as well as a factor common to phobia, panic and bulimia nervosa.[32]

Addiction may result from the interaction between genetic and environmental risk factors. One example of this is the interaction between the monoamine oxidase A (MAOA) gene and CSA. A recent study showed that among women who had experienced CSA those with the low activity MAOA variant were more likely to develop alcoholism compared to the women with the high activity variant who were more resilient to the effects of childhood adversity.[33]

Age and drinking patterns in women

Younger women (18–29 yrs) drink the most and tend to engage in heavy episodic drinking that can lead to severe adverse behavioral or social consequences. The 12-month prevalence of alcoholism is highest in this age group (10%) and declines with age.[3] Drinking in mid-life and elderly women is characterized by frequent light or moderate drinking.[21] Nevertheless, a substantial number of older women develop alcohol-related problems.

Drinking patterns and ethnicity

Some national (USA) data are available on drinking pattern differences between Caucasian, African American and Hispanic women. Abstention (approximately 50%) is higher among African American and Hispanic than Caucasian women. Caucasian women drink more over time and per occasion. As in men, the prevalence of alcoholism in women from all ethnic groups is highest in the young (18–29), and declines steadily with age.[3] The 12-month prevalence of alcoholism is highest in young Caucasian women (12%). In contrast, a large US survey of African

American women found that the prevalence of current drinking was highest among women aged 40–49 yrs.[34] It is possible that abstention and light drinking are more determined by cultural, social and historical characteristics than are problem drinking and alcoholism.[35]

Definitions: low-risk and problem drinking, alcoholism

The ceiling for low-risk alcohol use advocated by the US Government is one standard drink/day and not more than three drinks/occasion for women, and two standard drinks/day and no more than four drinks/occasion for men.[36] In the USA the standard drink is 14 gram of pure alcohol, equivalent to one 12 fl oz bottle of beer (5%), one 5 fl oz glass of wine (12%), or 1.5 fl oz of 80-proof distilled spirits.[36] In the UK the standard drink (unit) is 8 gram of pure alcohol and the ceiling for safe daily drinking is set at 3 to 4 units for men and 2 to 3 units for women. A meta-analysis of cohort studies evaluating the relationship between alcohol consumption and death from all causes found that the relative risk of death (due to cirrhosis, cancer and injury) increased significantly in women consuming 2 to 3 US standard drinks per day and men consuming 5 to 6 drinks per day.[37]

In some individuals, problem drinking progresses into alcoholism. The essential features of addiction are loss of control over consumption, compulsion to obtain the next stimulant, and continuation of abuse despite knowledge of negative health and social consequences (for a review of the diagnosis of alcoholism see Enoch and Goldman[5]). Prolonged heavy drinking may lead to long-lasting or permanent neurobiological changes, the essence of addiction, leading to craving and a loss of control over consumption. Tolerance and dependence are due to neuroadaptations.

Medical consequences of long-term, heavy drinking

The principal harmful effects of heavy drinking include liver pathology (hepatitis, hepatoma and cirrhosis), neurological complications and cancers of the mouth, larynx, esophagus and breast. Medical complications are likely to present in middle age in those alcoholics and smokers who started drinking and smoking in their youth.

Women achieve higher blood alcohol concentrations than men after the consumption of equivalent doses per body weight. The most likely explanation for this is that there is a lower volume of distribution of alcohol in women because the solubility of alcohol is greater in water than fat and women tend to have proportionally more fat and less body water than men. The higher blood alcohol concentration may cause greater organ toxicity than in men. Women tend to present with more severe liver disease (particularly alcoholic hepatitis) and do so after drinking less and over a shorter period of time than men. Women are more likely to die from cirrhosis.[38] The evidence is still inconclusive as to whether women's brains are more sensitive to the deleterious effects of alcohol; some studies have demonstrated that alcoholic women show greater (reversible) gray and white matter brain shrinkage than alcoholic men[39] but in other studies alcoholic women show no detectable deficits compared with healthy women.[40]

Alcohol intake is thought to be responsible for 6% of all cancer deaths worldwide.[41] Many studies report that moderate to heavy recent alcohol consumption increases the risk for breast cancer.[42,43] A meta-analysis of studies involving over 150,000 women showed an increased relative risk of breast cancer of 32% for an intake of 35 to 44 gram per day of alcohol, and the relative risk increased by 7% for each additional 10 gram per day alcohol intake.[44] The investigators concluded that if the observed relationship is causal then about 4% of the breast cancers in developed countries are alcohol related. A recent large meta-analysis has shown that the population attributable risk estimate is 0.9 to 2.4% in the USA and 3.2 to 8.8% in the UK, reflecting different drinking habits in the two countries.[45] Risk does not differ significantly by beverage type or menopausal status.[45] A prospective cohort study of nearly 45,000 postmenopausal women has shown that the relative risk is doubled when alcohol consumption is combined with hormone replacement therapy.[46] In contrast, smoking has little or no independent effect on the risk of developing breast cancer.[44]

Numerous case control, prospective studies and meta-analyses have demonstrated an association between alcohol consumption and colorectal cancer; there is a 15% increased risk of colon or rectal cancer for an increase of 100 gram of alcohol intake per week and 40% increased risk with regular consumption of around 50 gram per day.[47,48]

The multiple harmful effects of cigarette consumption are well known and will not be discussed further here. However, it should be noted that the effects of alcohol and cigarette smoking are synergistic in the development of oral, laryngeal, pharyngeal and esophageal cancers.

Beneficial effects of alcohol consumption

Before the age of 60, breast cancer is a more important cause of death than heart disease. Later on, the risk of heart disease exceeds that of breast cancer so the benefits of moderate drinking are more apparent. The consumption of at least one drink a day by mid-life and elderly women is associated with a 20% reduction in the risk of cardiovascular disease compared to non-drinkers.[49] In both sexes, differing ethnicities, and across numerous countries it has been shown that there is a U-shaped relationship between alcohol consumption and all-cause mortality, including in the elderly.[50]

Treatment

The treatment options that a family physician may discuss with a patient will depend on the severity of the alcohol problem, the presence of comorbid medical and psychosocial problems, the patient's motivation to change and also the patient's gender. There are sex differences not only in the causes and consequences of alcoholism but also in comorbidity, communication style, self-esteem, interpersonal relationships and societal roles. Mixed-gender treatment groups are usually composed primarily of men and may therefore ignore woman issues. For all these reasons, women might do better in integrated women-oriented treatment approaches (bearing in mind that woman alcoholics are not themselves a homogeneous group, e.g. they may differ in age, ethnicity, experience of abuse, symptom severity etc.). The treatment of woman alcoholics includes three unique categories:[51] (a) related woman biological issues (e.g. reproduction, menopause); (b) psychological issues more commonly associated with alcoholism in women than men (e.g. past sexual or physical abuse, poor self-esteem, guilt and shame); and (c) psychiatric comorbidity and multiple substance abuse. Treatment programs for women do exist; however, research on the impact of these services on both access and outcome is lacking. There is one controlled study of 200 women that demonstrated that woman alcoholics treated in a specialized woman unit of a psychiatric hospital showed better control of alcohol consumption and social adjustment than women treated in a mixed unit.[52]

Due to both increased comorbidity and the way that women articulate and rationalize their drinking problems, women are more likely than men to seek treatment in health and social service facilities than in alcoholism and chemical dependency services. However, the cultural constraints against the admission of a drinking problem (even to themselves) for middle-aged women are huge. Unlike men, women often view their heavy drinking as a coping mechanism and not a problem; the most frequent reasons given by women for seeking treatment are: depression, alcohol-related medical problems, interpersonal problems with spouse, partner or children, and, especially among mid-life women, the "empty nest" syndrome.[53] Therefore it may take longer for mid-life women's alcohol abuse to be recognized and treated.

Treatment of problem drinking; the use of brief intervention in family practice

The family physician can play a key role in recognizing problem drinking, together with comorbid conditions, and can often intervene successfully, particularly in the early stages.[36] Several formal screening instruments for problem drinking/alcoholism are available (reviewed in Enoch and Goldman[5]). Brief intervention is a short-term, counselling strategy based on motivational enhancement therapy, that concentrates on changing patient behavior and increasing patient compliance with therapy.[54] It is designed for health professionals who are not specialists in addiction. Brief intervention involves: (1) reviewing with the patient the quantity and frequency of current drinking and their personal causes of excessive drinking; (2) advising the patient to reduce or stop drinking and making them aware of their personal risks for alcohol-related problems; (3) discussing with them whether, or when, they will reduce or stop drinking and emphasizing their personal responsibility; (4) suggesting coping mechanisms, behavior modification, self-help groups (e.g. Alcoholics Anonymous); (5) establishing a drinking goal and the setting up of a drinking diary. For brief intervention to be successful it is very important for the physician to encourage self-motivation and optimism and to be non-judgmental and supportive. Brief

intervention has been shown to be effective for helping socially stable problem drinkers reduce or stop drinking, for motivating alcohol dependent patients to enter long-term alcohol treatment, and for treating some alcohol dependent patients in whom the goal is abstinence. It is generally only necessary to have four or fewer sessions, each ranging from a few minutes to an hour depending on the severity of the patient's alcohol problem.[54] It is not known whether this kind of intervention is equally effective in men and women and at all ages.

Treatment of alcohol dependence and abuse

A formal diagnosis of alcoholism can have enormous personal implications for a patient, therefore assessment should be detailed.[5] Alcohol abuse and dependence have a variable course characterized by periods of remission and relapse. There are three components to alcoholism: (a) physiological dependence (symptoms of withdrawal); (b) psychological dependence (alcohol used as self-medication); and (c) habit (the incorporation of drinking into the framework of daily living).

Alcohol dependence is treated in two stages: withdrawal and detoxification, followed by further interventions to prevent relapse.

Immediate treatment: detoxification and the control of alcohol withdrawal syndrome

In heavy, chronic drinkers, withdrawal symptoms begin 6 to 48 hours after the last drink, peak within 24 to 48 hours and gradually resolve within 5 to 7 days. The severity of withdrawal symptoms increases with each withdrawal episode. Severe withdrawal (grand mal convulsions, delerium tremens) occurs in 2 to 5% of heavy drinking chronic alcoholics. With treatment, mortality is about 1%, death usually being due to cardiovascular collapse or concurrent infection.

Benzodiazepines are widely used for treatment of withdrawal because they greatly reduce symptoms and the risk of seizure. However, benzodiazepines are sedating, produce cognitive impairment, are addictive, and may interact additively with alcohol. An alternative approach is to use non-sedating, non-addictive, anticonvulsant agents such as carbamazepine and valproic acid which have been used successfully for many years in Europe. These drugs have hematological side effects and liver toxicity so that patients have to be medically screened before use. Alcoholics should be admitted to hospital for detoxification if they are likely to have severe, life-threatening symptoms or have serious medical conditions, suicidal or homicidal tendencies or disruptive work or home situations.

Sustained treatment; prevention of relapse

Addictive substances acutely activate the HPA axis and this has been implicated in both positive and negative reinforcement of drug use. Chronic drug use leads to altered HPA axis homeostasis and this is thought to increase the risk of stress-induced relapse.[1] The HPA axis is modulated by sex hormones and it is not known whether the estrogen fluctuations experienced by perimenopausal women makes them more susceptible to stress-induced relapse; this seems unlikely since acute estrogen deficits have been correlated with normal stimulated cortisol production.[55]

There is considerable evidence that long-term neurobiological changes in the brains of alcoholics contribute to the persistence of craving. At any stage during recovery, relapse can be triggered by internal factors (craving for alcohol, depression, anxiety) or external factors (environmental triggers, social pressures, life events, taking drugs e.g. narcotics). Depression appears to be associated with relapse in women, but not in men. For both sexes the severity of alcoholism is a predictor of relapse but for women a measure of psychological functioning and social networks are predictive of outcome. Married men are less likely to relapse after treatment whereas for women, being married contributes to relapse in the short term.[56] Alcoholic women appear to receive less support from family and friends than do non-alcoholic women, both in childhood and adulthood.[53] The development of new, fulfilling social roles and an effective social support network (such as through Alcoholics Anonymous and Women for Sobriety) is an important aspect of alcoholism treatment for women.

The main elements of treatment for alcoholism are still psychosocial. These methods concentrate on helping alcoholics to understand, anticipate and prevent relapse. Relapse rates are still very high, however several promising drugs that can be used as adjuncts to psychosocial treatments are being developed.

Behavioral treatment approaches

No one behavioral approach has been shown to produce better results than another, therefore patient preference, cost considerations and availability of treatment will determine which approach is taken.

Alcoholics Anonymous (AA), Women for Sobriety and 12-step facilitation therapy

AA is a worldwide spiritual program that addresses people from all social strata. Group members share their experiences in a confidential environment and provide each other with help and support in order to maintain sobriety. AA and similar self-help groups follow 12 steps that alcoholics should work through during recovery. There are women-only AA groups. Twelve-step facilitation (TSF) is a formal treatment approach incorporating AA and similar 12-step programs.[57]

Women for Sobriety (WFS) is a rapidly expanding worldwide organization of women for women. The purpose is to help women recover from all aspects of addiction (physiological, mental and emotional) through the discovery of self, gained by sharing experiences, hopes and encouragement with other women in similar circumstances. The WFS "new life" program starts by accepting alcoholism as a disease, getting rid of negative thoughts (guilt, shame), creating and practicing a new, positive view of self, using new attitudes to enforce new behavior patterns, and making efforts to improve relationships and identify life's priorities.

Cognitive-behavioral therapy (CBT) and motivational enhancement therapy (MET)

The aim of CBT is to teach patients, by role play and rehearsal, to recognize and cope with high-risk situations for relapse, and to recognize and cope with craving.[58] MET is used to motivate patients to use their own resources to change their behavior and has been found to be most effective in those with high levels of anger.[59]

Pharmacotherapy of alcohol addiction

Only 30–60% of alcoholics maintain at least one year of abstinence with psychosocial therapies alone which is not much of an improvement over the more than 20% of alcoholics who achieve long-term sobriety even without active treatment. More effective therapies are clearly needed. New drugs are emerging that may complement psychosocial treatments. More research needs to be done to determine which therapies are most effective in which alcoholic subtypes and whether there are sex differences in treatment response. The treatment focus in the past has been on abstinence. However, it is being increasingly accepted that, although desirable, abstinence may be an unrealistic goal for many alcoholics and the focus has therefore broadened to include drinking reduction as a form of damage control.

Relapse prevention and drinking reduction

The most promising of these to date are the opioid antagonist, naltrexone (ReVia), and acamprosate (Campral), a glutamate antagonist, which have been shown to exert modest effects on the reduction of alcohol consumption. These drugs are likely to fore-shadow other pharmacotherapies which will target multiple neurotransmitters. Further studies are needed to identify the subgroups of alcoholics who may be most responsive to these drugs.

Several studies have shown that naltrexone, also used in the post detoxification treatment of heroin addicts, reduces alcohol consumption in both men and woman alcoholics and is moderately effective, when combined with psychosocial treatment, in reducing relapse to heavy drinking.[60,61] The effect of naltrexone on abstinence rates is less clear.[61] Naltrexone is recommended for the short-term treatment (12 weeks) of alcoholism and a long-acting injectible formulation (Vivitrol) is now available.[61] Taking naltrexone two hours prior to an anticipated high-risk situation reduces alcohol consumption in early problem drinkers.[62] Problem-drinking women appear to benefit more from targeted than daily naltrexone.[62] Acamprosate, used extensively in Europe and recently approved in the USA, appears to be safe and well tolerated and has a significant beneficial effect on abstinence maintenance in recently detoxified alcoholics.[61,63] Both naltrexone and acamprosate have been shown to be effective and at the present time there is little evidence to favor one drug over the other or to suggest that they should be used in combination.

Aversive pharmacotherapy

Disulfiram (Antabuse), a drug with a moderate record of adverse effects including hepatotoxicity, blocks the metabolism of acetaldehyde and causes the very

unpleasant flushing reaction if taken with alcohol. Outcomes with disulfiram are improved when the drug is taken under supervision.

Pharmacotherapy for comorbid conditions

Depression and anxiety can precipitate alcohol abuse but can also be a result of heavy drinking. It is important to take a careful history in order to identify the primary problem. Fluoxetine (Prozac), a serotonin re-uptake inhibitor, has been found to be effective in decreasing both depressive symptoms and the level of alcohol consumption in depressed alcoholics.[61]

Pharmacotherapy of nicotine addiction

The acute effects of smoking (calmness, alertness, and increased concentration) are positively reinforcing, whereas nicotine withdrawal symptoms (depressed mood, insomnia, irritability, anxiety, poor concentration, weight gain) are negatively reinforcing. Pharmacotherapy is an integral part of the treatment of nicotine dependence but is most effective with concurrent behavioral therapy. Both nicotine-replacement therapies and bupropion (Zyban) have been shown to approximately double long-term smoking cessation rates and have therefore been recommended as first-line therapy by the Agency for Healthcare Research and Quality.[64] Nicotine-replacement therapies (FDA approved) include 2 or 4 mg nicotine polacrilex gum, the nicotine patch, nicotine nasal spray, and the nicotine inhaler.[64,65] The choice of therapy can be individually tailored, depending on patient preference, side effects or the presence of other medical conditions. Sustained-release bupropion is an antidepressant medication.[65] Another antidepressant, nortriptyline, has recently been shown to be efficacious for smoking cessation.

Although nicotine-replacement therapies and bupropion significantly increase smoking cessation rates, many smokers still relapse – the one year quit rate remains low. There are limited or no research data regarding the success of smoking cessation therapies specific to gender or ethnicity. Further research needs to be done on treating specific populations, e.g. with comorbid diseases.

Treatment of alcoholic smokers

Studies indicate that alcohol consumption may be a risk factor for smoking relapse, partly because alcohol may increase craving for cigarettes. Likewise, smoking cues may promote craving for alcohol. Most alcoholic smokers state that they want to stop alcohol first and then cigarettes, however a substantial minority try both treatments simultaneously. It is not known which approach is the most efficacious.

Conclusion

Detecting and treating alcohol problems in mid-life women can be both challenging and complex because of the secrecy, the layers of comorbidity and the frequent undercurrent of (often suppressed) past adverse life events, particularly childhood sexual abuse. Nevertheless, family physicians are in a good position to diagnose and treat problem drinking because most adults visit their primary care physician at least once every two years and women in particular usually consult their physicians more frequently. In addition, there is often a trusting doctor–patient relationship, built up over years. Screening for alcohol problems needs to become routine in the same way that screening for smoking is now widespread. However, it may be harder for physicians to diagnose drinking problems in mid-life women, partly because they may assume that this group is low risk, partly because they may feel uncomfortable asking about a condition with a built-in social stigma, and partly because many middle-aged women prefer to keep their problem secret. This stigma may be erased over time with the aging of the current cohort of young women, amongst whom heavy drinking is socially acceptable. A holistic treatment approach needs to be taken, including management of comorbid conditions, counseling for previous emotional trauma, teaching of coping skills and the development of support networks, for example through AA and WFS.

References

1. Koob G. F. Alcoholism: allostasis and beyond. *Alcohol Clin Exp Res* 2003; **27**, 232–243.
2. Kessler R. C., Crum R. M., Warner L. A., *et al.* Lifetime co-occurrence of DSM-III-R alcohol abuse and dependence with other psychiatric disorders in the National Comorbidity Survey. *Arch Gen Psychiatry* 1997; **54**, 313–321.
3. Grant B. F., Dawson D. A., Stinson F. S., *et al.* The 12-month prevalence and trends in DSM-IV alcohol abuse and dependence: United States, 1991–1992 and 2001–2002. *Drug Alcohol Depend* 2004; **74**, 223–234.
4. Farrell M., Howes S., Bebbington P., *et al.* Nicotine, alcohol and drug dependence and psychiatric comorbidity. Results of a national household survey. *Br J Psychiatry* 2001; **179**, 432–437.
5. Enoch M.-A., Goldman D. Problem drinking and alcoholism: diagnosis and treatment. *Am Fam Physician* 2002; **65**, 441–450.
6. Fleming M. F. Strategies to increase alcohol screening in health care settings. *Alcohol Health Res World* 1997; **21**, 340–347.
7. Kessler R. C., McGonagle K. A., Zhao S., *et al.* Lifetime and 12-month prevalence of DSM-III-R psychiatric disorders in the United States: results from the National Comorbidity Survey. *Arch Gen Psychiatry* 1994; **51**, 8–19.
8. Graham K., Wilsnack S. C. The relationship between alcohol problems and use of tranquilizing drugs: longitudinal patterns among American women. *Addict Behav* 2000; **25**, 13–28.
9. Perkins K. A. Sex differences in nicotine versus non-nicotine reinforcement as determinants of tobacco smoking. *Exp Clin Psychopharmacol* 1996; **11**, 199–212.
10. National Institute on Alcohol Abuse and Alcoholism. Alcohol and tobacco. *Alcohol Alert* 1998; **39**, 1–4.
11. Enoch M.-A. Genetic and environmental influences on the development of alcoholism: resilience vs. risk. *Ann NY Acad Sci* 2006; **1094**, 193–201.
12. Stewart S. H., Karp J., Pihl R. O., Peterson R. A. Anxiety sensitivity and self-reported reasons for drug use. *J Subst Abuse* 1997; **9**, 223–240.
13. Winfield I., George L. K., Swartz M., *et al.* Sexual assault and psychiatric disorders among a community sample of women. *Am J Psychiatry* 1990; **147**, 335–341.
14. Wilsnack S. C., Vogeltanz N. D., Klassen A. D., Harris T. R. Childhood sexual abuse and women's substance abuse: national survey findings. *J Stud Alcohol* 1997; **58**, 264–271.
15. Widom C. S., Marmorstein N. R., White H. R. Childhood victimization and illicit drug use in middle adulthood. *Psychol Addict Behav* 2006; **20**, 394–403.
16. Vogeltanz N. D., Wilsnack S. C., Harris T. R. Prevalence and risk factors for childhood sexual abuse in women: national survey findings. *Child Abuse Negl* 1999; **23**, 579–592.
17. National Institute on Drug Abuse. Capsules. *Women and Drug Abuse* 1994; **6**, 2.
18. Heim C., Newport D. J., Heit S., *et al.* Pituitary-adrenal and autonomic responses to stress in women after sexual and physical abuse in childhood. *J Am Med Assoc* 2000; **284**, 592–597.

19. Wilsnack S. C., Wilsnack R. W. Drinking and problem drinking in US women. Patterns and recent trends. *Recent Dev Alcohol* 1995; **12**, 29–60.

20. Gomberg E. S. Risk factors for drinking over a woman's lifespan. *Alcohol Health Res World* 1994; **18**, 220–227.

21. Wilsnack S. C., Wilsnack R. W., Hiller-Sturmhofel S. How women drink: epidemiology of women's drinking and problem drinking. *Alcohol Health Res World* 1994; **18**, 173–180.

22. Heath A. C., Bucholz K. K., Madden P. A. F., *et al.* Genetic and environmental contributions to alcohol dependence risk in a national twin sample: consistency of findings in women and men. *Psychol Med* 1997; **27**, 1381–1396.

23. Ducci F., Enoch M.-A., Virkkunen M., *et al.* Increased anxiety and other similarities in temperament of alcoholics with and without antisocial personality disorder across three diverse populations. *Alcohol*, 2007; **41**(1), 3–12.

24. Madden P. A., Bucholz K. K., Dinwiddie S. H., *et al.* Nicotine withdrawal in women. *Addiction* 1997; **92**, 889–902.

25. Schuckit M. A., Smith T. L., Kalmijn J., *et al.* Response to alcohol in daughters of alcoholics: a pilot study and a comparison with sons of alcoholics. *Alcohol Alcohol* 2000; **35**, 242–248.

26. Goldman D., Oroszi G., Ducci F. The genetics of addictions: uncovering the genes. *Natl. Rev Genet* 2005; **6**, 521–532.

27. Kendler K. S., Neale M. C., Heath A. C., Kessler R. C., Eaves L. A twin-family study of alcoholism in women. *Am J Psychiatry* 1994; **151**, 707–715.

28. Prescott C. A., Aggen S. H., Kendler K. S. Sex differences in the source of genetic liability to alcohol abuse and dependence in a population-based sample of U.S. twins. *Alcohol Clin Exp Res* 1999; **23**, 1136–1144.

29. Prescott C. A., Kendler K. S. Genetic and environmental contributions to alcohol abuse and dependence in a population-based sample of men twins. *Am J Psychiatry* 1999; **156**, 34–40.

30. Hettema J. M., Corey L. A., Kendler K. S. A multivariate genetic analysis of the use of tobacco, alcohol and caffeine in a population-based sample of men and woman twins. *Drug Alcohol Depend* 1999; **57**, 69–78.

31. Goldman D., Bergen A. General and specific inheritance of substance abuse and alcoholism. *Arch Gen Psychiatry* 1998; **55**, 964–965.

32. Kendler K. S., Walters E. E., Neale M. C. The structure of the genetic and environmental risk factors for six major psychiatric disorders in women. *Arch Gen Psychiatry* 1995; **52**, 374–383.

33. Ducci F., Enoch M.-A., Hodgkinson C., *et al.* Interaction between a functional MAOA locus and childhood sexual abuse predicts alcoholism and antisocial personality disorder in adult women. *Mol Psychiatry* 2008; **13**, 334–347.

34. Rosenberg L., Palmer J. R., Rao R. S., Adams-Campbell L. L. Patterns and correlates of alcohol consumption among African-American women. *Ethn Dis* 2002; **12**, 548–554.

35. Caetano R. Drinking and alcohol-related problems among minority women. *Alcohol Health Res World* 1994; **18**, 233–241.

36. National Institute on Alcohol Abuse and Alcoholism. *Helping Patients Who Drink Too Much: A Clinician's Guide*, 2005. http://www.niaaa.nih.gov/guide.

37. Holman C. D., English D. R., Milne E., Winter M. G. Meta-analysis of alcohol and all-cause mortality: a validation of NHMRC recommendations. *Med J Aust* 1996; **164**, 141–145.

38. Day C. P. Who gets alcoholic liver disease: nature or nuture? *J R Coll Physicians Lond* 2000; **34**, 557–562.

39. Wuethrich B. Does alcohol damage woman brains more? *Science* 2001; **291**, 2077–2079.

40. Pfefferbaum A., Rosenbloom M., Deshmukh A., Sullivan E. Sex differences in the effects of alcohol on brain structure. *Am J Psychiatry* 2001; **158**, 188–197.

41. Danaei G., Vander Hoorn S., Lopez A. D., Murray C. J., Ezzati M., Comparative Risk Assessment Collaborating Group (Cancers). Causes of cancer in the world: comparative risk assessment of nine behavioural and environmental risk factors. *Lancet* 2005; **366**, 1784–1793.

42. Zhang S. M., Lee I. M., Manson J. E., *et al.* Alcohol consumption and breast cancer risk in the Women's Health Study. *Am J Epidemiol* 2007; **165**, 667–676.

43. Tjonneland A., Christensen J., Olsen A., *et al.* Alcohol intake and breast cancer risk: the European Prospective Investigation into Cancer and Nutrition (EPIC). *Cancer Causes Control* 2007; **18**, 361–373.

44. Hamajima N., Hirose K., Tajima K., *et al.* Alcohol, tobacco and breast cancer – collaborative reanalysis of individual data from 53 epidemiological studies, including 58,515 women with breast cancer and 95,067 women without the disease. *Br J Cancer* 2002; **87**, 1234–1245.

45. Key J., Hodgson S., Omar R. Z., *et al.* Meta-analysis of studies of alcohol and breast cancer with consideration of the methodological issues. *Cancer Causes Control* 2006; **17**, 759–770.

46. Chen W. Y., Colditz G. A., Rosner B., *et al.* Use of postmenopausal hormones, alcohol, and risk for invasive breast cancer. *Ann Intern Med* 2002; **137**, 798–804.

47. Moskal A., Norat T., Ferrari P., Riboli E. Alcohol intake and colorectal cancer risk: a dose-response meta-analysis of published cohort studies. *Int J Cancer* 2007; **120**, 664–671.

48. Cho E., Smith-Warner S. A., Ritz J., *et al.* Alcohol intake and colorectal cancer: a pooled analysis of 8 cohort studies. *Ann Intern Med* 2004; **140**, 603–613.

49. Thun M. J., Peto R., Lopez A. D., *et al.* Alcohol consumption and mortality among middle-aged and elderly U.S. adults. *New Engl J Med* 1997; **337**, 1705–1714.

50. Paganini-Hill A., Kawas C. H., Corrada M. M. Type of alcohol consumed, changes in intake over time and mortality: the Leisure World Cohort Study. *Age Ageing* 2007; **36**, 203–209.

51. Beckman L. J. Treatment needs of women with alcohol problems. *Alcohol Health Res World* 1994; **18**, 206–211.

52. Dahlgren L., Willander A. Are special treatment facilities for woman alcoholics needed? A controlled 2-year follow-up study from a specialized woman unit (EWA) versus a mixed men/woman treatment facility. *Alcohol Clin Exp Res* 1989; **13**, 499–504.

53. Gomberg E. S. Women and alcohol: use and abuse. *J Nerv Ment Dis* 1993; **181**, 211–219.

54. Fleming M., Manwell L. B. Brief intervention in primary care settings. *Alcohol Res Health* 1999; **23**, 128–137.

55. De Leo V., la Marca A., Talluri B., D'Antona D., Morgante G. Hypothalamo-pituitary-adrenal axis and adrenal function before and after ovariectomy in premenopausal women. *Eur J Endocrinol* 1998; **138**, 430–435.

56. Schneider K. M., Kviz F. J., Isola M. L., Filstead W. J. Evaluating multiple outcomes and gender differences in alcoholism treatment. *Addict Behav* 1995; **20**, 1–21.

57. Humphreys K. Professional interventions that facilitate 12-step self-help group involvement. *Alcohol Res Health* 1999; **23**, 93–98.

58. Longabaugh R., Morgenstern J. Cognitive-behavioral coping-skills therapy for alcohol dependence. *Alcohol Res Health* 1999; **23**, 78–85.

59. DiClemente C. C., Bellino L. E., Neavins T. M. Motivation for change and alcoholism treatment. *Alcohol Res Health* 1999; **23**, 86–92.

60. O'Malley S. S., Sinha R., Grilo C. M., *et al.* Naltrexone and cognitive behavioral coping skills therapy for the treatment of alcohol drinking and eating disorder features in alcohol-dependent women: a randomized controlled trial. *Alcohol Clin Exp Res* 2007; **31**, 625–634.

61. Soyka M., Roesner S. New pharmacological approaches for the treatment of alcoholism. *Expert Opin Pharmacother* 2006; **7**, 2341–2353.

62. Hernandez-Avila C. A., Song C., Kuo L., *et al.* Targeted versus daily naltrexone: secondary analysis of effects on average daily drinking. *Alcohol Clin Exp Res* 2006; **30**, 860–865.

63. Mann K., Lehert P., Morgan M. Y. The efficacy of acamprosate in the maintenance of abstinence in alcohol-dependent individuals: results of a meta-analysis. *Alcohol Clin Exp Res* 2004; **28**, 51–63.

64. Mallin R. Smoking cessation: integration of behavioral and drug therapies. *Am Fam Physician* 2002; **65**, 1107–1114.

65. Kranzler H. R., Amin H., Modesto-Lowe V., Oncken C. Pharmacologic treatments for drug and alcohol dependence. *Psychiatr Clin North Am* 1999; **22**, 401–423.

Useful websites

Alcoholics Anonymous
www.alcoholics-anonymous.org www.alcoholics-anonymous.org.uk

Local groups can be found in the phone directory under "Alcoholism" or call 212–870–3400 (USA), 0845–769–7555 (UK)

Women for Sobriety
www.womenforsobriety.org (215) 536 8026, 1–800–333–1606

Center for Substance Abuse Treatment 1–800–662–HELP for information about local US treatment programs

National Institute on Alcohol Abuse and Alcoholism www.niaaa.nih.gov Public Information Office 301–443–3860

National Clearinghouse for Alcohol and Drug Information http://ncadi.samhsa.gov 1–800–729–66

Institute of Alcohol Studies (UK) www.ias.org.uk 020 7222 4001

Al-Anon (for spouses/partners) and Alateen (for children of alcoholics) www.al-anon.alateen.org 1–888–425–2666

Common medical problems

Coronary heart disease

Meghan Walsh and Valerie Ulstad

Introduction

1. Coronary heart disease (CHD) is the single leading cause of death of American women.[1] In the USA alone, about half a million women die of cardiovascular disease each year. Based on 2003 data, CVD caused approximately one death a minute among women, which is more women than were claimed by the next five leading causes of death combined (cancer, COPD, Alzheimer's, diabetes and accidents).[1] The number of deaths caused by CHD is much higher than the breast cancer mortality in women at all ages.[2]

2. Despite the prevalence of CHD in women, few recognize it as a serious health threat. This underestimation of risk is partly caused by the lack of clinical cardiovascular research including, or reporting on, women, and partly caused by widely disseminated awareness of other illnesses, such as breast cancer.

3. The increasing prevalence of this disease and its burden on women has helped to increase the breadth of clinical evidence surrounding CHD and its prevention over the last decade. However, it is only in the last few years that a rigorous review of the literature and evidence-based preventive guidelines have started to develop specifically targeting women and CHD.[3]

CHD and women: research

1. Framingham Heart Study

This landmark study and the first long-term epidemiological study of its kind was designed originally to determine the risk factors most associated with CHD. In 1948, residents of Framingham, Massachusetts were randomly selected and invited to participate in the Framingham Heart Study. A total of 5209 men and women, primarily Caucasian, free of CHD, and between the ages of 28–62 years were enrolled and followed over the subsequent 50+ years.[4]

2. One of the most useful and important contributions of the Framingham Heart Study has been the development of a "risk score" for predicting the likelihood that an individual will develop CHD in the next 10 years.[5] Clinical CHD includes angina pectoris, myocardial infarction, cardiac ischemia without infarction, and death attributable to CHD. For younger patients (since age is weighted so heavily in the calculation) this should be used as a guide to consider a lifetime risk of cardiovascular disease. Most of all, it helps to highlight those risk factors that may be modified to decrease overall risk.

3. Risk factors and age are entered into the calculator and a percentage likelihood of disease is determined. A 20% or greater risk is considered "high risk" and aggressive risk modification should occur (Table 24.1). The risk estimating score sheets are only for persons without known heart disease.

4. The Nurses' Health Study (NHS) is the single largest cohort study of women. It began in 1976 and helped to first highlight CHD risk factors specific to women. It initially comprised a cohort of 121,700 women registered nurses, ages 30 to 55 years, who returned a mailed questionnaire and were followed for over 30 years. Through the years it has helped to determine the relationships of hormonal factors, a variety of nutrients, diabetes, exercise, and cigarette smoking with the subsequent risk of CHD.[6]

Table 24.1 Risk factors

Risk Group	Framingham global risk (10-year absolute CHD risk)
High risk	>20% (DM or previous MI included)
Intermediate risk	10% to 20%
Lower risk	<10%
Optimal risk	<10%

Note: Data extrapolated from Wilson P. W. F., D'Agostino R. B., Levy D., Belanger A. M., Silbershatz H., Kannel W. B. Prediction of coronary heart disease using risk factor categories. *Circulation* 1998; **97**, 1837–1847.

Risk factors (Table 24.2)

Non-modifiable risk factors for CHD

1. **Age**

   Age is the biggest risk factor for CHD. The onset of CHD in women lags about 10 years behind men.[1] The incidence of CHD in women aged 35–44 years is 1 per 1000, increasing to 4 per 1000 in women aged 45–54 years. By the sixth decade, the incidence of CHD is equal in women and men. One in four women older than age 65 years has CHD.[7]

2. **Race**

   Racial and ethnic disparities are quite pronounced in regards to CHD risk. CHD is a particularly important threat to African American women, who have a higher incidence of CHD and an earlier mortality from CHD than African American men, white women, and white men. Although mortality from CHD has declined among African American men and women over the years, the rate of decline has been slower than among white men and women.[8] The reasons for these differences remain unclear but may be related to differences in reporting, access to care, detection biases, and competing risks. In addition, higher prevalence of certain risk factors in black women (particularly diabetes and obesity) may explain their increased risk of CHD.[8]

3. Although most risk factors for CHD are similar in men and women, gender differences have been documented, particularly related to diabetes and dyslipidemia. As these differences have become more evident, more evidence-based guidelines (specifically for minority populations) are recommended.

4. **Family history**

   Family history is a risk factor for CHD. If a woman's first-degree male relative younger than 55 years of age, or first-degree female relative younger than 65 years of age developed clinically evident CHD or experienced unexplained death, her risk of CHD is increased. A family history of early heart disease in women relatives is a strong predictor for CHD.[9]

5. **Low socioeconomic status**

   Low socioeconomic status is significantly associated with the development of CHD in women. This is largely caused by the presence of associated risk factors including increased body mass index (BMI), physical inactivity, cigarette smoking, and elevated LDL cholesterol.[10]

Modifiable risk factors for CHD

1. **Hypertension**

   a. Nearly one in three American adults has hypertension.[11] A higher percentage of men, as compared to women, have hypertension until the peri/postmenopausal period when the number of women affected far exceeds that of men.[12]

   b. Unfortunately, the racial disparity in regards to hypertension is quite pronounced. JNC VII reports that as many as 20% of all deaths in hypertensive black women may be purely caused by high blood pressure.[11] Moreover, the underlying death rate from high blood pressure was nearly three times higher in black women than white women in 2003.[11]

   c. Hypertension strongly and independently increases the risk of CHD in women. Death from both ischemic heart disease and stroke increases progressively and linearly from blood pressure levels as low as 115 mmHg systolic and 75 mmHg diastolic upward. For every 20 mmHg systolic or 10 mmHg diastolic increase in BP, there is a doubling of mortality from both ischemic heart disease and stroke.[11]

   d. Because of the new data on lifetime risk of hypertension and the impressive increase in the risk of cardiovascular complications

Table 24.2 Using risk factor categories

Data extrapolated from Wilson P. W. F., D'Agostino R. B., Levy D., Belanger A. M., Silbershatz H., Kannel W. B. Prediction of coronary heart disease using risk factor categories. *Circulation* 1998; **97**, 1837–1847.

Framingham Point Score Estimate of 10-year risk for women

Age	Points
20–34	−7
35–39	−3
40–44	0
45–49	3
50–54	6
55–59	8
60–64	10
65–69	12
70–74	14
75–79	16

Total cholesterol (mg/dL)	Points				
	Age 20–39	Age 40–49	Age 50–59	Age 60–69	Age 70–79
<160	0	0	0	0	0
160–199	4	3	2	1	1
200–239	8	6	4	2	1
240–279	11	8	5	3	2
≥280	13	10	7	4	2

Smoking	Points				
	Age 20–39	Age 40–49	Age 50–59	Age 60–69	Age 70–79
Non-smoker	0	0	0	0	0
Smoker	9	7	4	2	1

HDL (mg/dL)	Points
≥60	−1
50–59	0
40–49	1
<40	2

Table 24.2 (cont.)

Systolic BP (mmHg)	Points	
	If untreated	If treated
<120	0	0
120–129	1	3
130–139	2	4
140–159	3	5
≥160	4	6

Point total	10-year risk %
<9	<1
9	1
10	1
11	1
12	1
13	2
14	2
15	3
16	4
17	5
18	6
19	8
20	11
21	14
22	17
23	22
24	27
≥25	≥30

10-year risk_____%

associated with levels of BP previously considered to be normal, the JNC VII report has introduced a new classification that includes the term "prehypertension" for those with BPs ranging from 120 to 139 mmHg systolic and/or 80 to 89 mmHg diastolic. This has helped to target those "at-risk" individuals with earlier interventions such as lifestyle changes and medical management

hoping to stave off the later complications of this disease.

e. Reducing blood pressure with medication, or by any means, decreases cardiovascular morbidity and mortality in women to the same extent as it does in men.[12]

2. **Dyslipidemia**

a. Elevated levels of total cholesterol, low-density lipoprotein (LDL) cholesterol, and triglycerides as well as low levels of high-density lipoprotein (HDL) cholesterol are risk factors for CHD in women.[13]

b. In women, LDL and total cholesterol levels increase after the age of 55 years and peak between 55 and 65 years of age, about a decade later than in men. The natural history of serum lipid levels and the risk of coronary artery disease reflect the influence of female hormones (and their decline after menopause) on raising HDL and lowering LDL levels.

c. Beginning at age 45, a higher percentage of women as compared to men have a total blood cholesterol of 200 mg/dL or higher.[14] An elevated serum cholesterol level in women is as predictive of later CHD events as it is in men.[15] A woman with a serum cholesterol level greater than 260 mg/dL has a 40% greater risk for CHD mortality compared to a woman with a cholesterol <200 mg/dL.[16]

d. **LDL cholesterol**

LDL is the major atherogenic lipoprotein in women. The higher the levels, the higher the CHD risk (ATP II). Although important, LDL levels do not predict CHD risk as strongly in women as they do in men.[15]

e. **HDL cholesterol**

HDL cholesterol, a stronger predictor of CHD risk in women than LDL, is second only to age as a predictor of death from cardiovascular disease among women.[17] Women with an HDL less than 50 mg/dL have an increased mortality (RR = 1.7) compared to women with an HDL over 50 mg/dL. An HDL level greater than 60 mg/dL is considered protective against CHD.[9]

f. **Triglycerides**

Elevated triglyceride levels have been shown to be an independent risk factor for CHD in women. The increased cardiovascular risk associated with elevated triglycerides appears to be higher in women (about 40% increase in CVD risk per 1 mmol/L increase in triglyceride level) than in men.[18,19]

g. The MRC/BHF Heart Protection Study was a randomized trial which assessed the effect of cholesterol lowering on CHD outcomes. Between 1994 and 1997, 20,536 participants (5082 women) with known CHD, other occlusive arterial disease, or diabetes were randomly assigned to simvastatin (40 mg daily) or identical placebo. The average length of follow-up was 5 years. Overall, among women with known CHD or at high risk for CHD, treatment with simvastatin significantly lowered cardiovascular event rates by approximately 25%, regardless of pretreatment cholesterol levels.[20]

h. Unfortunately, many of the clinical trials of lipid-lowering treatments have not included or reported on women, and therefore current evidence for benefits in women is insufficient. Although the MRC/BHF Heart Protection Study demonstrated that statins used in high risk patients are effective in reducing CHD mortality, non-fatal MI, and revascularization by 20–30%, statin use has not been shown to affect overall mortality. Currently, for women without cardiovascular disease, lipid lowering has not been shown to affect total or CHD mortality.[13]

i. **Treatment**

According to ATP III, patients with an absolute 10-year risk of >20% for developing clinical coronary disease are considered candidates for very aggressive therapy. This includes an LDL cholesterol treatment goal of <100 mg/dL and a recommendation to initiate drug therapy at an LDL level of >130 mg/dL. Patients with diabetes are also considered candidates for aggressive therapy, whether or not clinical coronary disease is present, because their absolute risk for major events is also very high. For patients with an estimated absolute risk of 10–20%, somewhat less aggressive therapy is recommended, although the guidelines do suggest pharmacotherapy, if needed, to keep LDL levels <130 mg/dL.[21]

3. Overall, the Framingham criteria should be utilized to assess a woman's overall risk for CHD, and decisions regarding lipid lowering made based on this global risk. Generally, women found to be at intermediate or high 10-year CHD risks should be treated accordingly. The Institute for Clinical Systems Improvement (ICSI) has provided a treatment algorithm for lipid management that encompasses the most up to date lipid management guidelines, see Figure 24.1.[22]

4. **Cigarette smoking**

a. Smoking is the single biggest cause of CHD in young and middle-aged women, accounting for up to half of all coronary deaths.[23]

b. Among Americans age 18 and older, 20 million women (18.5%) are smokers.[24] Ethnic differences again occur: nearly one-third of American Indian/Alaskan Native women are smokers, one-fifth of non-Hispanic whites, and one-tenth of Hispanics.[24]

c. Cigarette smoking has a strong dose-response effect. A woman who smokes one to four cigarettes per day is twice as likely to have an acute myocardial infarction as a non-smoker, while a woman who smokes more than 45 cigarettes per day has a risk that is 11 times higher than that of a non-smoker.[23] On average, women who smoke have their first MI 19 years earlier than women who do not smoke.[25]

d. Following smoking cessation, the cardiac risk falls to the level of a non-smoker within three to five years (the risk of lung cancer takes much longer to drop back to baseline). This finding is independent of the amount smoked, the age of quitting or the duration of the smoking habit.[26]

e. Not only does smoking contribute to overall CHD risk, but it can add mortality risk after a myocardial infarction as well. Mortality was reduced by 65% among women who stopped smoking after their MI, compared to persons who continued to smoke.[27]

267

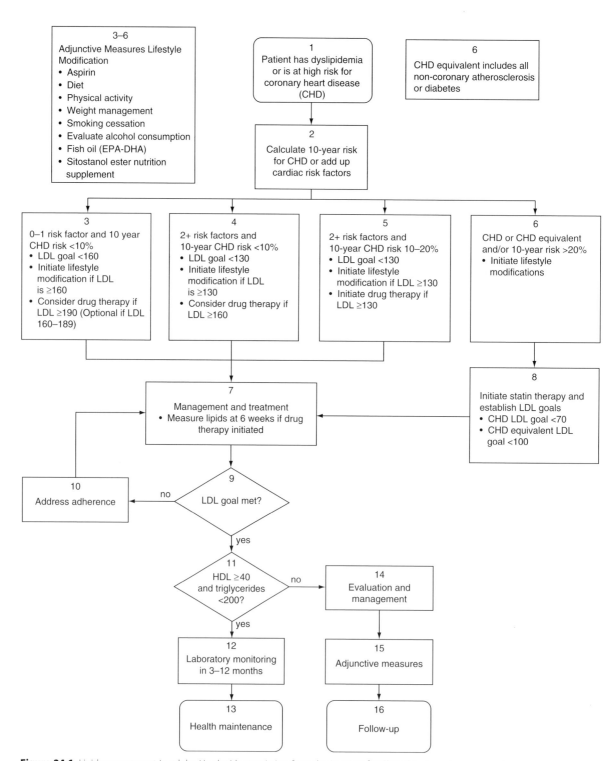

Figure 24.1 Lipid management in adults. Used with permission from the Institute for Clinical Systems Improvement. Copyright © 2007 by Institute for Clinical Systems Improvement.

5. **Diabetes mellitus**

   a. Diabetes is the fourth leading cause of death among black women and third among Hispanic women aged 45 to 74 years and American Indian women aged 65 to 74 years. Approximately half of all deaths in persons with non-insulin dependent diabetes mellitus are caused by heart disease, the majority of which is ischemic heart disease.[28]

   b. Diabetes is associated with a threefold to sevenfold elevation in CHD risk among women.[29]

   c. Women with diabetes constitute the only subgroup in which CHD mortality has not improved over time; in two time periods (between 1971 and 1975, and between 1982 and 1984), CHD mortality decreased in men with and without diabetes and in women without diabetes but increased by 23% in women with diabetes.[30]

   d. Diabetes mellitus is considered a coronary risk equivalent in the updated ATP III guidelines; therefore, associated cardiovascular risk factors must be aggressively modified in these patients.

   e. Diabetes is a more potent risk factor for CHD in women than in men and negates the gender-protective effect in the age of CHD onset.[6]

6. **Metabolic syndrome (Table 24.3)**

   a. Several CHD risk factors tend to cluster together: central obesity, high blood pressure, increased blood glucose, and dyslipidemia (low HDL, high triglycerides).

   b. Metabolic syndrome has a prevalence of 20–24% of the US population and 40–45% among those >60 years of age.[31]

   c. People with metabolic syndrome are twice as likely to die from, and three times as likely to have a heart attack or stroke, compared to people without the syndrome.[32] Despite this increased risk, these patients often register as "low risk" on the Framingham score if they are younger in age.

   d. There is no specialized treatment for metabolic syndrome at this stage, but patients with this diagnosis should have any associated risk factors aggressively modified.

Table 24.3 The International Diabetes Federation Definition: metabolic syndrome, women

International Diabetes Federation. *The IDF Consensus Worldwide Definition of the Metabolic Syndrome,* http://www.idf.org/webdata/docs/IDF_Metasyndrome_definition.pdf2005.

Central obesity: waist circumference ≥80 cm for women and any two of the following four factors

(1) Elevated triglycerides: ≥150 mg/dL (or on treatment)

(2) Decreased HDL: women <50 mg/dL (or on treatment)

(3) Elevated blood pressure: ≥130/85 mmHg (or on treatment)

(4) Elevated fasting plasma glucose: ≥100 mg/dL, or previously diagnosed type II DM

7. **Physical activity**

   a. Physically active women have a significant graded reduction in CHD risk as compared with sedentary women.[33]

   b. Physical inactivity contributes to obesity and is an independent risk factor for myocardial infarction.[34]

   c. Data from the National Center for Health Statistics indicate that 43% of white women and 65% of women of color do not get enough physical exercise.[35]

   d. All-cause mortality is lower in physically fit women and higher levels of fitness have been shown to offer a greater mortality benefit for women than for men.[36]

   e. The NHS indicates that moderate-intensity physical activity three days a week, such as the equivalent of walking briskly (at 3–4 miles/hour or 4–6.8 km/hour), is associated with a 50% reduction in risk of myocardial infarction.[37]

8. **Obesity**

   a. Obesity is epidemic in many western nations. Currently about one-third of adult women in America (or 34 million) are classified as obese.[38]

   b. There is a direct positive association between obesity and the risk of CHD in women. Although obesity is associated with diabetes mellitus, lipid abnormalities, and hypertension, an independent effect of obesity persists even after adjustment for known cardiovascular risk factors.[39]

c. Even women who were mildly to moderately overweight (BMI 25–28.9) had nearly twice the risk of CHD compared with lean women.[40] Moreover, the risk of CHD rises steeply among women whose waist-to-hip ratio is higher than 0.8.[41]

d. The most effective treatment for obesity in women remains in question, and unfortunately, exercise appears to be less effective in promoting weight loss in women than in men.[42]

CHD risk reduction: medical management

1. **Hormone replacement therapy**

   a. The gradual decrease in estrogen levels related to menopause has been implicated in the rise of CHD risk occurring with advancing age in women. The large, observational Nurses' Health Study showed a lower incidence of CHD events and all-cause mortality in hormone replacement therapy (HRT) users than non-users.[43] As a result, a series of studies questioned whether supplemental estrogen with or without progesterone might have a protective effect against the development of CHD.

   b. The "grandmother" of all clinical trials associating HRT and CHD is the PEPI trial, published in 1995.[44] This randomized, double-blind, placebo-controlled trial included 875 postmenopausal women randomized to one of five regimens of either placebo, estrogen alone, or varying doses of estrogen + progesterone. They were followed for three years and found that all active treatment groups had increased HDL, decreased LDL, and higher triglyceride levels compared to placebo. Although the lipid profiles improved in treated women, it remained in question whether this also translated to decreased risk of CHD.

   c. The HERS trial became the first randomized, double-blind, placebo-controlled secondary prevention trial to study the effect of HRT on cardiovascular disease outcomes (MI, CABG, revascularization or coronary artery narrowing.)[45] Nearly 3000 postmenopausal women (age <80 years) with a history of CHD were randomized to placebo or a fixed dose of estrogen and progesterone. They were followed for four years and surprisingly no difference was seen between the treatment and the placebo group in the combined endpoint of non-fatal MI or CHD death. Unfortunately, the treatment group did show a threefold increased risk of venothromboembolic disease.

   d. Finally, the largest ever randomized clinical trial, the Women's Health Initiative (WHI), randomized over 16,000 women to placebo or to a combined estrogen-progestin HRT. After only 5.2 years of follow-up the HRT treatment arm was halted caused by the increased incidence of CVD (22%) and breast cancer (26%) in women treated with combination HRT.[46]

   e. The HRT discussion is far from over. The aforementioned trials raised many more questions than they have answered. For instance, the age differences of study participants, timing of initiation of HRT (peri- or postmenopausal), dosage, drug combination, preparation (oral versus transdermal) or underlying genetic effects may play a role in the risk or benefit of HRT as it applies to CHD. A recent meta-analysis performed by Salpeter *et al.* pooled the data from 23 trials and separated odds ratios for CHD events for younger women (mean time from menopause ≤10 years or age <60 years) from older women (mean time from menopause >10 years or age >60 years).[47] It was found that HRT reduces the risk of CHD events in younger postmenopausal women, but increases them in older women. It is therefore biologically plausible that HRT may be able to slow progression of atherosclerosis in the perimenopausal woman without CHD. Furthermore, the addition of statin lipid therapy with HRT may counteract the deleterious effects of HRT on CHD, and this is currently under further investigation.

   f. Overall, evidence-based guidelines for CHD prevention in women were released by the

American Heart Association in 2004 and recommended that HRT should neither be initiated nor continued for prevention of CVD in postmenopausal women.[48]

2. **Lipid-lowering therapy with statins**

   a. Current ATP III guidelines for CHD prevention recommend target LDL levels of <100 mg/dL to <160 mg/dL depending on the presence of CHD risk factors or CHD itself. Although lifestyle modifications remain the recommended starting point, many patients require drug therapy to reach these targets. Statins are extremely effective at lowering LDL levels and are therefore recommended as first line drug therapy.[49]

   b. The effect of statins on cholesterol metabolism includes lowering LDL and triglycerides, as well as increasing HDL. Moreover, there is considerable evidence to suggest that they also down-regulate inflammatory markers, inhibit vascular smooth muscle cell proliferation, and modulate endothelial dysfunction, all of which contribute to CHD.[50]

   c. The more efficacious statins, atorvastatin and rosuvastatin, induce the greatest changes in LDL with reductions of 37%–51% (10–80 mg) and 46%–55% (10–40 mg), respectively.[51] These reductions are similar in both men and women.

3. **Aspirin**

   a. **Primary prevention**

      The updated 2007 American Heart Association guidelines state that all women at "high risk" (10-year CHD risk >20%) should be taking daily aspirin (75–325 mg) unless there is a compelling reason not to (e.g., history of bleeding stomach ulcers). "At risk" women (10-year CHD risk 10–20%) 65 and older should be considered for aspirin therapy if the benefits outweigh the risks. Most of all, avoid aspirin therapy in healthy women less than age 65.[52]

   b. This aspirin recommendation is based largely on the impressive 44% reduction in risk of acute MI seen in the Physician's Health Study among male physicians aged 40 to 90 taking daily aspirin.[53] After about five years of a

scheduled 12 year trial, the independent Data and Safety Monitoring Board unanimously recommended early termination of the aspirin component due primarily to this statistically significant reduction in first MI.[53]

   c. The Women's Health Study (WHS) compared low-dose aspirin (100 mg on alternate days) with placebo in 39,876 apparently healthy women health care providers and found that after a mean duration of about 10 years, aspirin lowered the risk of a first non-fatal stroke by 19% but had no significant effect on first non-fatal myocardial infarction, cardiovascular mortality, or all-cause mortality. Subgroup analysis among women 65 years and older demonstrated that aspirin significantly reduced the risk of a first MI by about one-third, a reduction virtually identical to the findings in the primary prevention trials of men.[54]

   d. **Secondary prevention**

      Aspirin reduces the incidence of subsequent MI, stroke, and death from cardiovascular causes by 25% in women and men with established vascular disease.[55]

   e. Aspirin has been shown to have benefit in women and men with evolving MI.[56] Guidelines published in 2004 from the ACC/AHA and the ACCP, which are consistent with the data from randomized trials, recommend that aspirin should be given in an initial dose of 162 to 325 mg to all patients unless there is a contraindication. (If the preparation is enteric coated, the first tablet should be crushed or chewed to achieve a rapid clinical antithrombotic effect.)[57,58]

   f. The optimum dose of aspirin for chemoprevention is not known. Primary and secondary prevention trials have demonstrated benefits with a variety of regimens, including 75 mg per day, 100 mg per day, and 325 mg every other day. Doses of approximately 75 mg per day appear as effective as higher doses; whether doses below 75 mg per day are effective has not been established. Enteric-coated or buffered preparations do not clearly reduce adverse gastrointestinal effects of aspirin.[59]

271

g. Although adherence to primary and secondary prevention recommendations for aspirin is improving, it remains an underutilized therapy. While 60 to 84% of patients in the USA hospitalized for unstable angina or an MI receive aspirin, it is less frequently used in outpatients with coronary artery disease or diabetes, an important subgroup.[60] One study of 10,942 visits to cardiologists or primary care physicians by patients with coronary disease found that, for the period of 1993 to 1996, aspirin use was only 26%.[61]

4. **Vitamin E**

   a. The Nurses' Health Study found that supplementation with at least 100 IU of vitamin E per day was associated with a lower risk of CHD.[62] Unfortunately the few randomized controlled trials performed have not found a benefit of supplementation with vitamin E for primary prevention of CHD.[63]

   b. Regarding secondary prevention, the Heart Protection Study randomized 20,536 patients who had a history of CHD, vascular disease, or diabetes mellitus to five years of antioxidant vitamin supplementation (vitamin E 600 mg (900 IU), vitamin C 250 mg, and beta-carotene 20 mg) or placebo. Supplementation had no effect on cardiovascular mortality and non-fatal myocardial infarction.[64]

5. **Chest pain in women**

   Chest pain is second only to abdominal pain as the most common reason for an emergency room visit annually. Approximately 1–4% of patients who present to an ER with what is actually an acute MI are discharged in error.[65,66] Unfortunately, these are the patients who most often present with atypical symptoms and thus a worse prognosis.

   a. An MI can present in a myriad of ways. Although chest pain is the most common symptom associated with MI in both men and women, up to 25% of patients may present with other symptoms such as shortness of breath, back pain or dizziness.[67,68]

   b. Angina is the clinical manifestation of myocardial ischemia caused by an imbalance

Table 24.4 Characteristics of typical and atypical angina pectoris

Douglas P. S., Ginsberg G. S., The evaluation of chest pain in women. *N Engl J Med* 1996; **334**, 1311–1315, with permission.
Typical
Substernal*
Characterized by a burning, heavy, or squeezing feeling
Precipitated by exertion* or emotion
Promptly relieved by rest or nitroglycerin*
Atypical
Located in the left chest, abdomen, back, or arm in the absence of mid-chest pain
Sharp or fleeting
Repeated, very prolonged
Unrelated to exercise
Not relieved by rest or nitroglycerin
Relieved by antacids
Characterized by palpitations without chest pain

between myocardial oxygen supply and demand. Any activity that increases the workload of the heart can precipitate angina in a person with a significant (>70%) stenosis in a coronary artery.

   c. Angina pectoris is characterized by substernal discomfort that may radiate to the neck or left arm, but it can be perceived anywhere between the xyphoid process and the ears. Angina is a disagreeable pressure-like sensation. During history-taking, some real cardiac chest pain can be missed by asking patients if they are having "pain" rather than "pressure."

   d. Douglas and Ginsberg have helped to highlight the differences between typical angina and atypical symptoms (see Table 24.4).

   e. There are several symptoms that significantly lower the likelihood of ischemia: pleuritic or reproducible pain, stabbing pain, pain radiating to lower extremities or pain that has lasted longer than 48 hours.[69]

f. Atypical pain is more common in women than in men, because of the higher prevalence among women of less common causes of ischemia, such as vasospastic and microvascular angina.[70]

g. The constellation of symptoms associated with MI has its basis on research performed largely on men. As a result, if women have symptoms that do not fall into the "normal" pattern, they may delay seeking help. There are several reasons why women's symptoms may differ from men's.

   i. Women have smaller coronary artery lumens (independent of body size) as well as less collateral circulation that may add to anginal complaints.[71] This anatomic difference may alter the symptom complex, contributing to greater ischemia especially in times of stress. In fact, the Myocardial Infarction Triage and Intervention (MITI) trial demonstrated notable gender differences in symptoms of acute MI: women tended to experience significantly more upper abdominal pain, dyspnea, nausea, and fatigue than did men in the study population. Conversely, men complained of diaphoresis more often than did women.[72]

   ii. While women with CAD are just as likely to have exertional angina as men, such women are more likely to experience angina at rest, during sleep or with mental stress.[73]

   iii. Psychosocial influences also play a role in MI presentation. Depression is three times more common in women than in men. Some studies have shown that depressed patients reported more intense and frequent anginal pain than non-depressed patients.[74,75] Furthermore, depression may affect the development, progression and outcomes of CHD.[76]

h. Overall, women are at a greater disadvantage than men in relation to chest pain and outcomes for acute MI for a myriad of reasons:

   i. Presenting symptoms in women differ and therefore a delay in diagnosis may occur.[77]

   ii. Women have been shown to delay seeking medical care when their cardiac symptoms do not match their (or the public's) expectation.

Table 24.5 Indications and contraindications for stress testing

Tak T., Gutierrez R. Comparing stress testing methods: available techniques and their use in CAD evaluation. *Postgraduate Med* 2004; **115**, 61–70, with permission.

Indications

Chest pain evaluation

Prognosis and severity of coronary artery disease

Screening for CHD

Evaluation of therapy

CHF evaluation

Contraindications

Unstable angina or acute MI

Acute myocarditis or pericarditis

Rapid atrial or ventricular dysrhythmias

Symptomatic or severe aortic stenosis

Acute illness, severe anemia, or infection

Acute aortic dissection

Hyperthyroidism

Suspected left main disease

   iii. Women are treated with less intensive therapies thus treatment differs as compared to men.[78]

   iv. All of these factors result in higher case fatality rates in the hospital, at 30 days, and one year after MI for women as compared to men.[79,80,81]

Risk stratification with stress testing (Table 24.5)

1. Stress testing should be utilized when the diagnosis of CAD is uncertain. The clinician's estimation of the likelihood of obstructive CAD is based on the patient's history (age, gender, and symptoms), physical exam, and initial testing. When a patient presents with definite anginal symptoms, the likelihood of disease is so high that the result of the stress test does not change the probability of disease. Diagnostic testing is the most valuable, therefore, when the probability of disease is intermediate, and the result of the test can greatly affect the disease outcome.[82]

2. Classic angina may be difficult to identify accurately, but criteria have been established to help classify a collection of symptoms into one of three categories: typical angina, atypical angina, or non-specific chest pain. Each of these classifications in turn is associated with a likelihood of obstructive CAD. The Coronary Artery Surgery Study (CASS) prospectively enrolled 20,000 patients with chest pain (19% women, aged 30–70 years), and performed coronary angiography to determine CHD prevalence with the various chest pain presentations.[83] Results were as follows.

   a. **Typical angina**

      Substernal chest discomfort that is precipitated by exertion, relieved by rest or nitroglycerine in less than 10 minutes, and radiates to the shoulder, jaw or ulnar aspect of left arm. Significant CHD was found in 72% of women in this category.

   b. **Atypical chest pain**

      This has many features of angina but the patterns were not classic, such as unusual radiation or suboptimal relief with nitroglycerine. Significant CHD was found in 36% of women in this category.

   c. **Non-specific pain**

      This has none of the features of typical angina. Significant disease was found in 6% of women in this category.

3. The stress electrocardiogram (ECG) or graded exercise test is a relatively inexpensive test that is widely available and often used as the next step in the evaluation of chest pain. Unfortunately, the specificity for stress testing for significant CHD is much less in women. For example, women are 5 to 20 times more likely to have a false positive stress test than men.[84]

4. Exercise-induced ST-segment depression is a less sensitive result in women than in men, which reflects both a lower prevalence of severe CAD and the inability of many women to exercise to maximum aerobic capacity.[85] Women also tend to release greater amounts of catecholamines during exercise than men, which is thought to potentiate coronary vasoconstriction and augment the incidence of false-positive test results.[86]

5. In postmenopausal women with typical angina, if the baseline ECG is normal, a treadmill ECG is probably the test of choice. Since the pretest probability of an important obstruction is fairly high (72%), a positive test will further increase the likelihood that the woman has an important coronary lesion. However, the addition of some form of imaging to exercise stress testing markedly improves test accuracy in women thus many providers will go directly to an imaging modality first.[87]

6. In premenopausal women, however, the strategy changes. The likelihood of a significant coronary lesion is much lower (depending on other cardiac risk factors) and therefore a stress test using another imaging modality such as echocardiogram or nuclear imaging should be the first step towards further risk stratification.[88] For example, in the woman with atypical angina with a normal baseline electrocardiogram, there is a 36% pretest probability of an important coronary lesion. A positive regular treadmill test enhances the post test probability to only 40–50%.

7. Women have a low false-negative rate in exercise stress testing, which suggests that routine testing reliably rules out CAD in women with negative results.[89] Therefore, in a low-risk, premenopausal patient, a negative exercise test (regular or with imaging) is powerful in excluding significant CHD because the low pretest probability is further lowered by the negative test.[90]

8. Any woman who has the inability to exercise or walk on a treadmill may still have a stress imaging study performed using a pharmacological stress such as dipyridamole, dobutamine, or adenosine. This includes women with underlying left bundle branch blocks (LBBB) as artifactual perfusion defects can occur with exercise testing in these patients.

9. Interestingly, the prognostic value of exercise testing in asymptomatic women seems to derive more from the fitness outcomes that arise in these tests rather than the electrocardiographic changes that appear during them. A total of 2994 asymptomatic North American women, aged 30 to 80 years, without known cardiovascular disease were given near-maximal Bruce treadmill stress tests from 1972–1976 and followed for 20 years.

Exercise capacity, low heart rate recovery (HRR), and not achieving target heart rate were independently associated with increased all-cause and cardiovascular mortality in these women. There was no increased cardiovascular death risk for exercise-induced ST-segment depression. After adjusting for multiple other risk factors, women who were below the median for both exercise capacity and HRR had a 3.5-fold increased risk of cardiovascular death.[91]

10. Syndrome X, defined as exertional angina, a positive response to exercise testing and angiographically normal coronary arteries, occurs predominantly in postmenopausal women. Although chest pain may be typical for angina, conventional antianginal therapy may not successfully treat symptoms. Long-term survival rates are not reduced in women with syndrome X.[92]

Acute myocardial infarction

1. Women tend to have their MIs at older ages than men, with a higher case fatality rate.[93]

2. The National Registry of Myocardial Infarction (NRMI) Investigators data from 1990–1993 demonstrates that thrombolytic therapy was used more frequently in men than in women of all ages.[94]

3. The international GUSTO-I trial demonstrated that women were older than men when presenting with acute MI. Women took longer to present to the hospital and experienced longer delays than men to diagnosis and treatment with thrombolytic therapy. Women had higher mortality than men in every age category, with a 15% greater risk of dying than men and higher rates of post-MI complications including CHF, re-infarction, shock, and serious bleeding.[95]

4. However, the use of invasive diagnostic procedures in the GUSTO-I trial in patients with acute MI was similar in women and men and a small but significant difference was seen in the rates of revascularization.[95]

5. Hochman et al. looked at the clinical presentation and outcomes of 3662 women and 8480 men with acute coronary syndromes.[96] Outcomes varied by sex depending upon the type of acute coronary syndrome. Women were more likely than men to have unstable angina rather than

acute myocardial infarction. Women with unstable angina had a better prognosis than their male counterparts. This often occurs because an ST-elevation MI often reflects little to no flow in the coronary artery whereas a non-ST-elevation MI may involve continued flow to the myocardium with only minimal myocardial damage. Women with acute MI and ST-segment elevation had similar outcomes to men. Among patients with MI, a smaller percentage of women than men presented with ST-segment elevation.

Treatment and revascularization

1. Virtually all single-center and large-scale multicenter trials have reported that in comparison to men, women undergoing CABG or PCI have more comorbid disease, are older, are smaller in size, and have a higher prevalence of hypertension, diabetes mellitus, hypercholesterolemia, peripheral vascular disease, and unstable angina, as well as more severe angina.[97,98,99] As a result of these comorbidities, they have had worse outcomes following these interventions as compared to men.

2. Despite smaller vessel size in women, coronary lesion morphology and distribution is similar to that in men, except that women tend to have more ostial lesions.[100] Among patients undergoing contemporary PCI, stent usage is similar in women and men after adjusting for vessel size.[101] In comparison with men, however, women tend to be treated less often with platelet glycoprotein IIb/IIIa receptor antagonists, despite similar efficacy in women and men.[102]

3. Although techniques and medications have improved over the years, sex differences in in-hospital mortality after CABG have persisted and have been notably consistent over the past 20 years. On average, in-hospital mortality is two times higher in women in comparison with men, and stratification according to age reveals a more pronounced difference in younger women.[98,106] In addition, women have a higher incidence of periprocedural morbid events, such as stroke and bleeding, in comparison with men.[97,103] These differences may relate to older age at presentation, comorbidities or vessel size, to name a few.

275

4. Optimal revascularization strategies for women are just beginning to evolve. After hospital discharge, adjusted survival at 5 years after CABG and adjusted survival at 1 and 4 years after PCI have been shown to be similar in women and men.[101,104]

5. In the Bypass Angioplasty Revascularization Investigation (BARI) trial, survival at 5 years was no different in women and men overall and was no different in women treated with CABG or balloon angioplasty.[100]

6. It is nearly impossible to discuss revascularization without mentioning stents and the rising concern over in-stent re-stenosis and thrombosis. Re-narrowing at the angioplasty site, or re-stenosis, occurs in as many as 50% of patients following percutaneous transluminal coronary angioplasty. Diabetes mellitus and chronic renal insufficiency appear to be the two most dominant clinical factors that predispose patients to re-stenosis. As a result of this complication, the bare metal stent was created which could stent a blocked artery while also decreasing the risk of re-stenosis by nearly 50%.

7. In 2003 the drug-eluting stent was approved by the FDA. Several clinical trials (RAVEL & SIRIUS) demonstrated significantly reduced in-stent re-stenosis rates (0% to 3%) and in-segment or vessel re-stenosis rates (9%) in the drug-eluting stents, compared to 33% in the bare-metal stent arm. Stent thrombosis, major clinical events, and aneurysms at the site of the stent placement were similar in the two treatment groups.[105,106] Although re-stenosis rates were improved with drug-eluting stents, the cost of these was three times that of the bare metal stent.

8. Subacute stent thrombosis is a rare but much more dangerous complication after coronary stent placement. It usually occurs before endothelialization has been completed. For bare-metal stents, this process takes a few weeks; the newer, drug-eluting stents inhibit re-stenosis by inhibiting fibroblast proliferation, but they also tend to delay the endothelialization process thereby increasing the risk for thrombosis formation.[107] As a result, patients who have had drug-eluting stents are prescribed aspirin and clopidogrel therapy for at least 6 months, and perhaps will even extend to lifetime therapy as more research arises. Drug-eluting stents and the duration of clopidogrel therapy remain extremely controversial topics.

Conclusion

CHD in women remains a premier public health priority. As our population ages and comorbidities in women continue to rise, CHD is likely to remain a concern for all women long into the future. Risk factor modification and emphasis on healthy lifestyles in younger women are the cornerstones of prevention. Health care providers need to be aware of gender differences in presentation, prognosis, and responsiveness to treatment of CHD in order to optimize patient care. Because CHD disproportionately affects women and minorities, we need to push for more research and improved evidence-based guidelines for these groups.

References

1. Heart disease and stroke statistics – 2006 update: a report from the American Heart Association Statistics Committee and Stroke Statistics Subcommittee. *Circulation* 2006; **113**(6), e85–151.

2. Wingo P. A., Calle E. E., McTiernan A. How does breast cancer mortality compare with that of other cancers and cardiovascular diseases at different ages in US women? *J Womens Health Gend Based Med* 2000; **9**, 999–1000.

3. Mosca L., Appel L. J., *et al.* Evidence-based guidelines for cardiovascular disease prevention in women; AHA scientific statement, consensus panel statement. *Circulation* 2004; **99**, 2480–2484.

4. Dawber T. R., Kannel W. B., Revotskie N., Stokes J. I., Kagan A., Gordon T. Some factors associated with the development of coronary heart disease; six years' follow-up experience in the Framingham Study. *Am J Public Health* 1959; **49**, 1349–1356.

5. Wilson P. W. F., D'Agostino R. B., Levy D., Belanger A. M., Silbershatz H., Kannel W. B. Prediction of coronary heart disease using risk factor categories. *Circulation* 1998; **97**, 1837–1847.

6. Rich-Edwards J. W., Manson J. E., Hennekens C. H., Buring J. E. The primary prevention of coronary heart disease in women. *N Engl J Med* 1995; **332**, 1758–1766.

7. Bush T. L. The epidemiology of cardiovascular disease in postmenopausal women. *Ann NY Acad Sci* 1990; **592**, 263–271.

8. Mosca L., Manson J. E., Sutherland S. E., *et al.* Cardiovascular disease in women. A statement for healthcare professionals from the American Heart Association. *Circulation* 1997; **96**, 2468–2482.

9. NCEP. Summary of Second Report of the National Cholesterol Education Program (NCEP) Expert Panel on Detection, Evaluation, and Treatment of High Blood Cholesterol in Adults (adult treatment panel II). *J Am Med Assoc* 1993; **269**, 3015–3023.

10. Winkelby M. A., Kraemer H. C., Ahn D. K., Varady A. N. Ethnic and socioeconomic differences in cardiovascular disease risk factors. *J Am Med Assoc* 1998; **280**, 356–362.

11. Joint National Committee on the Detection, Evaluation, and Treatment of Blood Pressure. The seventh report of the Joint National Committee on Prevention, Detection, Evaluation, and Treatment of High Blood Pressure. *Hypertension* 2003; **42**, 1206.

12. Gueyffier F., Boutitie F., Boissel J. P., *et al.* Effect of antihypertensive drug treatment on cardiovascular outcomes in women and men: a meta-analysis of individual patient data from randomized controlled trials. *Ann Intern Med* 1997; **126**, 761–767.

13. Walsh J. M. E., Pignone M. Drug treatment of hyperlipidemia in women. *J Am Med Assoc* 2004; **291**, 2243–2252.

14. Ford E. S., *et al.* Serum cholesterol concentrations and awareness, treatment, and control of hypercholesterolemia among US adults: findings from the National Health and Nutrition Survey, 1999 to 2000. *Circulation* 2003; **107**, 2185–2189.

15. Manolio T. A., Pearson T. A., Wengber N. K., *et al.* Cholesterol and heart disease in older persons and women. *Ann Epidemiol* 1992; **2**, 161–176.

16. Bass K. M., Newschaffer C. H., Klag M. J., Bush T. L. Plasma lipoprotein levels as predictors of cardiovascular death in women. *Arch Intern Med* 1993; **153**, 2209–2216.

17. Jacobs D. R. Jr., Meban I. L., Bangdiwala S. I., Criqui M. H., Tyroler H. A. High-density lipoprotein cholesterol as a predictor of cardiovascular disease mortality in men and women: the follow-up study of the Lipid Research Clinic Prevalence Study. *Am J Epidemiol* 1990; **131**, 32–47.

18. Hokanson J. E., Austin M. A. Plasma triglyceride level is a risk factor for cardiovascular disease independent of high-density lipoprotein cholesterol level: a meta-analysis of population-based prospective studies. *J Cardiovasc Risk* 1996; **3**(2), 213–219.

19. Austin M. A., Hokanson J. E., Edwards K. L. Hypertriglyceridemia as a cardiovascular risk factor. *Am J Cardiol* 1998; **81**(4A), 7B–12B.

20. Heart Protection Study Collaborative Group. MRC/ BHF Heart Protection Study of cholesterol lowering with simvastatin in 20,538 high-risk individuals: a randomized placebo controlled trial. *Lancet* 2002; **360**, 7–22.

21. NCEP. Executive Summary of the Third Report of the National Cholesterol Education Program (NCEP) Expert Panel on Detection, Evaluation, and Treatment of High Blood Cholesterol in Adults (adult treatment panel III). *J Am Med Assoc* 2001; **285**, 2486–2497.

22. Institute for Clinical Systems Improvement (ICSI). *Lipid Management in Adults*, Bloomington, MN: ICSI, 2006.

23. Willett W. C., Green A., Stampfer M. J., *et al.* Relative and absolute excess risk of coronary heart disease among women who smoke cigarettes. *N Engl J Med* 1987; **317**, 1303–1309.

24. *National Health Interview Survey (NHIS)*, January–June 2006. Bethesda, MD: National Center for Health Statistics.

25. Hansen E. F., Andersen L. T., Von Eyben F. E. Cigarette smoking and age at first acute myocardial infarction, and influence of gender and extent of smoking. *Am J Cardiol* 1993; **71**, 1439–1442.

26. Rosenberg L., Palmer J. R., Shapiro S. Decline in the risk of myocardial infarction among women who stop smoking. *N Engl J Med* 1990; **322**, 213–217.

27. Wilson K., Gibson N., Willan A., Cook D. Effect of smoking cessation on mortality after myocardial infarction: meta-analysis of cohort studies. *Arch Intern Med* 2000; **160**(7), 939–944.

28. Geiss L. S., Herman W. H., Smith P. J. Mortality in non-insulin-dependent diabetes. In *Diabetes in America*, National Institutes of Health, National Institute of Diabetes and Digestive and Kidney Disease, 1995, pp. 249–250.

29. Manson J. E., Spelsberg A. Risk modification in the diabetic patient. In Manson J. E., Ridker P. M., Gaziano J. M., Hennekens C. H., eds., *Prevention of Myocardial Infarction*, New York: Oxford University Press, 1996, pp. 241–273.

30. Gu K., *et al.* Diabetes and decline in heart disease mortality in US adults. *J Am Med Assoc* 1999; **281**, 1291–1297.

31. Centers for Disease Control and Prevention. *The Third National Health and Nutrition Examination Survey (NHANES III 1988–94) Reference Manuals and Reports.* Bethesda, MD: National Center for Health Statistics, 1996.

32. Hunt K. J., Resendez R. G., Williams K., *et al.* National Cholesterol Education Program versus World Health Organization metabolic syndrome in relation to all-cause and cardiovascular mortality in the San Antonio Heart Study. *Circulation* 2004; **110**, 1251–1257.

33. Kushi L. H., Fee R. M., Folsom A. R., Mink P. J., Anderson K. E., Sellers T. A. Physical activity and mortality in postmenopausal women. *J Am Med Assoc* 1997; **277**, 1287–1292.

34. Stampfer M. J., Hu F. B., Manson J. E., Rimm E. B., Willett W. C. Primary prevention of coronary heart disease in women through diet and lifestyle. *N Engl J Med* 2000; **343**, 16–22.

35. National Center for Health Statistics, http://www.cdc.gov/nchs/products/pubs/pubd/hestats/3and4/sedentary.htm, accessed 12/06.

36. Blair S. N., Kohl H. W. III, Paffenbarger R. S. Jr., Clark D. G., Cooper K. H., Gibbons L. W. Physical fitness and all-cause mortality; a prospective study of healthy men and women. *J Am Med Assoc* 1989; **262**, 2395–2401.

37. Colditz G. A., Coakley E. Weight, weight gain, activity, and major illnesses: the Nurses' Health Study. *Int J Sports Med* 1997; **18**(suppl 3), S162–S170.

38. Kuczmarski R. J., Flegal K. M., Campbell S. M., Johnson C. L. Increasing prevalence of overweight among US adults: the National Health and Nutrition Examination Surveys, 1960 to 1991. *J Am Med Assoc* 1994; **272**, 205–211.

39. Manson J. E., Stampfer M. J., Colditz G. A., *et al.* A prospective study of obesity and the risk of coronary heart disease in women. *N Engl J Med* 1990; **322**, 882–889.

40. Kaplan N. M. The deadly quartet: upper body obesity, glucose intolerance, hypertriglyceridemia, and hypertension. *Arch Intern Med* 1989; **149**, 1514–1520.

41. Bjorntorp P. Regional patterns of fat distribution. *Ann Intern Med* 1985; **103**, 994–995.

42. Gleim G. W. Exercise is not an effective weight loss modality in women. *J Am Coll Nutr* 1993; **12**, 363–367.

43. Grodstein F., Manson J. E., Colditz G. A., Willett W. C., Speizer F. E., Stampfer J. M. A prospective, observational study on hormone therapy and primary prevention of cardiovascular disease. *Ann Intern Med* 2000; **133**, 933–941.

44 Writing Group for the PEPI Trial. Effects of estrogen or estrogen/progestin regimens on heart disease risk factors in women. The Postmenopausal Estrogen/Progestin Interventions (PEPI) trial. *J Am Med Assoc* 1995; **273**, 199–208.

45. Hully S., Grady D., Bush T., *et al.* Randomized trial of estrogen plus progestin for secondary prevention of coronary heart disease in postmenopausal women: Heart and Estrogen/Progestin Replacement Study (HERS) Research Group. *J Am Med Assoc* 1998; **280**, 605–613.

46. Writing Group for the Women's Health Initiative Investigators. Risks and benefits of estrogen plus progestin in healthy postmenopausal women: principal results from the Women's Health Initiative randomized controlled trial. *J Am Med Assoc* 2002; **288**, 321–333.

47. Salpeter S. R., Walsh J. E., Greyber E., Salpeter E. E. Coronary heart disease events associated with hormone therapy in younger and older women, a meta-analysis. *J Gen Intern Med* 2006; **21**(4), 363–366.

48. Mosca L., Appel L. J., Benjamin E. J., *et al.* Evidence-based guidelines for cardiovascular disease prevention in women. *Circulation* 2004; **109**, 672–693.

49. Clearfield M. Coronary heart disease risk reduction in postmenopausal women: the role of statin therapy and hormone replacement therapy. *Prev Cardiol* 2004; 7, 131–136.

50. Liao J. Beyond lipid lowering: the role of statins in vascular protection. *Int J Cardiol* 2002; **86**, 5–18.

51. Jones P. H., Davidson M. H., Stein E. A., *et al.* Comparison of the efficacy and safety of rosuvastatin versus atorvastatin, simvastatin, and pravastatin across doses (STELLAR) trial. *Am J Cardiol* 2003; **92**, 152–160.

52. Mosca L., Banka C. L., Benjamin E. J., *et al.*, for the American Heart Association Expert Panel/Writing Group. Evidence-based guidelines for cardiovascular disease prevention in women: 2007 update. *Circulation.* American Heart Association website, available at http://circ.ahajournals.org/cgi/reprint/CIRCULATIONAHA.

53. The Steering Committee of the Physicians' Health Study Research Group. Final report from the aspirin component of the ongoing Physicians' Health Study. *N Engl J Med* 1989; **321**, 129–135.

54. Ridker P. M., Cook M. R., Lee I.-M., *et al.* A randomized trial of low-dose aspirin in the primary prevention of cardiovascular disease in women. *N Engl J Med* 2005; **352**(13), 1293–1304.

55. Antiplatelet Trialists' Collaboration. Collaborative overview of randomized trials of antiplatelet therapy. Prevention of death, myocardial infarction, and stroke by prolonged antiplatelet therapy in various categories of patients. *Br Med J* 1994; **308**, 81–106.

56. ISIS-2 (Second International Study of Infarct Survival) Collaborative Group. Randomised trial of intravenous streptokinase, oral aspirin, both, or neither among 17,187 cases of suspected acute myocardial infarction: ISIS-2. *Lancet* 1988; **2**, 349.

57. Harrington R. A., Becker R. C., Ezekowitz M., *et al.* Antithrombotic therapy for coronary artery disease: the Seventh ACCP Conference on Antithrombotic and Thrombolytic Therapy. *Chest* 2004; **126**, 513S.

58. Braunwald E., Antman E., Beasley J., *et al.* ACC/AHA 2002 guideline update for the management of patients with unstable angina and non-ST-segment elevation myocardial infarction. Available at www.acc.org/qualityandscience/clinical/statements.htm, accessed 12/23/06.

59. Hayden M., Pignone M., Phillips C., Mulrow C. Aspirin for the primary prevention of cardiovascular events: a summary of the evidence for the US Preventive Services Task Force. *Ann Intern Med* 2002; **136**, 161–172.

60. Krumholz H. M., Philbin D. M. Jr., Wang Y., *et al.* Trends in the quality of care for Medicare beneficiaries admitted to the hospital with unstable angina. *J Am Coll Cardiol* 1998; **31**, 957.

61. Stafford R. S. Aspirin use is low among United States outpatients with coronary artery disease. *Circulation* 2000; **101**, 1097.

62. Stampfer M. J., Hennekens C. H., Manson J. E., *et al.* Vitamin E consumption and the risk of coronary disease in women. *N Engl J Med* 1993; **328**, 1444.

63. de Gaetano, G. Low-dose aspirin and vitamin E in people at cardiovascular risk: a randomised trial in general practice. Collaborative Group of the Primary Prevention Project. *Lancet* 2001; **357**, 89.

64. MRC/BHF Heart Protection Study of antioxidant vitamin supplementation in 20536 high-risk individuals: a randomised placebo-controlled trial. *Lancet* 2002; **360**, 23.

65. McCarthy B. C., Beshansky J. R., D'Agostino R. B., Selker H. P. Missed diagnoses of acute myocardial infarction in the emergency department: results from a multicenter study. *Ann Emerg Med* 1993; **22**, 579–582.

66. Pope J. H., Aufderheide T. P., Ruthazer R., Woolard R. H., Feldman J. A., Beshanky J. R., *et al.* Missed diagnoses of acute cardiac ischemia in the emergency department. *N Engl J Med* 2000; **342**, 1163–1170.

67. Goldberg R., Goff D., Cooper L., Luepker R., Zapka H., Bittner V., *et al.* Age and sex differences in presentation of symptoms among patients with acute coronary disease: the REACT trial. *Coron Artery Dis* 2000; **11**, 399–407.

68. Milner K. A., Funk M., Richards S., Wilmes R. M., Vaccarino V., Krumholz H. M. Gender differences in symptom presentation association with coronary heart disease. *Am J Cardiol* 1999: **84**, 396–399.

69. Goldman L., Cook E. F., Brand D. A., Lee T. H., Rouan G. W., Weisberg M. C., *et al.* A computer protocol to predict myocardial infarction in emergency department patients with chest pain. *N Engl J Med* 1988; **318**, 797–803.

70. Sullivan A. K., Holdright D. R., Wright C. A., *et al.* Chest pain in women: clinical, investigative, and prognostic features. *Br Med J* 1994; **308**, 883–886.

71. Sheifer S. E., Canos M. R., Weinfurt K. P., Arora U. K., Mendelsohn F. O., Gersh B. J., Weissman N. J. Sex differences in coronary artery size assessed by intravascular ultrasound. *Am Heart J* 2000; **139**, 649–653.

72. Kudenchuk P. J., Maynard C., Martin J. S., Wirkus M., Weaver W. D. Comparison of presentation, treatment, and outcome of acute myocardial infarction in men versus women (the Myocardial Infarction Triage and Intervention Registry). *Am J Cardiol* 1996; **78**, 9–14.

73. Pepine C. J. Angina pectoris in a contemporary population: characterstcs and therapeutic implications. TIDES Investigators. *Cardiovasc Drugs Ther* 1998; **12**(Supp 3), 211–216.

74. Legato M. J. Gender-specific physiology: how real is it? How important is it? *Int J fertil* 1997; **42**(1), 19–29.

75. Light K. C., Herbst M. C., Bragdon E. E., Hinderliter A. L., Koch G. G., Davis M. R., *et al.* Depression and type A behavior pattern in patients with coronary artery disease: relationships to painful versus silent myocardial ischemia and B-endorphin responses during exercise. *Psychosom Med* 1991; **53**, 669–683.

76. Carney R. M., Blumenthal J. A., Stein P. K., Watkins L., Catellier D., Berkman L. F., *et al.* Depression, heart rate variability, and acute myocardial infarction. *Circulation* 2001; **104**, 2024–2028.

77. Ayanian J. Z., Epstein A. M. Differences in the use of procedures between women and men hospitalized for coronary heart disease. *N Engl J Med* 1991; **325**(4), 221–225.

78. Roger V. L., Farkouh M. E., Weston S. A., Reeder G. S., Jacobsen S. J., Zinsmeister A. R., *et al.* Sex differences in evaluation and outcome of unstable angina. *J Am Med Assoc* 2000; **283**(5), 646–652.

79. Mehta R. H., Montoye C. K., Faul J., *et al.* Enhancing quality of care for acute myocardial infarction: shifting the focus of improvement form key indicators to process of care and tool use. *J Am Coll Cardiol* 2004; **43**, 2166–2173.

80. Mehta R. H., Montoye C. K., Gallogly M., *et al.* Improving quality of care for acute myocardial infarction: the Guidelines Applied in Practice (GAP) initiative. *J Am Med Assoc* 2002; **287**, 1269–1276.

81. Ryan T. J., Antman E. M., Brooks N. H., *et al.* 1999 Update: ACC/AHA guidelines for the management of patients with acute myocardial infarction: executive

summary and recommendations: a report of the American College of Cardiology/American Heart Association Task Force on Practice Guidelines (Committee on Management of Acute Myocardial Infarction). *Circulation* 1999; **100**, 1016–1030.

82. ACC/AHA 2002 Guideline Update for Exercise Testing: a Report of the American College of Cardiology/AHA Task Force on Practice Guidelines. www.americanheart.org.

83. Chaitman B. R., Bourassa M. G., Davis K., *et al.* Angiographic prevalence of high risk coronary artery disease in patient subsets (CASS). *Circulation* 1981; **64**, 360–367.

84. Miller D. D. Noninvasive diagnosis of CAD in women. *J Myocard Ischem* 1995; 7, 263–268.

85. Schlant R. C., Blomqvist C. G., Brandenburg R. O., *et al.* Guidelines for exercise testing: a report of the Joint American College of Cardiology/American Heart Association Task Force on Assessment of Cardiovascular Procedures (Subcommittee on Exercise Testing). *Circulation* 1986; **74**(3), 653–667A.

86. Clark P. I., Glasser S. P., Lyman G. H., *et al.* Relation of results of exercise stress tests in young women to phases of the menstrual cycle. *Am J Cardiol* 1988; **61**(1), 197–199.

87. Hung J., Chaitman B. R., Lam J., *et al.* Noninvasive diagnostic test choices for the evaluation of coronary artery disease in women: a multivariate comparison of cardiac fluoroscopy, exercise electrocardiography and exercise thallium myocardial perfusion scintigraphy. *J Am Coll Cardiol* 1984; **4**(1), 8–16.

88. Marwick T. H., Anderson T., Williams M. J., *et al.* Exercise echocardiography is an accurate and cost-effective technique for detection of coronary artery disease in women. *J Am Coll Cardiol* 1995; **26**, 335–341.

89. Weiner D. A., Ryan T. J., Parsons L., *et al.* Long-term prognostic value of exercise testing in men and women from the Coronary Artery Surgery Study (CASS) registry. *Am J Cardiol* 1995; **75**(14), 865–870.

90. Pratt C. M., Francis J. M., Divine G. W., Young J. B. Exercise testing in women with chest pain. Are there additional exerice characteristics that predict true positive test results? *Chest* 1989; **95**, 139–144.

91. Mora S., Redberg R. F., Cui Y., Whiteman M. K., Flaws J. A., Sharrett A. R., Blumenthal R. S. Ability of exercise testing to predict cardiovascular and all-cause death in asymptomatic women: a 20-year follow-up of the lipid research clinics prevalence study. *J Am Med Assoc* 2003; **290**, 1600–1607.

92. Kaski J. C., Rosano G. M. C., Collins P., Nihoyannopoulos P., Maseri A., Poole-Wilson P. A. Cardiac syndrome X: clinical characteristics and

left ventricular function. *J Am Coll Cardiol* 1995; **25**, 807–814.

93. Vaccarino V., Parsons L., Every N. R., Barron H. V., Krumholz H. M. Sex-based differences in early mortality after myocardial infarction. *N Engl J Med* 1999; **341**, 217–225.

94. Chandra N. C., Rogers W. J., Tiefenbrunn, A. J., *et al.* for the National Registry of Myocardial Infarction (NRMI) Investigators. High MI mortality in women: gender or age? *JACC* 1993; **21**(Suppl A), 347A.

95. Weaver W. D., White H. D., Wilcox R. G., *et al.* Comparisons of characteristics and outcomes among women and men with acute MI treated with thrombolytic therapy. *J Am Med Assoc* 1996; **275**, 777–782.

96. Hochman J. S., Tamis J. E., Thompson T. D., *et al.* Sex, clinical presentation, and outcome in patients with acute coronary syndromes. *N Engl J Med* 1999; **341**, 226–232.

97. O'Connor G. T., Morton J. R., Diehl M. J., *et al.* Differences between men and women in hospital mortality associated with coronary artery bypass graft surgery. *Circulation* 1993; **88**, 2104–2110.

98. Vaccarino V., Abramson J. L., Veledar E., *et al.* Sex differences in hospital mortality after coronary artery bypass surgery: evidence for a higher mortality in younger women. *Circulation* 2002; **105**, 1176–1181.

99. Jacobs A. K. Coronary revascularization in women in 2003: sex revisited. *Circulation* 2003; **107**, 375.

100. Jacobs A. K., Kelsey S. F., Brooks M. M., *et al.* Better outcome for women compared with men undergoing coronary revascularization a report from the Bypass Angioplasty Revascularization Investigation (BARI). *Circulation* 1998; **98**, 1279–1285.

101. Jacobs A. K., Johnston J. M., Haviland A., *et al.* Improved outcomes for women undergoing contemporary percutaneous coronary intervention: a report from the National Heart, Lung, and Blood Institute Dynamic Registry. *J Am Coll Cardiol* 2002; **39**, 1606–1614.

102. Cho L., Topol E. J., Balog C., *et al.* Clinical benefit of glycoprotein IIb/IIIa blockade with abciximab is independent of gender: pooled analysis from EPIC, EPILOG and EPISTENT trials. *J Am Coll Cardiol* 2000; **36**, 381–386.

103. Hogue C. W. Jr., Barzilai B., Pieper K. S., *et al.* Sex differences in neurological outcomes and mortality after cardiac surgery: a Society of Thoracic Surgery National Database report. *Circulation* 2001; **103**, 2133–2137.

104. Herlitz J., Brandrup-Wognsen G., Karlson B. W., *et al.* Mortality, risk indicators of death, mode of death and

symptoms of angina pectoris during 5 years after coronary artery bypass grafting in men and women. *J Intern Med* 2000; **247**, 500–506.

105. Morice M.-C., Serruys P. W., Sousa J. E., *et al.* A randomized comparison of a sirolimus-eluting stent with a standard stent for coronary revascularization. *N Engl J Med* 2002; **346**, 1173–780.

106. Moses J. W., Leon M. B., Popma J. J., *et al.* Sirolimus-eluting stents versus standard stents in patients with stenosis in a native coronary artery. *N Engl J Med* 2003; **349**, 1315–1323.

107. Sousa J. E., Costa M. A., Abizaid A., *et al.* Lack of neointimal proliferation after implantation of sirolimus-coated stents in human coronary arteries: a quantitative coronary angiography and three-dimensional intravascular ultrasound study. *Circulation* 2001; **103**, 192–195.

Diabetes in mid-life women

Phillippa J. Miranda and Diana McNeill

A 51-year-old woman with type 2 diabetes for five years is managed with metformin, diet, and exercise. She notes worsening hyperglycemia, but attention to diet and exercise does not seem to improve glycemic control as it has in the past. She mentions to her physician that she has missed her last two menstrual periods and seems to be a "bit more edgy." She wonders if there is a correlation between her worsening diabetes control and her menstrual changes.

Definitions

1. Diabetes mellitus refers to a group of common metabolic disorders characterized by hyperglycemia. Diabetes may be type 1 (juvenile onset or insulin-dependent diabetes mellitus, IDDM), type 2 (adult onset or non-insulin dependent diabetes mellitus, NIDDM), or gestational (during pregnancy).
2. In type 1 diabetes, which accounts for about 5–10% of cases, hyperglycemia is caused by an absolute deficiency of insulin secretion.
3. In type 2 diabetes which accounts for about 90–95% of cases, hyperglycemia is caused by a combination of insulin resistance and inadequate compensatory insulin secretory response, with a relative, not absolute, insulin deficiency.
4. Gestational diabetes occurs in 2–5% of all pregnancies, and although it usually resolves after pregnancy, women with a history of gestational diabetes have a 20–50% chance of developing type 2 diabetes within the next 5–10 years.[1]
5. The most common type of diabetes in mid-life is type 2 diabetes, often caused by a combination of inherited and environmental factors and lifestyle choices. Type 2 diabetes is associated with numerous metabolic abnormalities including

reduced insulin secretion, increased hepatic glucose production, decreased glucose uptake by muscle and adipose tissue, and dyslipidemia. These metabolic abnormalities underlie the complications of diabetes, including heart attack, stroke, blindness, end-stage renal disease, and lower extremity amputation.
6. With type 2 diabetes, there may be a long period without clinical symptoms but with elevated insulin levels and mild-moderate hyperglycemia, which can result in damage to target tissues before diabetes is diagnosed.

Epidemiology

1. The incidence and prevalence of diabetes are increasing worldwide. Using World Health Organization (WHO) diagnostic criteria, the worldwide prevalence of diabetes in adults was estimated to be 4.0% (135 million people) in 1995, rising to 5.4% (300 million people) by 2025.
2. Diabetes is more prevalent in developed countries; the countries with the largest number of people with diabetes are India, China, and the USA. Notably, there are more women than men with diabetes, especially in developed countries.[2]
3. Diabetes is also more prevalent in older age groups. According to the Centers for Disease Control and Prevention (CDC), the total prevalence of diabetes in the USA in 2002 was 6.3% of the total population (18.2 million people) for all ages and 18.3% of the population age 60 and older.[2]
4. Individuals with diabetes also experience more morbidity and mortality than individuals without diabetes. In a cohort of US adults aged 25–74 years, the 5.1% of subjects who had diabetes

Handbook of Women's Health, second edition, ed. Jo Ann Rosenfeld. Published by Cambridge University Press.
© Cambridge University Press 2009.

experienced 10.6% of the observed mortality. Median life expectancy was 8 years lower for those age 55–64 years with diabetes and 4 years lower for those age 65–74 years with diabetes compared to those without diabetes.[3]

5. In addition to the high rates of diabetes and associated mortality, mid-life women should be concerned about diabetes due to the implications for the management of menopause. This chapter will examine the diagnosis, prevention, and management of diabetes in mid-life women.

Clinical course

Signs and symptoms

1. In mid life, type 2 diabetes is the most common type of diabetes. The diagnosis of type 2 diabetes is made based on symptoms of hyperglycemia and the measurement of elevated blood glucose readings.

2. The classic symptoms of significant hyperglycemia include polyuria, polydipsia, weight loss, polyphagia, and blurred vision. Hyperglycemia may also cause fatigue, vaginitis, or other non-specific symptoms, which may be attributed to menopause. If the onset of hyperglycemia is gradual, there may not be any symptoms, thus delaying the diagnosis of diabetes.

Screening of asymptomatic individuals

1. Since hyperglycemia can be asymptomatic, those individuals at increased risk for diabetes should be screened at regular intervals. Individuals at increased risk for type 2 diabetes include those with increasing age, obesity, and lack of physical activity.

2. Obesity is a major contributing factor to insulin resistance and diminished pancreatic cell reserve capacity in type 2 diabetes. Even those patients who are not overweight by standard criteria may have an increased percentage of body fat and/or an abnormal distribution of body fat, predominantly in the abdominal viscera, placing them at increased risk for developing diabetes.

3. Additional risk factors for type 2 diabetes include prior gestational (pregnancy-related) diabetes or delivery of a baby weighing over 9 pounds, hypertension, dyslipidemia, family history of type 2 diabetes, and certain racial and ethnic groups (Table 25.1).

Table 25.1 Risk factors associated with type 2 diabetes

Increasing age

Obesity (BMI over 25 kg/m^2)

Lack of physical activity

Prior gestational (pregnancy-related) diabetes

Delivery of a baby weighing over 9 pounds

Hypertension

Dyslipidemia

Family history of type 2 diabetes

4. Screening for type 2 diabetes is important because there are at least 5.2 million individuals with undiagnosed type 2 diabetes in the USA based on CDC estimates in 2002.[1] Undiagnosed diabetes is still clinically significant, as retinopathy may develop before the diagnosis of diabetes is made. Furthermore, coronary heart disease, stroke, and peripheral vascular disease are common in those with undiagnosed diabetes.

5. Thus, early detection of diabetes in those at risk has significant potential to impact morbidity and mortality from the disease. The ADA recommends that testing for diabetes in asymptomatic individuals should be considered for those age 45 years and older and should be repeated every three years.[4]

6. In addition, testing should be considered at a younger age or more frequently if the woman is overweight (BMI>25 kg/m^2), has a first-degree relative with diabetes, is a member of a high-risk ethnic population, has been diagnosed with gestational diabetes, or delivered a baby weighing over 9 lbs, has hypertension with BP $\geq$140/90 mmHg, HDL cholesterol $\leq$35 mg/dL, and/or triglycerides $\geq$250 mg/dL; or pre-diabetes, impaired glucose tolerance, or impaired fasting glucose.

7. Testing may be performed using an oral glucose tolerance test (OGTT) or fasting plasma glucose (FPG); however, FPG is preferred because of ease of testing, convenience, acceptability to patients, and lower cost.

Diagnostic criteria

1. Diagnostic criteria and classification schemes for diabetes have been proposed and published by the ADA and WHO.[5,6] In January 2002, the ADA

Table 25.2 ADA criteria for diagnosis of diabetes

Symptoms of diabetes (polyuria, polydipsia, or unexplained weight loss) plus random plasma glucose ≥200 mg/dL (11.1 mmol/L)

Fasting (no calories for at least 8 hours) plasma glucose ≥266 mg/dL (7.0 mmol/L)

2-hour plasma glucose ≥200 mg/dL (11.1 mmol/L) during an OGTT, with a 75-gram glucose load, per WHO guidelines

Note: Data from ADA. Standards of medical care in diabetes – 2006. *Diabetes Care* 2006; **29**(S1), S4–S42.

Table 25.3 Target levels of blood glucose readings

Time of day	Plasma	Whole blood
Preprandial glucose	90–130 (5.0–7.2)	80–260 (4.4–6.7)
1–2 hour postprandial glucose	<180 (<10.0)	<180 (<10.0)
Bedtime glucose	110–260 (6.1–8.3)	100–140 (5.5–7.8)

Note: Values are given in mg/dL, with mmol/L in parentheses.

published revised criteria for the diagnosis of diabetes, which state that diabetes can be diagnosed by any one of three criteria (Table 25.2).

2. In the absence of unequivocal hyperglycemia with metabolic decompensation, criteria should be confirmed by repeat testing on a different day. The OGTT is not recommended for routine clinical use, but may be necessary when diabetes is suspected despite normal fasting plasma glucose.[5]

3. The ADA does not recommend glycosylated hemoglobin (hemoglobin A1c, HbA1c) for the diagnosis of diabetes. Even though HbA1c is a reliable marker of glycemia over a period of approximately 2–3 months, this test should not be used to diagnose diabetes because too many different methods are used for the measurement of HbA1c, and the correlations between fasting plasma glucose, 2-hour post-load glucose, and HbA1c are imperfect.

4. In recent years, the levels at which plasma glucose is considered diagnostic of diabetes have been revised downwards. The cut-off point of a 2-hour post-load glucose over 200 mg/dL (11.1 mmol/L) has been shown to mark that level of hyperglycemia at which the prevalence of microvascular complications considered specific for diabetes increases dramatically.[5]

5. The fasting plasma glucose (FPG) has been revised down from 140 mg/dL (7.8 mmol/L) to 266 mg/dL (7.0 mmol/L) as this value better reflects the same degree of hyperglycemia responsible for the 2-hour post-load glucose of over 200 mg/dL (11.1 mmol/L) on an OGTT.

Blood glucose target levels

1. For the individual with diabetes, monitoring of blood glucose levels by the patient and the

health care provider is necessary to achieve glycemic control. Based on findings from the diabetes Control and Complications Trial (DCCT), self-monitoring of blood glucose (SMBG) is recommended for most individuals with diabetes. The routine use of home blood glucose meters has replaced the use of urine glucose testing, which was previously the only method of home testing available to patients.

2. Target pre-prandial, postprandial, and bedtime blood glucose levels, based on ADA recommendations, are given in Table 25.3.[7]

3. In addition to SMBG data, HbA1c is recommended for monitoring response to diabetes therapy. HbA1c testing should be performed at initial assessment and then as part of continuing care in all patients with diabetes. Because the HbA1c test reflects an average blood glucose over 2–3 months, testing every three months is required to determine if glycemic control departs from the target range.

4. Expert opinion recommends HbA1c testing at least twice a year in patients meeting treatment goals, and more frequently for those not at goal or whose therapy has changed. Although reference ranges vary by lab and method used for measuring HbA1c, normal individuals without diabetes usually have HbA1c readings of 4–6%, corresponding to blood glucose levels of 60–260 mg/dL (3.3–6.7 mmol/L).

5. For patients in general with diabetes, the ADA recommends a target level for HbA1c of less than 7%, which corresponds to a blood glucose level of 260 mg/dL (8.3 mmol/L); however, for the individual patient, the ADA recommends a HbA1c goal "as close to normal (<6%) as possible without significant hypoglycemia".[8]

Prevention of diabetes

1. In April 2002, the ADA published a position statement on the prevention or delay of type 2 diabetes, and these recommendations were restated in the 2006 ADA position statement entitled "Standards of Medical Care in Diabetes – 2006."[8,9] These statements review the evidence for the benefits of prevention, who to screen, and how to implement prevention programs.

2. Screening should occur during the regular office visit with either FPG or 2-hour OGTT. If impaired glucose tolerance (IGT, defined by glucose $\geq$140 mg/dL but <200 mg/dL on OGTT) or impaired fasting glucose (IFG, defined by FPG level of $\geq$100 mg/dL but <266 mg/dL) is found, intervention should include counseling for weight loss and increase in physical activity.

3. Goals should be modest weight loss (5–10% body weight) and modest physical activity (30 minutes per day). Follow-up counseling is vital, with rescreening for diabetes every 1–2 years.

4. Additional interventions to reduce other cardiovascular risk factors (tobacco use, hypertension, and dyslipidemia) are appropriate, but drug therapy for glycemic control is not routinely recommended to treat IGT or IFG until more conclusive evidence is available.

5. In addition, individuals at high risk for diabetes need to become aware of the benefits of weight loss and increased physical activity, and health care providers should encourage these healthy lifestyle choices at every opportunity.

Risk factors

1. Risk factors for the development of type 2 diabetes include obesity, physical inactivity, age, and family history of type 2 diabetes. The Nurses' Health Study found that obesity, specifically adult weight change, was a risk factor for diabetes. In this prospective cohort study, more than 114,000 women aged 30 to 55 years in eleven US states were followed for 14 years, during which time 2204 cases of diabetes were diagnosed. Compared with women with a BMI less than 22 kg/m^2, women of average weight (BMI 24–24.9 kg/m^2) had a relative risk for developing diabetes of 5.0 (95% CI 3.6 to 6.6), and obese women (BMI over 31.0 kg/m^2) had a relative risk of 40.0 or greater.

This study also confirmed that family history is a predictor of risk for diabetes; however, family history did not alter the risks associated with weight gain.[10]

2. Another risk factor for type 2 diabetes is physical inactivity. The Iowa Women's Health Study Cohort was used to examine the relationship between physical activity and new diabetes in postmenopausal women. A series of mailed questionnaires were sent to a cohort of 34,257 postmenopausal women aged 55 to 69 years to assess the 26-year incidence of diabetes and level of physical activity. After adjusting for age, education, smoking, alcohol, estrogen use, diet, and family history, women who reported any physical activity had a relative risk of diabetes of 0.69 compared to sedentary women. When further adjusted for obesity, the relative risk reduction with physical activity decreased to 0.86. Any level of physical activity decreased diabetes risk; however, with increasing frequency or intensity of exercise, the diabetes risk showed an incremental decrease.[11]

Diabetes prevention program

1. Type 2 diabetes is a preventable disease if obesity and physical inactivity are modified with lifestyle changes for both men and women. The Diabetes Prevention Program (DPP) Research Group conducted a large randomized controlled trial to directly compare the effect of lifestyle modification to medical therapy with metformin to prevent diabetes.[12] In this study, more than 3200 US adults at high risk for the development of type 2 diabetes were randomized to standard lifestyle recommendations plus placebo, standard lifestyle recommendations plus metformin, a biguanide antihyperglycemic agent, or an intensive lifestyle modification program with goals of at least 7% weight loss and 260 minutes of physical activity per week. The participants had a mean age of 51 years, had a mean BMI of 34.0 kg/m^2, were 68% women, and were 45% minorities. Over the 2.8-year follow-up period, the intensive lifestyle modification group had a 58% reduction in the incidence of diabetes, while the metformin group had a 31% reduction as compared to placebo. In subgroup analysis, metformin was less effective in those $\geq$60 years old or with

BMI<30, but metformin was as effective as lifestyle modification in those age 24–44 or with BMI ≥ 35. In order to prevent one case of diabetes during three years, seven people would have to undertake intensive lifestyle modification.

2. This study demonstrates that either intensive lifestyle modification or metformin can reduce the incidence of type 2 diabetes in men and women who are at increased risk of diabetes.

Menopause and diabetes
Type 2 diabetes and menopause

1. Menopause is defined as the cessation of menses for one year, while erratic menses that can occur prior to that time is known as perimenopause. As the population ages, estimates suggest that by the year 2026, 45% of all women will be 45 years or older, an age often associated with changes in the menstrual cycle.[13]

2. The decrease in endogenous estrogen that occurs with the onset of menopause can be associated with:
   a. fluctuations in sex hormone levels and increased relative androgen levels, which can contribute to increased fasting glucose;
   b. increasing hepatic glucose production leading to increased fasting glucose;
   c. increased body fat, particularly central intra-abdominal fat, which can lead to increased insulin resistance and cardiovascular risk;[14] and
   d. other changes in insulin metabolism and resistance.[15] All of these physiological changes can affect glycemic control in the menopausal woman with diabetes.

3. Evidence about the effects of hormone replacement therapy (HRT) used for the management of menopausal symptoms on glycemic control is inconclusive and conflicting. In the Postmenopausal Estrogen/Progestin Intervention (PEPI) Trial, combination treatment with estrogen plus medroxyprogesterone increased two-hour postprandial glucose levels.[16]

4. Other studies have shown that estrogen alone may improve diabetes control in postmenopausal women by decreasing relative androgen levels, since androgens contribute to insulin resistance,

as seen in patients with polycystic ovary syndrome.[17]

5. In the United Kingdom Prospective Diabetes Study (UKPDS), the seminal study of glycemic control in patients with type 2 diabetes, HbA1c improved by 0.5% in patients using hormone replacement (HRT) compared to those who did not. While this change may seem small, it is consistent with a 10% reduction in any diabetes complication and a 7% decrease in myocardial infarction for those taking HRT.[18]

6. The UKPDS results were further supported in an observational study of 26,435 women with type 2 diabetes who were members of a health maintenance organization. In the 25% who were using HRT, HRT use was independently associated with a decreased HbA1c, whether the HRT contained a progestin or not.[19]

7. A major confounding factor in these studies is that women who consider HRT are more likely to modify other aspects of their health by monitoring their blood glucose more often, exercising more regularly, and attempting weight management and control.

8. Randomized studies were needed, and two randomized, placebo-controlled trials (the Heart and Estrogen/Progestin Replacement Study (HERS) and the Women's Health Initiative (WHI) were undertaken to address the questions surrounding HRT and the primary and secondary prevention of cardiovascular disease (CVD). In HERS, treatment with oral conjugated equine estrogen plus medroxyprogesterone acetate did not reduce the overall rate of CVD events during the 4-year follow-up period; however, in women with coronary disease, HRT reduced the incidence of diabetes by 35%.[20,21] In WHI, 16,608 postmenopausal women with a uterus, of whom only 4.4% had diabetes at baseline, were randomized to placebo versus conjugated equine estrogen (0.625 mg) plus medroxyprogesterone acetate (2.5 mg). After 5.2 years, the trial was stopped due to concerns that the risks of invasive breast cancer and cardiovascular events outweighed the benefits of decreased colorectal cancer and improved bone health.[22,23]

9. The finding of an increased rate of cardiovascular events with HRT use was particularly important for women with diabetes, as they have an

increased cardiovascular risk compared to women without diabetes regardless of menopausal status.[24] Although the WHI has offered health care workers and patients an opportunity to discuss the relative risks and benefits of HRT on an individual basis, controversy about the use of HRT generated by the data from the WHI has made recommendations about hormone replacement in the woman with diabetes less clear.

10. At present, the only indication for use of HRT is for the management of menopausal symptoms, including hot flashes, vaginal dryness, and mood and sleep disturbances. Women with diabetes who experience these symptoms should only consider HRT after an informed discussion with their health care provider and a complete evaluation of their cardiac risk status and modification of any cardiac risk factors. Furthermore, evidence clearly indicates that HRT should be avoided in the first year after myocardial infarction.[25]

11. In addition to cardiovascular disease prevention and glycemic control, what else should the mid-life woman with diabetes be told about the management of her health? Issues for the menopausal woman with diabetes include bone health and the risk of osteoporosis, depression, and macrovascular and microvascular complications of diabetes.

12. Bone health should be assessed and a bone density evaluation should be considered for women over 50 years old or any woman with increased risk of osteoporosis from chronic thyroid hormone replacement, smoking, low body mass index, or a family history of osteoporosis.[26]

13. Depression is more common in women with diabetes, and depression also increases in postmenopausal women. Since anxiety and depression can adversely affect glycemic control, stress management and pharmacological treatment of severe depression may have a positive effect on glycemic control.[27]

Type 1 diabetes and menopause

1. The relationship between type 1 diabetes and menopause is even more complex, as menopause in patients with type 1 diabetes may occur at a younger age.[28]

2. Genetic factors, including haplotypes found in association with the DR4 haplotype (more common in type 1 diabetes), may increase the risk of early menopause two-fold. The long-term effects of premature menopause, beside a shorter time for childbearing, include a higher risk of cardiovascular disease, dyslipidemia, and osteoporosis. Early menopause may occur in women with type 1 diabetes from autoimmune premature ovarian failure (similar to the autoimmune thyroiditis seen more commonly in patients with type 1 diabetes) and from hypothalamic dysfunction in the setting of poorly controlled diabetes.

3. Health care providers should routinely ask women about their menstrual history to aid in the early detection of premature menopause in these women.

Glycemic control: therapeutic interventions

1. Once the diagnosis of diabetes has been made, each individual needs a diabetes management plan to control the disease and prevent complications. The diabetes management plan should include the following components: education about the disease; instruction in home self-blood glucose monitoring; diet counseling and nutritional modification; exercise; and medications, if needed.

2. Oral diabetes medications, which can be used alone or in combination, include sulfonylureas, biguanides, thiazolidinediones, and others. New diabetes medications include the oral agent Sitagliptin and the two injectable medications – Pramlintide and Exenatide.

3. Options for insulin therapy have increased in recent years with the introduction of insulin analogs (insulin lispro, insulin aspart, insulin glargine, and insulin determir) and rapid-acting inhaled insulin (Exubera).

Education

1. Education of the individual with diabetes about the disease and its management is the most important intervention in the diabetes management plan. Certified Diabetes Educators (CDEs) are excellent resources to provide diabetes education. Education may be provided through group classes, one-on-one counseling sessions, or

both. The goal of education is to provide knowledge and understanding of the disease in order to improve motivation and compliance with other therapies, and thus improve outcomes and quality of life.

2. Education programs should include basic disease information and blood glucose targets; practical advice to implement lifestyle changes, including diet and exercise; instruction in home blood glucose monitoring; and education on prevention of complications. Each of these topics is discussed in more detail below.

Diet

1. Diet therapy is central to the management of type 2 diabetes. Frequently, type 2 diabetes coexists with obesity, and a reduction in calorie intake will not only facilitate weight loss but also improve metabolic parameters by decreasing insulin resistance, reducing hepatic glucose output, and enhancing insulin secretion from the pancreas.

2. As little as a 5–10% reduction in body weight may significantly improve glycemic control. A well-balanced diet with a moderate calorie restriction (500–1000 less calories per day) in combination with behavioral modification and education is a safe and effective method for improving metabolic control.

3. Because of the complexity of nutritional issues, the ADA recommends that a registered dietitian who is knowledgeable about diabetes management and education provide medical nutrition therapy. All diabetes caregivers should be familiar with medical nutrition therapy and supportive of patient efforts to make lifestyle changes. Some specific nutritional recommendations are listed in Table 25.4.[29]

4. For individuals with diabetes, carbohydrate and monounsaturated fat together should provide 60–70% of energy intake while saturated fat should be <7% of total calories. There is no evidence to suggest that the usual protein intake of 26–20% should be modified, as long as renal function is normal; however, protein intake should be limited to the recommended daily allowance (RDA) of 0.8 g/kg in the setting of any degree of chronic kidney disease to reduce the risk of worsening nephropathy (see Chapter 3).

Table 25.4 Nutrition guidelines for persons with diabetes

Total amount of carbohydrate is more important than source or type of carbohydrate

Good carbohydrate sources include whole grains, fruits, vegetables, and low-fat milk

Sucrose does not need to be restricted because it does not increase glycemia more than starch, but should be substituted for other carbohydrates

Less than 7% of energy should come from saturated fats

Dietary cholesterol should be less than 300mg per day

Non-nutritive sweeteners are safe when consumed in recommended amounts

Notes: Data from ADA. Evidence-based nutrition principles and recommendations for the treatment and prevention of diabetes and related complications. *Diabetes Care* 2002; **25**(S1): S50–S60, and ADA. Standards of medical care in diabetes – 2006. *Diabetes Care* 2006; **29**(S1), S4–S42.

Exercise

1. Middle-aged and older adults with diabetes should be encouraged to exercise and be physically active, as the potential health benefits of exercise for the individual with type 2 diabetes are substantial[30,31] (see Chapter 4). Analysis of data from the Nurses' Health Study showed that among women with diabetes, increased physical activity including regular walking was associated with fewer cardiovascular events.[32]

2. Exercise may improve insulin sensitivity and help normalize blood glucose levels. Evidence also suggests that the progressive decline in fitness and strength seen with aging can be mitigated with regular exercise, leading to an improved quality of life.

3. Although exercise is an important component of therapy in diabetes, the risks and benefits of exercise must be understood and analyzed for a given patient. Before beginning an exercise program, each individual with diabetes should undergo a complete medical evaluation to screen for vascular disease with diagnostic studies, as appropriate.

4. The history and physical examination should focus on the heart and blood vessels, eyes, kidneys, and nervous system. For those planning to participate in low-intensity exercise, such as walking, the physician should use clinical judgment in deciding whether a cardiac/exercise stress test is warranted. For those planning

Table 25.5 Oral agents and (non-insulin) injectables for treatment of type 2 diabetes

Sulfonylureas	Biguanides	TZDs	Other orals	Injectables
Glipizide	Metformin	Pioglitazone	Acarbose	Pramlintide
Glyburide		Rosiglitazone	Miglitol	Exenatide
Glimepiride			Repaglinide	
			Nateglinide	
			Sitagliptin	

a moderate to high-intensity exercise program, an exercise electrocardiogram or cardiac stress test is recommended for the following individuals:

a. known or suspected coronary artery disease;
b. older than age 30 years with type 1 diabetes;
c. more than 26 year history of type 1 diabetes; or
d. older than 35 years old with type 2 diabetes.[30]

5. A thorough ophthalmologic examination is also recommended, as impaired vision increases the risk of injury, and proliferative retinopathy increases the risk of retinal or vitreous hemorrhage during certain activities.

6. The ADA recommends a gradual increase in the duration and frequency of physical activity to 30–45 minutes of moderate aerobic activity, 3–5 days per week with a goal of at least 260 minutes per week. Evidence from the Diabetes Prevention Program, discussed above, supports the recommendation of 30 minutes of moderate physical activity at least 5 days per week (260 minutes/week). Aerobic exercise is recommended, with precautionary measures taken if the activity involves the feet. For those individuals with loss of protective sensation in the feet, recommended exercises include swimming, bicycling, rowing, chair exercises, arm exercises, and other non-weight-bearing exercise.

7. Regardless of the activity, exercise should include a proper warm-up and cool-down period. Warm-up should include 5–10 minutes of low-intensity aerobic activity followed by 5–10 minutes of gentle muscle stretching. After the exercise activity is complete, a cool-down period of 5–10 minutes should be performed at a lower-intensity level to gradually bring the heart rate down to pre-exercise level.

8. As for anyone who exercises, proper hydration is essential, especially if exercising in extreme

temperatures. Individuals with diabetes should wear a diabetes identification bracelet or tag that is clearly visible when exercising.

Home blood glucose monitoring

1. Monitoring of blood glucose levels by the patient and the health care provider is a cornerstone of diabetes care. With the development of home blood glucose meters, the management of diabetes has changed dramatically. Based on findings from the DCCT, self-monitoring of blood glucose (SMBG) is recommended for individuals with diabetes to facilitate reaching goals for blood glucose levels.[33]

2. The optimal frequency of blood glucose monitoring in type 2 diabetes is not known, and the role of SMBG in diet-controlled type 2 diabetes is not known. SMBG is recommended for all insulin-treated patients with diabetes, and the frequency of monitoring should be increased when adding or modifying any diabetes therapy, with insulin or oral hypoglycemic agents. Patients need instruction in SMBG including:

a. the use of the blood glucose meter;
b. goal blood glucose levels (see Table 25.3);
c. how to interpret and use SMBG data to modify diet, exercise, or medical regimen to maintain adequate glycemic control; and
d. recording blood glucose data in a logbook format that can be reviewed to determine patterns of abnormal blood glucose levels that can be corrected with changes to the diabetes management plan.

Medications

A summary of oral medications used to treat diabetes is given in Table 25.5.

Oral agents: sulfonylureas

1. In the mid-1960s, the first generation of sulfonylureas were used to treat type 2 diabetes. Although use of sulfonylureas declined after tolbutamide was shown to increase cardiovascular risk in the University Group Diabetes Program (UGDP) study, a second generation of sulfonylureas with more potency and fewer side effects has emerged and are widely used. The second-generation sulfonylureas include glipizide, glyburide, and glimepiride.

2. The mechanism of action of these compounds involves binding to the ATP-dependent potassium channel of the pancreatic beta-cell, leading to sustained depolarization, calcium ion influx, and increased insulin secretion. The sulfonylureas have been shown to lower fasting plasma glucose by 50–70 mg/dL and lower HbA1c by 0.8–1.7%.

3. Despite these typical improvements in glycemic control, 20–25% of patients will have primary failure in obtaining glycemic control with sulfonylurea therapy, while an additional 5–10% per year will experience secondary failure to maintain glycemic control.[34]

4. Initiation of sulfonylurea therapy should be considered if a patient has failed to achieve adequate blood glucose control with diet and exercise. Recommended doses and frequency of dosing vary by specific drug, but for many of these agents best results are obtained when taken 26 to 30 minutes before meals.

5. The most common side effect from sulfonylurea therapy is hypoglycemia, which may be life threatening. Because these drugs are metabolized by the liver and kidneys, they should be used with caution in patients with hepatic or renal dysfunction, which may increase the risk of hypoglycemia.

Oral agents: biguanides

1. Metformin is the only biguanide currently available for clinical use. The mechanism of action of metformin, although incompletely understood, involves decreased hepatic glucose output, improved insulin sensitivity, and decreased gastrointestinal glucose absorption. The effects on hepatic glucose output appear to be the most important in reducing fasting plasma glucose and HbA1c.

2. Metformin reduces fasting plasma glucose by 22–26% and reduces HbA1c by 1.2–1.7%, without the risk of hypoglycemia seen with sulfonylureas.

3. Although 5–10% of patients do not tolerate metformin due to gastrointestinal side effects, 80–90% of patients show improvement in overall glycemic control. The most serious potential side effect from metformin therapy is lactic acidosis, with an estimated incidence of 0.03 cases per 1000 patient-years.

4. Contraindications to metformin therapy include renal dysfunction (creatinine>1.5 mg/dL), hepatic dysfunction, alcohol abuse, cardiac disease, peripheral vascular disease, pulmonary disease, and intercurrent illness. Metformin therapy should be temporarily discontinued when intravenous contrast studies are planned, as a transient decrease in renal clearance could lead to increased risk of lactic acidosis.

Oral agents: thiazolidinediones

1. Thiazolidinediones (TZDs) are peroxisome proliferator-activated receptor (PPAR)-gamma ligands and enhance insulin sensitivity directly to improve glycemic control. Pioglitazone and Rosiglitazone are the two members of this class that are currently available for clinical use. The mechanism of action of TZDs is incompletely understood, but involves decreased insulin resistance in peripheral tissues and increased insulin-stimulated glucose uptake in skeletal muscle. Controlled studies have shown that both Rosiglitazone and Pioglitazone reduce HbA1c by 1.5–1.6%.

2. Side effects of TZDs include weight gain, edema, and anemia. Given the liver toxicity associated with Troglitazone, which was withdrawn from clinical use, the FDA recommends periodic monitoring of liver function tests for all patients receiving TZDs. Patients with congestive heart failure and hepatic impairment should not receive TZDs. Several weeks of therapy are necessary to see improvement in glycemic control.

3. These medications may be used alone or in combination with other agents; however, only Pioglitazone is approved for use with insulin.[35]

Other oral agents

1. The alpha-glucosidase inhibitors, Acarbose and Miglitol, decrease the rate of breakdown of dietary

polysaccharides to delay the absorption of glucose from the gut, and thus decrease the postprandial glucose rise. These agents reduce fasting plasma glucose by 25–35 mg/dL and reduce HbA1c by 0.4–0.7%.

2. However, for patients who consume less than 50% of calories as carbohydrates, there is little benefit on glycemic control.

3. The non-sulfonylurea insulin secretagogs (Meglitinides) have similar action to sulfonylureas and act by stimulating insulin production from the pancreas to control postprandial hyperglycemia. The two members of this class are the benzoic acid derivative Repaglinide and the phenylalanine derivative Nateglinide.

4. The newest oral agent for management of type 2 diabetes is Sitagliptin phosphate, which was approved by the FDA in October 2006. Sitagliptin is a DPP-4 (dipeptidyl peptidase 4) inhibitor which enhances the body's ability to lower elevated blood glucose by blocking the enzyme DPP-4 which breaks down the proteins that trigger insulin release. When used as monotherapy, Sitagliptin lowers HbA1c by 0.6–1.4%. This medication can be used as monotherapy or in combination with metformin or TZDs. The most common side effects are stuffy or runny nose, sore throat, upper respiratory infection, and headache.

Injectable medications (other than insulin)

1. Pramlintide is a synthetic (man-made) hormone that resembles human amylin, a hormone produced by the pancreas and released into the blood after meals to help regulate blood glucose. Amylin slows the rate of glucose absorption from the intestine and reduces hepatic glucose output by inhibiting the action of glucagon. In addition, amylin modulates the rate of gastric emptying, thus reducing appetite and increasing sensations of satiety.

2. Pramlintide, which was FDA approved in March 2005, is given as a twice daily subcutaneous injection with meals and is approved to be used in combination with insulin in the treatment of both type 1 and type 2 diabetes.

3. The most common side effect of Pramlintide is nausea. When taken in combination with insulin and/or a sulfonylurea, Pramlintide has been

associated with an increased risk of severe insulin-induced hypoglycemia. Therefore, appropriate patient selection and education is very important, and dose reduction of concurrent diabetes medications, particularly pre-meal doses of short-acting insulin, is recommended.

4. Exenatide belongs to a class of drugs called incretin mimetics because these drugs mimic the effects of incretins, which are hormones produced and released into the blood by the intestine in response to food. Exenatide is a synthetic (man-made) hormone that resembles and acts like human-glucagon-like peptide-1 (GLP-1), which increases the secretion of insulin from the pancreas, slows absorption of glucose from the intestine, and reduces the action of glucagon. Exenatide, which was FDA approved in April 2005, is given as a subcutaneous injection twice per day, and results in HbA1c lowering of 0.4–0.9%.

5. An additional advantage of Exenatide is a moderate weight loss of about 8–9 pounds after one year of therapy.

6. The most common side effects with Exenatide are nausea, vomiting, diarrhea, feeling jittery, dizziness, headache, and dyspepsia. When given in combination with a sulfonylurea or a sulfonylurea and metformin, the risk of hypoglycemia is increased compared to placebo; therefore, dose reduction of these concurrent medications should be considered.

Insulin: types available and profiles

1. Individuals with type 2 diabetes usually experience a progressive decline in endogenous insulin production as the duration of diabetes increases. Thus, many people with type 2 diabetes may become insulin requiring.

2. Insulin supplementation in type 2 diabetes may be necessary either on a temporary basis for stress-induced hyperglycemia or permanently after failure of oral agents to maintain adequate glycemic control.

3. There are a variety of insulin preparations that are currently available, including human insulins and insulin analogs. Animal insulins, such as pork or beef insulin, are no longer routinely used in clinical practice. Each type of insulin has a unique profile of action, including onset of effect, time of peak effect, and duration of action (see Table 25.6).

Table 25.6 Insulins and insulin analogs

Class	Onset	Peak	Duration	Members
Rapid acting	5–26 mins	1–2 hrs	4–6 hrs	Lispro (Humalog)
				Aspart (Novolog)
				Exubera (inhaled)
Short acting	30–60 mins	2–4 hrs	6–10 hrs	Regular
Intermediate acting	1–2 hrs	4–8 hrs	10–20 hrs	NPH
				Lente
Long acting	2–4 hrs	10–30 hrs	16–20 hrs	Ultralente
Very long acting ("peakless")	1–2 hrs	flat	24 hrs	Glargine (Lantus)
				Detemir (Levemir)

Note: In addition to the insulins listed here, a variety of insulin mixtures, such as 70/30 or 75/25, which contain a combination of long and short/rapid acting insulins, are also available and are widely used.

4. The profile of action is dependent on absorption from the subcutaneous site of injection into the circulation. The timing of insulin injections and choice of type and dose of insulin must be made on an individual basis using home blood glucose monitoring data and HbA1c as a guide.

5. Individuals with type 1 diabetes always require insulin therapy alone. For individuals with type 2 diabetes who do not reach a target HbA1c of less than 7.0% with a single oral agent or insulin, combination therapy can be helpful.

6. The use of an oral agent, in particular an insulin sensitizer such as metformin or a TZD, in combination with insulin may improve glycemic control and decrease insulin requirements. Depending on the level of glycemic control achieved and patient willingness and ability to use a multi-injection regimen, an intensive insulin regimen with 3–4 insulin injections per day may be appropriate.

7. Referral to an endocrinologist for assistance with diabetes management is appropriate for patients with polypharmacy, continued poor glycemic control, progressive diabetic complications including hypoglycemia, or insulin pump therapy.

Diabetes complications

1. The complications of diabetes develop over many years and include microvascular disease (neuropathy, retinopathy, and nephropathy) and macrovascular disease (myocardial infarction, stroke, and peripheral vascular disease). Given the chronicity of diabetes, the increasing evidence that improving glycemic control in type 1 diabetes (DCCT)[36] and type 2 diabetes (UKPDS)[37] can decrease microvascular complications and ameliorate macrovascular complications has been encouraging.

2. Prevention and management of diabetes complications now are part of the standard of care in the management of all patients with diabetes.

3. Cardiovascular disease (CVD) remains the major cause of morbidity and mortality for all patients with diabetes. Women with diabetes are five times more likely to develop coronary artery disease than women without diabetes.[13]

4. The protective effect of female gender against cardiovascular disease before menopause is not present for any woman with diabetes. The clinical presentation of heart disease may be atypical in the woman with diabetes. Fatigue, decreased exercise tolerance, or dyspepsia may be anginal equivalent symptoms in the woman with diabetes.

5. Routine evaluation with exercise stress testing may have up to a 54% false-positive rate in women, so other cardiac evaluation such as a stress nuclear perfusion study or stress echo may be necessary.[38] Interventions for CVD may also be more difficult in the setting of diabetes and in women.

6. Small vessel disease, which is less amenable to surgery and percutaneous stenting, is more common in diabetes. Furthermore, cardiac revascularization procedures may be more difficult in women with diabetes due to the smaller size of coronary blood vessels in women compared to men.

7. Cardiovascular risk factor modification is critical for women with diabetes. The Strong Heart Study showed that compared to men with diabetes, women with diabetes had greater adverse differences in levels of several CVD risk factors.[39]

8. Risk factor modification should address smoking cessation, aspirin use, blood pressure control (with consideration of an ACE inhibitor or an angiotensin receptor blocking agent), and aggressive lipid management.

9. Dyslipidemia in women is a powerful contributing factor to the macrovascular complications of diabetes, in particular the increasing cardiovascular morbidity and mortality. Subset analysis has shown that goal LDL cholesterol of less than 100 mg/dL and triglycerides less than 200 mg/dL impact cardiovascular events in women with diabetes. In addition to diet and exercise, lipid-lowering medications such as the HMG CoA reductase inhibitors (to lower LDL) or fibric acid derivatives (to lower triglycerides) may be necessary to achieve target lipid levels.

10. Microvascular disease affecting the eyes, kidneys, and feet can be devastating for the patient with diabetes. Annual dilated ophthalmology exam, urine screening for protein or microalbumin, as well as a careful foot examination at each health care visit can help detect complications early, allowing for stabilization and improved outcomes. Preventive care suggestions in the management of diabetes are outlined in Table 25.7.

11. Diabetes complications appear to be related to level of glycemic control. The UKPDS showed a 14% reduction in all-cause mortality for every 1% lowering in HbA1c.[18] HbA1c averaging less than 7% is associated with fewer long-term microvascular complications than HbA1c levels over 7%. With aggressive glucose lowering to meet HbA1c targets and prevent vascular complications, increasing frequency and severity of hypoglycemia can occur and should also be considered a diabetes complication.

Table 25.7 Preventive care in diabetes

Serum blood glucose monitoring
HbA1c at least twice a year (target less than 7%)
Blood pressure target less than 130/80 mmHg
Annual test for urine microalbumin if urinalysis negative for protein
Annual dilated eye exam
Smoking cessation
Laboratory testing for lipid abnormalities, at least annually (target LDL <100)
Aspirin therapy (adult diabetes patients with macrovascular disease or age >40 years old)
Medical nutrition therapy
Regular physical activity (goal of 30–45 minutes at moderate intensity 3–5 times/week, for total of at least 260 minutes per week)
Annual influenza vaccine
Lifetime pneumococcal vaccine (once)

12. One option to help achieve target HbA1c with less hypoglycemia is to monitor 2-hour postprandial glucose levels, with target level under 180 mg/dL (10.0 mmol/L).

Summary

1. The development of diabetes at mid life can make the management of both menopausal symptoms and diabetes more difficult. Good glycemic control, thorough education, self blood glucose monitoring, diet and exercise, as well as medications, are important to minimize the increased health risks associated with diabetes.

2. Since the complications of diabetes including heart attack, stroke, blindness, end-stage renal disease, and lower extremity amputation are more prevalent with advancing age and duration of diabetes, mid-life women with diabetes must advocate for their own health care management. Working with their health care providers, women with diabetes can participate in health care maintenance behavior that can prevent or identify diabetes and its complications earlier.

3. As research toward understanding the cause and finding the cure for all types of diabetes continues,

prevention and early treatment of diabetes is crucial to improve outcomes and quality of life for all who live with this disease.

Take-home points

- Physiological changes of menopause can worsen glycemic control.
- Use of HRT in menopausal women with diabetes remains controversial.
- Women with diabetes are at increased risk for cardiovascular disease, which is the leading cause of death in menopausal women with diabetes.
- Osteoporosis and depression need to be addressed in the menopausal woman with diabetes.
- Diabetes management plan should include education, self blood glucose monitoring, diet and exercise, as well as medications and insulin, if necessary.

> *For the 51-year-old woman with type 2 diabetes and symptoms suggestive of perimenopause, her worsening diabetes control is likely related to her menstrual changes. If her glycemic control remains inadequate with current diet, exercise, and metformin therapy, she may require additional therapy with a second medication or insulin. She should work with her health care provider to assess and modify any risk factors for cardiovascular disease. She should also discuss her individual risks and benefits from HRT with her health care provider, and the decision to use HRT or not should be reassessed on a regular basis, as more evidence becomes available.*

References

1. Centers for Disease Control and Prevention. *National Diabetes Fact Sheet: General Information and National Estimates on Diabetes in the United States, revised edition, 2003.* Atlanta, GA: US Departmental of Health and Human Services, Centers for Disease Control and Prevention, 2004.

2. King H., Aubert R. E., Herman W. H. Global burden of diabetes, 1995–2025. *Diabetes Care* 1998; **21**(9), 1414–1431.

3. Gu K., Cowie C. C., Harris M. I. Mortality in adults with and without diabetes in a national cohort of the U.S. population, 1971–1993. *Diabetes Care* 1998; **21**(7), 1138–1145.

4. American Diabetes Association. Screening for diabetes. *Diabetes Care* 2002; **25**(S1), S21–S24.

5. The Expert Committee on the Diagnosis and Classification of Diabetes Mellitus. Report of the Expert Committee on the Diagnosis and Classification of Diabetes Mellitus. *Diabetes Care* 2002; **25**(S1), S5–S20.

6. World Health Organization. *Diabetes Mellitus: Report of a WHO Study Group*, Technical Report Series, no. 726, Geneva: World Health Organization, 1985.

7. American Diabetes Association. Standards of medical care for patients with diabetes mellitus. *Diabetes Care* 2002; **25**(S1), S33–S49.

8. American Diabetes Association. Standards of medical care in diabetes – 2006. *Diabetes Care* 2006; **29**(S1), S4–S42.

9. American Diabetes Association and NIDDK. The prevention or delay of type 2 diabetes. *Diabetes Care* 2002; **25**(4), 742–749.

10. Colditz G. A., Willett W. C., Rotnitzky A., Manson J. E. Weight gain as a risk factor for clinical diabetes mellitus in women. *Ann Intern Med* 1995; **262**(7), 481–486.

11. Folsom A. R., Kushi L. H., Hong C. P. Physical activity and incident diabetes mellitus in postmenopausal women. *Am J Public Health* 2000; **90**(1), 134–138.

12. Knowler W. C., Barret-Connor E., Fowler S. E., Hamman R. F., Lachin J. M., Walker E. A., Nathan D. M. Reduction in the incidence of type 2 diabetes with lifestyle intervention or metformin. *New Engl J Med* 2002; **346**(6), 393–403.

13. Poirier L., Coburn K. *Women and Diabetes*, Alexandria, VA: American Diabetes Association, 1997.

14. Samaras K., Hayward C., Sullivan D., Kelly R., Campbell L. Effects of postmenopausal hormone replacement therapy on central abdominal fat, glycemic control, lipid metabolism, and vascular factors in type 2 diabetes. *Diabetes Care* 1999; **22**(9), 1401–1407.

15. Matthews K. A., Meilahn E., Kuller L. H., Kelsey S. F., Caggiula A. W., Wing R. R. Menopause and risk factors for coronary heart disease. *New Engl J Med* 1989; **321**, 641–646.

16. The Writing Group for the PEPI Trial. Effects of estrogen or estrogen/progestin regimens on heart disease risk factors in postmenopausal women: the Postmenopausal Estrogen/Progestin Intervention (PEPI) Trial. *J Am Med Assoc* 1995; **263**, 199–208.

17. Andersson B., Mattsson L. A., Hahn I., Marin P., Lapidus L., Holm G., Bengtsson B.-A., Bjorntorp P. Estrogen replacement therapy decreases hyperandrogenicity and improves glucose homeostasis

and plasma lipids in postmenopausal women with noninsulin-dependent diabetes. *J Clin Endocrinol Metab* 1997; **82**, 638–643.

18. Stratton I. M., Adler A. I., Neil H. A., Matthews D. R., Manley S. E., Cull C. A., Hadden D., Turner R. C., Holman R. R. Association of glycaemia with macrovascular and microvascular complications of type 2 diabetes (UKPDS 35): prospective observational study. *Br Med J* 2000; **321**, 405–426.

19. Ferrara A., Karter A., Ackerson L., Liu J., Selby J. Hormone replacement therapy is associated with better glycaemic control in women with type 2 diabetes. *Diabetes Care* 2001; **24**(7), 1144–1260.

20. Hulley S., Grady D., Bush T., Furberg C., Herrington D., Riggs B., Vittinghoff E. Randomized trial of estrogen plus progestin for secondary prevention of coronary heart disease in postmenopausal women. *J Am Med Assoc* 1998; **280**(7), 605–613.

21. Kanaya A. M., Herrington D., Vittinghoff E., Lin F., Grady D., Bittner V., Cauley J. A., Barrett-Connor E. Glycemic effects of postmenopausal hormone therapy: the Heart and Estrogen/Progestin Replacement study. *Ann Intern Med* 2003; **138**, 1–9.

22. Writing Group for the Women's Health Initiative Investigators. Risks and benefits of estrogen plus progestin in healthy postmenopausal women. *J Am Med Assoc* 2002; **288**(3), 321–333.

23. Manson J. E., Hsia J., Johnson K. C., Rossouw J. E., Assaf A. R., Lasser N. L., Trevisan M., Black H. R., Heckbert S. R., Detrano R., Strickland O. L., Wong N. D., Crouse J. R., Stein E., Cushman M. Estrogen plus progestin and the risk of coronary heart disease. *N Eng J Med* 2003; **349**(6), 523–534.

24. Hu F. B., Stampfer M. J., Solomon C. G., Liu S., Willett W. C., Speizer F. E., Nathan D. M., Manson J. E. The impact of diabetes mellitus on mortality from all causes and coronary heart disease in women. *Arch Intern Med* 2001; **161**, 1717–1723.

25. Grady D., HERS Research Group. Cardiovascular disease outcomes during 6.8 years of hormone therapy. *J Am Med Assoc* 2002; **288**(1), 49–57.

26. Osteoporosis Prevention, Diagnosis, and Therapy. NIH Consensus Statement Online, **17**(1), 1–36, March 26–29, 2000.

27. Surwit R., Van Tilburg M., Zucker N., McCaskill C., Parekh P., Feinglos M., Edwards C., Williams P., Lane J. Stress management improves long-term glycemic control in type 2 diabetes. *Diabetes Care* 2002; **25**(1), 30–34.

28. Dorman J., Steenkiste A., Foley T., Strotmeyer E., Burke J., Kuller L., Kwoh C. Menopause in type 1

diabetic women: is it premature? *Diabetes* 2001; **50**, 1857–1862.

29. American Diabetes Association. Evidence-based nutrition principles and recommendations for the treatment and prevention of diabetes and related complications. *Diabetes Care* 2002; **25**(S1), S50–S60.

30. American Diabetes Association. Diabetes mellitus and exercise. *Diabetes Care* 2002; **25**(S1), S64–S68.

31. Devlin J. T., Ruderman N., eds. *The Health Professional's Guide to Diabetes and Exercise* Alexandria VA: American Diabetes Association, 1995.

32. Hu F. B., Stampfer M. J., Solomon C., Liu S., Colditz G. A., Speizer F. E., Willett W. C., Manson J. E. Physical activity and risk for cardiovascular events in diabetic women. *Ann Intern Med* 2001; **134**, 96–105.

33. American Diabetes Association. Implications of the diabetes control and complications trial. *Diabetes Care* 2002; **25**(S1), S25–S26.

34. Feinglos M. N., Bethel M. A., Treatment of type 2 diabetes mellitus. *Med Clinics North Am* 1998; **82**(4), 757–790.

35. Inzucchi S. E., Oral antihyperglycemic therapy for type 2 diabetes, scientific review. *J Am Med Assoc* 2002; **287**(3), 360–372.

36. Diabetes Control and Complications Trial Research Group. The effect of intensive treatment of diabetes on the development and progression of long-term complications in insulin-dependent diabetes mellitus. *New Engl J Med* 1993; **329**, 977–986.

37. UK Prospective Diabetes Study Group. Intensive blood glucose control with sulfonylureas or insulin compared with conventional treatment and risk of complications in patients with type 2 diabetes (UKPDS 33). *Lancet* 1998; **352**, 837–853.

38. Koerbel G., Korytkowski M. Coronary heart disease in women with diabetes. *Diabetes Spectrum* 2003; **16**(3), 148–263.

39. Howard B., Cowan L., Go O., Welty T., Robbins D., Lee E. Adverse effects of diabetes on multiple cardiovascular disease risk factors in women. *Diabetes Care* 1998; **21**(6), 2658–2665.

Additional references

www.diabetes.org – American Diabetes Association

www.endo-society.org – The Endocrine Society

www.mayoclinic.com – information on diabetes and menopause

www.cdc.gov/diabetes/index.htm – Centers for Disease Control and Prevention, general information on diabetes and links to other diabetes-related websites and resources

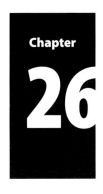

Chapter

26

Thyroid disorders

William J. Hueston

Introduction

Thyroid disorders comprise a wide range of problems that affect the normal functioning of the thyroid gland. These conditions can be grouped into several large categories that include inflammatory diseases of the thyroid (i.e. thyroiditis), autoimmune stimulation of the thyroid (Graves' disease), benign thyroid nodular diseases, and thyroid cancers. While the manifestations of thyroid disease are usually obvious if the presentation is classic, subtle changes in thyroid function, especially in the elderly, can lead to confusion about the diagnosis and treatment for complications of the thyroid condition rather than the underlying thyroid problem. Since thyroid disorders are the second most common endocrine disorder after diabetes, primary care physicians will encounter many individuals with these problems.

Epidemiology
Occurrence

1. Thyroid disease affects 1 out of 200 adults (0.5%), but is more commonly seen in the elderly and in women.[1,2] By the time adults reach older ages, approximately 5% have a thyroid abnormality, most commonly, hypothyroidism.
2. Another 10% to 20% of women over the age of 60 have laboratory abnormalities consistent with subclinical hypothyroidism.

Gender risk

1. The risk of thyroid disease in women is 10 times higher than that in men. For example, about 2% of the female adult population has been hyperthyroid during their lifetime compared to 0.2% of men.[1]

Thyroid nodules also are more common in women than in men.

Relative frequency

1. Hypothyroidism is more common than hyperthyroidism, nodular disease, or thyroid cancer.
2. Thyroid nodules occur in between 4 and 8% of all individuals and, like other thyroid problems, increase in incidence with age. While nodules are more common in women, thyroid carcinoma is more common in women than in men.[3] However, thyroid cancer represents a higher percentage of cancer deaths in men (0.24%) than in women (0.16%).[4]

Clinical presentation
Hypothyroidism

1. Patients with hypothyroidism generally present with a constellation of symptoms that include lethargy, weight gain, hair loss, dry skin, slowed mentation or forgetfulness, and a depressed affect. However, because the presenting symptoms are multiple or often non-specific, clinicians need to have a high index of suspicion to diagnose this illness. In older patients, hypothyroidism can be confused with Alzheimer's or other conditions that cause dementia.
2. In women, hypothyroidism is often confused with depression.
3. Physical findings that can occur with hypothyroidism include a low blood pressure and bradycardia, non-pitting edema, generalized hair thinning along with hair loss in the outer third of

Handbook of Women's Health, second edition, ed. Jo Ann Rosenfeld. Published by Cambridge University Press.
© Cambridge University Press 2009.

297

the eyebrows, skin drying, and a diminished relaxation phase of reflexes.

4. Subclinical hypothyroidism is defined as an elevated TSH in the presence of normal thyroid hormone levels. This is seen most commonly in women and may or may not be associated with symptoms such as lethargy or depression.

Hyperthyroidism

1. Hyperthyroidism usually presents with progressing nervousness, tremor, palpitations or an irregular heart rate when atrial fibrillation is present, weight loss, dyspnea on exertion, and difficulty concentrating.

2. Physical findings include a rapid pulse and elevated blood pressure with the systolic increasing to a greater extent than diastolic creating a wide pulse-pressure hypertension. Additionally, cardiac dysrythmias such as atrial fibrillation may be evident on examination. A resting tremor may be noted on physical examination.

Thyroid storm (thyroid crisis)

1. Thyroid storm represents an acute hypermetabolic state associated with sudden release of large amounts of thyroid hormone. This occurs more often in Graves' disease, but can occur in acute thyroiditis conditions or in thyroid cancers.

2. Individuals with thyroid storm present with cardiac compromise including heart failure or atrial fibrillation along with confusion, fever, restlessness, and sometimes with acute psychotic-like symptoms.

3. Physical examination shows tachycardia, elevated blood pressure, and sometimes fever. Cardiac dysrhythmias may be present or may develop. They will have other signs of high output heart failure (dyspnea on exertion, peripheral vasoconstriction) and may exhibit signs of cardiac or cerebral ischemia.

4. Thyroid storm is a medical crisis requiring prompt attention and reversal of the metabolic demands from the acute hyperthyroidism.

Thyroid nodules

1. Most thyroid nodules are asymptomatic and found on routine health examinations of women.

Because of increasing use of ultrasound for the evaluation of head and neck problems, an increasing number of small nodules are being discovered as incidental findings on ultrasound.

2. In rare cases, the nodule may be very large and compressing nearby structures, but most benign nodules grow slowly. Small nodules under 4 cm in size are rarely malignant.

3. Nodules usually do not produce symptoms of hypo- or hyperthyroidism, but autonomously functioning adenomas may cause hyperthyroidism. In this situation, the adenoma is not under the control of TSH and continues to produce thyroid hormone despite inappropriately high levels.

Laboratory and radiological evaluation
Blood levels of circulating thyroid hormone

1. Both T4 and T3 are highly protein bound. These hormones bind to a number of serum proteins including thyroid binding globulin (TBG) which has a special affinity for T4 and T3. Under normal circumstances, 99% of T4 and 97% of T3 is protein bound.

2. Congenital absences of TBG occur, appearing in genetic patterns. In these patients, both total T4 and T3 levels are extremely low, although patients are usually euthyroid.

3. Other physiological conditions that alter serum proteins can influence total thyroid hormone levels while total free thyroid remains normal. The high ratio of bound to free thyroid hormones means that measurements of total T4 and T3 may not reflect levels of free thyroid hormone.

4. Radioimmunoassays (RIA) that measure free T3 are available that can avoid confusion over bound and free hormone levels. In addition, total T4 measurements can be paired with a test that measures bound levels of T4, called the T3 resin uptake test or T3RU. The combination of these two tests, often termed the free thyroid index or sometimes referred to as a T7, can offer better indications of thyroid status in patients.

Thyroid stimulating hormone (TSH) levels

1. Measuring the amount of TSH in the blood can assess thyroid function, in most hypo- or hyperthyroid individuals. Since, in normal

individuals, TSH rises with low free thyroid levels and falls when free thyroid is elevated, it is an alternative measure for actual circulating levels of the free thyroid hormones.

2. However, when the cause of the thyroid dysfunction is abnormal production of TSH, the test may be misleading. In the case of secondary hypothyroidism, i.e. thyroid deficiency due to low levels of TSH production, both TSH and thyroid hormones levels will be low.

3. In most circumstances it is not necessary to measure both TSH and thyroid hormones. Only when the TSH level appears to contradict the clinical appearance of the patient, such as a low TSH in a patient suspected of hypothyroidism, should thyroid hormone testing be done.

Thyroid releasing hormone (TRH) stimulation testing

1. If pituitary dysfunction is suspected, further evaluation of the anterior pituitary function can be performed using a TRH stimulation test. In this test, TSH levels are determined before and after administration of intravenous TRH. In normal circumstances, infusion of TRH results in a modest rise in TSH. With pituitary dysfunction, the TSH response is absent or blunted. If an exaggerated rise in TSH is noted, this indicates that the pituitary is normal and that the lack of production of TSH reflects an abnormality in TRH production in the hypothalamus.

Other blood tests

Other diagnostic tests for the thyroid include measurement of thyroid antibodies. These antibodies are found in Graves' disease and usually cause stimulation of the thyroid gland resulting in hyperthyroidism.

Radionucleotide thyroid scanning

1. Radionucleotide scanning of the thyroid provides both a direct image of the thyroid and an indication of thyroid functioning. Imaging is performed using an isotope of either technetium (^{99}TcM) or iodine (^{123}I). These radionucleotides are taken up by the active thyroid and, in the case of ^{123}I, incorporated into thyroid hormone.

2. ^{99}TcM is preferred over radio-labeled iodine for scanning for a couple of reasons. First, the radiation dose from ^{99}TcM is much lower than that delivered by ^{123}I. Second, uptake of radioactive iodine is altered by the use of thyroid suppressing medications. This means that patients who have had their hyperthyroidism controlled by thyroid suppressing drugs must have their medications withdrawn before an adequate scan can be completed. Use of ^{99}TcM is not affected by thyroid suppressing medications, avoiding any risk to the patient from the temporary discontinuation of their medications.[5]

3. Imaging of the thyroid after the administration of one of these agents allows visualization of active and inactive areas of the thyroid as well as an indication of the level of activity in that area of the thyroid gland. Similarly, thyroid nodules can be localized and determined to be thyroid producing ("hot" nodules) or non-thyroid hormone producing ("cold" nodules).

Ultrasound

Ultrasound is used primarily as a confirmatory test following the visualization of a non-functioning nodule on thyroid scans. In the presence of a cold nodule, ultrasound can be used to differentiate a hypoechoic nodule which raises suspicion for a thyroid cancer from a solid non-functioning nodule which is usually a "burned out" adenoma and a thyroid cyst which is rarely malignant. Ultrasound also can be used as a screening tool to evaluate patients at high risk for thyroid cancers which includes patients with previous head and neck irradiation or those with family histories of endocrine neoplasia syndrome.

MRI

1. When a thyroid mass is suspected, but cannot be differentiated from other possible neck masses, MRI is the test of choice. MRI provides excellent resolution among neck structures such as the thyroid, muscle, and lymphoid tissue.

2. MRI can be used to determine what structures are involved and, if a thyroid cancer is suspected, evaluate the extent of involvement of adjacent structures.

3. In contrast to MRI, CT provides poor differentiation among the soft tissues of the neck

and has little advantage over ultrasound despite considerable differences in the cost.

Diagnosis and management of thyroid disorders

Thyroiditis

Thyroiditis encompasses a number of unrelated clinical conditions that involve either autoimmune, infectious, or unknown insults to the thyroid. Symptoms may include painless or tender enlargement of the thyroid, hyper- or hypothyroid symptoms, and even fever and other stigmata of invasive bacterial infections.

1. **Chronic lymphocytic (Hashimoto's) thyroiditis**
    a. Hashimoto's thyroiditis is the most common type of thyroiditis and is seen most often in middle-aged women. The prevalence of Hashimoto's has increased dramatically in the USA in the last 50 years.
    b. It presents with non-painful enlargement of the thyroid.
    c. About 20% of patients presenting with Hashimoto's will already be hypothyroid either clinically or on measurement of TSH. Patients with Hashimoto's often go on to develop hypothyroidism, but progression is generally slow.
    d. Hashimoto's is an autoimmune disease; 95% of patients will have anti-thyroid perixodase (formerly known as anti-microsomal) antibodies in their serum.

2. **Subacute lymphocytic (painless or silent) thyroiditis**
    a. Subacute lymphocytic thyroiditis is also autoimmune mediated, but the immune insult is usually more transient.
    b. Patients with subacute lymphocytic thyroiditis often have fairly acute enlargement of the thyroid without tenderness (hence, the label "painless").
    c. Autoimmune inflammation of the thyroid may result in the release of preformed thyroid hormone resulting in a period of hyperthyroidism. Following this hyperthyroid phase, patients may become hypothyroid as the injured thyroid undergoes repair.
    d. Fewer than 10% of patients will have permanent hypothyroidism.

3. **Subacute granulomatous (giant cell thyroiditis or deQuervain's) thyroiditis**
    a. Subacute granulomatous thyroiditis is similar to subacute lymphocytic thyroiditis, except it is not autoimmune mediated, but is believed to arise from a viral infection. In subacute granulomatous thyroiditis, patients usually have a viral illness preceding their symptoms and the thyroid enlargement is mildly painful.
    b. The clinical presentation of subacute granulomatous thyroiditis is similar to subacute lymphocytic thyroiditis with a hyperthyroid stage followed by euthyroid or hypothyroid periods.
    c. Acute inflammation in the thyroid may be treated with aspirin or other non-steroid anti-inflammatory agents or, in severe cases, with prednisone. Usually steroids administered at 40 mg a day result in a rapid reduction in thyroid pain and after a week the steroids can be tapered over 2 to 4 weeks. However, prednisone withdrawal may result in a rebound in thyroid swelling and tenderness in approximately 20% of patients. Anti-inflammatorys may provide symptomatic benefit, but there is little evidence that anti-inflammatory treatment reduces the duration of the inflammatory process or changes the long-term likelihood of hypothyroidism.[6]
    d. Approximately 10% of patients will require permanent thyroid replacement.

4. **Suppurative thyroiditis**
    a. Suppurative thyroiditis is an acute bacterial infection of the thyroid gland usually with *Staphylococcus aureus*, *Streptococcus pyogenes* (group A strep), or *Streptococcus pneumoniae*. It is a rare condition with only 224 cases reported between 1900 and 1980.[6] However, thyroid infection with opportunistic organisms such as cytomegalovirus, *Mycobacterium avium-intercellulare* complex, and *Pneumocystis carinii* has become more common in patients with HIV and other immunosuppressive disorders.[6]
    b. Patients have a tender, swollen thyroid, fever, elevated white blood cell count and other manifestations of an acute bacterial illness. Occasionally thyroid abscesses can develop.

c. Suppurative thyroiditis is treated like any other acute, serious bacterial infection. Parenteral administration of antibiotics to cover the likely organisms (*Staphylococcus aureus* and *Streptococcus* spp.) is indicated.

d. Fluctuence may signal abscess formation. Abscesses can be confirmed by ultrasound (if large) or by thyroid scanning (if small). These should be surgically drained.

e. Unless extensive damage to the thyroid has occurred, patients usually have normal thyroid function following clearance of the acute infection.

5. **Invasive fibrous (Reidel's) thyroiditis**

a. This condition presents with a gradually enlarging, firm but non-tender thyroid. In this condition, thyroid tissue is infiltrated with dense fibrous tissue that causes a hard, woody goiter.

b. Patients are usually euthyroid although a small minority can develop hypothyroidism over time.

c. Occasionally, because the large, firm thyroid may be uncomfortable or compress nearby structures, surgical removal of the thyroid is warranted. Otherwise, monitoring for symptoms of hypothyroidism is all that is needed.

Hypothyroidism

1. **Etiology**

Most hypothyroidism is idiopathic. Many of these cases are most likely end-stage Hashimoto's thyroiditis that has resulted in a dysfunctional thyroid.

2. **Evaluation of hypothyroidism**

The most important aspect of evaluation is to differentiate primary hypothyroidism (thyroid failure) from secondary hypothyroidism (pituitary insufficiency). If the TSH is high, primary hypothyroidism is present. If the TSH is low but the thyroid hormones are also low, further examination of pituitary function is warranted.

3. **Imaging and other studies**

Unless secondary hypothyroidism is suspected, no imaging or blood tests are necessary.

4. **Treatment of hypothyroidism**

Treatment is simple and inexpensive. Treatment should start with 50 mcg (0.050 mg) of thyroid replacement daily. After one month's use, a repeat TSH is performed. If it is still elevated, the dosage is titrated up slowly. Usually 100–125 mcg is the daily dose needed.

Subclinical hypothyroidism

1. **Etiology**

Many patients, especially elderly women, will have elevations in TSH but normal thyroid hormones. These findings may represent either early thyroid failure or normal changes of ageing.

2. **Evaluation**

About half of the patients with subclinical hypothyroidism have anti-thyroid antibodies present. These patients are more likely to progress to overt hypothyroidism. About 10% of patients with subclinical hypothyroidism will progress to overt hypothyroidism within 3 years; periodic assessment of thyroid status is recommended to follow these patients.

3. **Treatment**

Management of patients with subclinical hypothyrioidism is controversial. Large population studies have shown that elderly patients with this condition do not have more rapid physical or intellectual decline and are at no increased risk of death. Treatment of asymptomatic patients is probably not useful. However, patients with neurocognitive symptoms (depression, fatigue, etc.) may benefit from thyroid replacement.[7]

Hyperthyroidism/Graves' disease

1. **Etiology**

Hyperthyroidism usually is caused by either Graves' disease, acute thyroiditis, or an autonomous thyroid nodule. Graves' disease is the most common cause of hyperthyroidism.

2. Graves' disease is an autoimmune disorder caused by IgG antibodies that bind to TSH receptors and initiate the production and release of thyroid hormone. Like most of the autoimmune conditions noted in thyroiditis, Graves' disease is more common in women.

Table 26.1 Treatment of hyperthyroidism

Treatment	Best in which patients	Dose	Comments
Radioactive iodine	1. Adult patients who are not pregnant		Some experts initially treat Graves' disease with oral suppressive therapy until eye disease is stabilized
	2. Radioactive iodine should not be used in children or breastfeeding mothers		
Anti-thyroid medication	1. Pregnant women	1. PTU must be given in divided doses (two or three times a day)	1. Anti-thyroid drugs are well tolerated and successful
	2. Women in whom there is a concern that the administration of radioactive iodine in patients with active ophthalmopathy may accelerate progression of eye disease	2. Methimazole and carbimazole can be administered once a day	2. The most serious side effect of these drugs is agranulocytosis that occurs in 3 per 10,000 patients per year
	3. Adolescents where Graves' disease may go into spontaneous remission after 6 to 18 months of therapy		3. PTU is the favored treatment in pregnant or potentially pregnant women
Surgery	1. Women in whom medication and radioactive iodine ablation are not acceptable treatment strategies		1. After 1 year show that approximately 80% of patients will be euthyroid, 20% may be hypothyroid, and 1% remain hyperthyroid
	2. Patients with a large goiter that compresses nearby structures or is disfiguring		2. Recurrence of hyperthyroid occurs at a rate of 1 to 3% per year
			3. Complications of surgery include damage to the superior laryngeal nerve (1–2% of cases) and possible hypocalcemia from inadvertent removal of parathyroid tissue

3. In addition to the hyperthyroid symptoms noted above, approximately 50% of patients with Graves' disease also exhibit exophthalmos. Thyroid hormones will be elevated, with a corresponding low TSH.
4. On thyroid scan, diffuse increased uptake of radiolabeled iodine will be found; this distinguishes Graves' disease from thyroid producing nodules.
5. The single diagnostic test that differentiates Graves' disease from other causes of hyperthyroidism is the detection of thyroid-receptor antibodies, specific for Graves' disease.
6. There are three approaches available to treat Graves' disease (Table 26.1).

   a. Radioactive iodine is the treatment of choice for Graves' disease in adult patients who are not pregnant. Radioactive iodine should not be used in children or breastfeeding mothers. There is also concern that the administration of radioactive iodine in patients with active ophthalmopathy may accelerate progression of eye disease. For this reason, some experts initially treat Graves' disease with oral suppressive therapy until eye disease is stabilized.

b. Anti-thyroid drugs are well tolerated and successful at blocking the production and release of thyroid hormone in patients with Graves' disease. These drugs work by blocking the organification of iodine. Propylthiouracil (PTU) also prevents peripheral conversion of T4 to the more active T3. PTU must be given in divided doses (two or three times a day), whereas methimazole and carbimazole can be administered once a day. The most serious side effect of these drugs is agranulocytosis that occurs in 3 per 10,000 patients per year. All of these drugs are relatively safe in pregnancy, but associations of carbimazole with aplasia cutis and the decreased release of PTU in breast milk make PTU the favored treatment in pregnant or potentially pregnant women. Anti-thyroid drugs are especially useful in adolescents where Graves' disease may go into spontaneous remission after 6 to 18 months of therapy.

c. Surgery is reserved for women where medication and radioactive iodine ablation are not acceptable treatment strategies or where a large goiter is present that compresses nearby structures or is disfiguring. Surgical results for Graves' disease after 1 year show that approximately 80% of patients will be euthyroid, 20% may be hypothyroid, and 1% remain hyperthyroid. Recurrence of hyperthyroid occurs at a rate of 1 to 3% per year. Complications of surgery include damage to the superior laryngeal nerve (1–2% of cases) and possible hypocalcemia from inadvertent removal of parathyroid tissue.

Thyroid storm

1. Thyroid storm is an acute event related to the release of large amounts of thyroid hormone in a short period of time. This condition is usually seen with acute onset of Graves' disease, but also may be encountered with abrupt onset of thyroiditis or in stable patients who are under physiologic stress such as with severe infections, surgery, or trauma.

2. The URGENT treatment of thyroid storm is essential to prevent cardiac ischemic

complications. Administration of high doses of PTU (100 mg every 6 hours) to quickly block thyroid production and reduce peripheral conversion of T4 to T3 and high doses of beta-blockers (propranalol 1–5 mg IV or 20–80 mg orally every 4 hours) are the optimal strategy to control symptoms of thyrotoxicosis and prevent complications. Iodine supplementation (SSKI or Logol's solution) can be used to block thyroid hormone release. Hydrocortisone (200–300 mg/day) is also used to prevent possible adrenal crisis.

Thyroid nodules

1. Solitary thyroid nodules are usually asymptomatic and are discovered primarily during a routine medical examination or during ultrasound for other head and neck problems. Incidental thyroid nodules are common: up to 50% of patients at autopsy are found to have an undetected thyroid nodule.

2. An exception to this is an autonomous nodule that produces thyroid hormone without TSH control in which symptoms of hyperthyroidism are frequently present.

3. The most common type of nodule is a simple colloid cyst (about 40%). Other types of nodules include adenomas, carcinomas (see below), metastatic disease from breast, kidney or prostate tumors, lymphomas, or benign neoplasms such as a neurofibroma, hamartoma, or teratoma.

4. On examination, most benign nodules are soft and cystic or may be tender. Cervical lymph nodes should not be enlarged.

5. Evaluation of nodules should include radionucleotide scanning and a TSH.[8] Radionucleotide scanning may reveal a functioning nodule or, in the case of an autonomous adenoma, may reveal a "hot" nodule with suppression of the remainder of the thyroid. In some instances, an adenoma may "burn out" and appear "cold."

6. **Cold nodules**

Since non-functioning nodules may represent thyroid cancers, further evaluation with fine needle biopsy is recommended. Fine needle aspiration is also indicated for nodules that are suspicious on ultrasound based on the nodule size, margins, location or echogenecity. In cystic nodules, no further treatment is necessary and evaluation can proceed based on the TSH.

7. **Functioning nodules**

For functional nodules, an attempt at suppression with exogenous thyroid is indicated to determine whether the nodule is under the control of TSH. Functioning adenomas that respond to TSH will suppress after administration of exogenous thyroid. Women with these types of nodules can be controlled with small doses of thyroid hormones.

8. **Autonomously functioning nodules**

Autonomous nodules do not suppress and may cause symptoms of hyperthyroidism. These nodules may need to be treated with anti-thyroid medications or radioactive iodine. For large nodules, surgical excision may be considered.

Thyroid cancers

1. Thyroid cancers are more common in women than in men. Thyroid cancer is more common in patients with familial colonic polyposis and hamartomas (Cowden's syndrome). Previous breast, renal, or central nervous system malignancy also increases the risk for a primary thyroid cancer.
2. Two classes of primary thyroid cancer exist: medullary cancer (10% of all cancers) and adenocarcinomas.

   a. Nodules suggestive of thyroid cancer are often hard and fixed and may involve adjacent cervical tissue. Nodules larger than 4 cm should also be suspected of being malignant.
   b. Paralysis of the vocal cords and/or cervical lymphadenopathy are other concerning signs.
   c. Definitive diagnosis should be made with thyroid biopsy. Most often this can be achieved through a fine needle aspiration biopsy.
   d. Adenocarcinomas are the most common type of thyroid cancer and can be subcategorized into four different groups: papillary (60% of all cancers), follicular (25%), medullary, Hurthle cell, and anaplastic carcinomas (<5%).

      i. Papillary carcinoma is the most common but least aggressive form of thyroid cancer. Follicular cancers with some papillary components also behave like papillary carcinomas. These tumors tend to remain

in the thyroid gland and, if they do spread, metastasize only to local lymph nodes.

      ii. Follicular cancer, on the other hand, metastasizes to lung and bone. These two kinds of cancer combined have a 97% cure rate when treated with surgery, radioactive iodine and thyroid suppression.
      iii. In contrast, anaplastic thyroid tumors have a very bad prognosis. This is a very aggressive tumor that rapidly invades adjacent tissue. Surgery, chemotherapy, and iodine radiation are usually ineffective at preventing metastases. Patients rarely survive more than 6 months from diagnosis.

   e. Medullary carcinoma is also aggressive and often part of the multiple endocrine neoplasia (MEN) syndrome. Surgical resection may initially control symptoms, but is not curative. Other chemotherapeutic agents can help slow the spread of disease.
   f. Non-Hodgkin's lymphoma (NHL) of the thyroid is increasing in incidence. There is a relationship between chronic lymphocytic (Hashimoto's) thyroiditis and NHL, so as the prevalence of chronic lymphocytic thyroid disease increases, NHL should increase as well. This type of tumor should be suspected when patients with chronic lymphocytic thyroiditis develop superimposed thyroid nodules. Surgery is the primary therapeutic option with supplemental radiation and chemotherapy.

Special populations
Pregnancy

1. Pregnant women often have a goiter and have elevated T4 levels with normal TSH levels. Thyroid levels may be difficult to diagnose during pregnancy.
2. Mild hyperthyroidism in pregnancy can mimic hyperemesis gravidarum and women with intractable vomiting may need TSH levels checked.
3. Women with any question of hypothyroidism in pregnancy must be treated with adequate to high levels of thyroid replacement to prevent cretinism in the infant. Two to three months postpartum,

the woman can then be assessed to determine thyroid levels.

4. Pregnant women with hyperthyroidism should be treated with PTU (Table 26.1).

Women on OCPs

Women on OCPs often have both a slightly enlarged thyroid or goiter and, although euthyroid, an elevated T4 with normal TSH, as in pregnancy.

Postpartum thyroiditis

1. Postpartum thyroiditis occurs in between 2 and 17% of all women in the first 6 months after delivery.
2. The symptoms of hypothyroidism may mimic those of normal new motherhood (tiredness, weight gain, lethargy) or postpartum depression.
3. The etiology of the thyroiditis is believed to be autoimmune and the clinical features are similar to chronic lymphocytic (Hashimoto's) thyroiditis.
4. In contrast to Hashimoto's, a large percentage of women (40%) remain hypothyroid after the onset postpartum.

Adolescents and children

1. A goiter can be found in 1–3% of healthy teenage girls on routine health examinations. Many of these represent subclinical Graves' disease or chronic lymphocytic thyroiditis.
2. As noted earlier, Graves' disease in adolescent girls tends to resolve spontaneously. Symptomatic treatment with anti-thyroid medications for 6 to 18 months may provide time for remission to occur. Most remissions are permanent.
3. Chronic lymphocytic thyroiditis is more common than Graves' disease in adolescents, but rarely causes hyper- or hypothryoidism. Anti-peroxidase antibodies usually disappear after about 2 years signaling a resolution of the thyroiditis.

Elderly women

1. Thyroid disease increases with age. Between 8 and 12% of older women have hypothyroidism.
2. The symptoms of hypothyroidism in older women can easily be confused with or complicate other disorders such as depression, dementia, and congestive heart failure.

3. To confuse matters further, individuals with hyperthyroidism in older age groups can behave as if they are hypothyroid with lethargy and confusion. The only clue to the hyperthyroid state may be the development of new onset atrial fibrillation.

Thyroid medications and drug interactions

Several potential drug interactions complicate the use of thyroid replacement in individuals with comorbid conditions. These include interactions with the following.

1. **Coumadin**

   Coumadin effect is enhanced with increases in thyroid doses.

2. **Oral hypoglycemics**

   The effect of these agents is blunted by increases in thyroid dose.

3. **Estrogens**

   Administration of hormone replacement with estrogens increases thyroid binding and may require higher doses of thyroid hormone.

4. **Clofibrate**

   This may reduce thyroid hormone absorption.

Screening for thyroid abnormalities

The US Preventive Services Task Force does not recommend screening for thyroid disease. If screening is being considered, older women who comprise the population with the greatest risk of asymptomatic disease should be targeted.

References

1. Turnbridge W. M., Evered D. C., Hall R., *et al.* The spectrum of thyroid disease in a community: the Wickham survey. *Clin Endocrinol* 1977; **7**, 481–493.
2. Sawin C. R., Castelli W. P., Hershman J. P., McNamara P., Bacharach P. The aging thyroid. Thyroid deficiency in the Framingham study. *Arch Intern Med* 1985; **145**, 1386–1388.
3. dos Santos Silva I., Swerdlow A. J. Sex differences in the risks of hormone-dependent cancers. *Am J Epidemiol* 1993; **138**, 10–28.
4. Boring C. C., Squires T. S., Tong T. Cancer statistics, 1993. *CA Cancer J Clin* 1993; **43**, 7–26.5.

5. Shamma F. N., Abrahams J. J. Imaging in endocrine disorders. *J Reprod Med* 1995; **37**, 39–45.

6. Farwell A. P., Braverman L. E. Inflammatory thyroid disorders. *Otolaryngol Clin North Am* 1996; **29**, 541–556.

7. Gussekloo J., van Exel E., deCraen A. J. M., *et al.* Thyroid status, disability and cognitive function, and survival in old age. *J Am Med Assoc* 2004; **292**, 2591–2599.

8. AACE/AME Task Force on Thyroid Nodules. Medical guidelines for clinical practice for the diagnosis and management of thyroid nodules. *Endocrine Pract* 2006; **12**, 63–102.

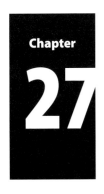

Hypertension and stroke

Jo Ann Rosenfeld

Hypertension

1. Hypertension is the most important risk factor in the development of CHD, myocardial infarction (MI), diabetes, and stroke. Hypertensive women are four times more likely than age-matched controls to develop CHD. The treatment of hypertension has and is leading to a remarkable decrease in the incidence of MI and stroke.

2. Hypertension increases with age. The Framingham Heart Study found that 55-year-old normotensive individuals have a 90% risk for developing hypertension.[1]

Epidemiology and natural history

1. Unfortunately not everyone who has hypertension has been diagnosed. Fewer receive treatment and fewer are in good control, although this has improved in the past years.

2. Because of more effective treatment of hypertension, the mortality and morbidity of stroke and MI have declined. Age-adjusted rates of death declined by 60% from stroke and 53% for CHD.

3. The Joint National Committee on Detection, Evaluation and Treatment of Hypertension VII states:

   The relationship between BP and risk of cardiovascular disease (CVD) events is continuous, consistent, and independent of other risk factors. The higher the BP, the greater the chance of myocardial infarction, heart failure (HF), stroke, and kidney disease. For individuals aged 40 to 70 years, each increment of 20 mm Hg in systolic BP or 10 mm Hg in diastolic BP doubles the risk of CVD across the entire BP range from 115/75 to 185/115 mm Hg.[2,3]

4. More women than men have hypertension. In women older than age 50 years, there has been a reduction in stroke mortality. One-half of the reduction of stroke in white women, and two-thirds of the reduction of stroke in African-American women can be attributed to improvement in hypertensive control. More men in the USA older than age 45 than women have higher blood pressure levels. However, by age 60–69 men and women have similar blood pressure levels, and by age 70 women have higher blood pressure levels than men.[4]

5. Untreated hypertension can worsen a woman's quality of life. Surveys of untreated hypertensive women found that cognitive and sleep functions and sense of well-being were inversely related to diagnosis, degree, and duration of hypertension. Women who were hypertensive reported poorer social activity and poorer physical health status.[5]

Diagnosis

1. Diagnosis of hypertension should occur on two separate occasions. Both arms should be measured at least for the first few times. Two high readings establish the diagnosis of hypertension.

2. The cuff should be two-thirds the height of the arm.

3. How best to diagnose and monitor blood pressure levels is under investigation. Blood pressure readings taken at home, by nurses or ambulatory blood pressure machines may be more reflective of actual blood pressure.

4. Approximately 10% of individuals have "white coat hypertension" (WCH), episodic elevation in blood pressure when taken by a health professional. WCH

Handbook of Women's Health, second edition, ed. Jo Ann Rosenfeld. Published by Cambridge University Press.
© Cambridge University Press 2009.

is more common in men than women, and is not always benign. It is associated with an increase in left ventricular mass and left ventricular hypertrophy.

Evaluation

1. The evaluation needed for hypertension is minimal, because most individuals have primary or essential hypertension (Table 27.1).
2. Treatable causes of hypertension, although rare, are listed in Table 27.2. They should be suspected with new, sudden, or very high, hard-to-control hypertension. Signs that should indicate a more intensive evaluation are listed in Table 27.3. Drug causes of hypertension are listed in Table 27.4.
3. A creatinine clearance for determination of renal function, 24 hour urine for protein and uric acid, glycosolated hemoglobin level, drug screens, echocardiography and specific tests for endocrinopathies may be needed.
4. With a diagnosis of hypertension, a complete evaluation for other risk factors for heart disease including diabetes and hyperlipidemia is important. Many experts support the treatment of diabetes and lipid abnormalities with lifestyle changes and even medication in individuals with hypertension who may not have the overt disease yet.

Treatment

1. **Gender disparities**

   Most trials of treatment have primarily or exclusively studied men. When studies showed improvement of men with treatment of hypertension, similar analyses were accomplished for women. The INDANA (individual data analysis of antihypertensive trials) examined the results of more than 20,000 women and men in seven drug RCTs, some double and some single blind. Treatment !significantly and statistically improved the risk for all major coronary events, fatal coronary events and stroke for men, but not for coronary events or total mortality in women, perhaps because the rates of these events were lower in women. However, treatment of hypertension did reduce the incidence of stroke, fatal strokes and cardiovascular events in women.[6]

2. A French study found that in a population in which few were treated adequately, being older and being a man were two risk factors for worse hypertensive control.[7]

Table 27.1 Minimal laboratory evaluation for new patients with hypertension

Blood

    Electrolytes

    Complete blood count

    BUN and creatinine

    Glucose (fasting, if possible)

    Cholesterol and triglycerides

Urine analysis

Electrocardiogram

Table 27.2 Causes of secondary hypertension

Alcohol abuse

Renal parenchymal disease

Renovascular hypertension

Endocrinopathies

    Pheochromocytoma

    Cushing's disease

    Primary aldoneronism

Drug use – ephedra, diet pills, phenylpropaline, etc.

Table 27.3 Indications for more intensive evaluation for possible secondary hypertension

Hypertension that is difficult to control

Early onset of hypertension, especially in a woman younger than age 30

Rapid progression or sudden worsening of hypertension

Weight loss or truncal obesity

A rapid rise in BUN or creatinine while on an ACEI

Hypokalemia

Abnormal urine analysis including proteinuria, creatinine, or infection

Hyperglycemia

3. Lifestyle modifications are the first treatment for hypertension.

   a. A low salt, low cholesterol diet can improve blood pressure and decrease cardiovascular morbidity and mortality.

   b. The change in sodium intake does not have to be large to be effective. Removing the salt

Table 27.4 Drug causes of hypertension

Non-steroidal anti-inflammatory drugs

Oral contraceptives

Adrenal steroids

Cocaine, amphetamines, other illicit drugs

Cyclosporine and tacrolimus

Sympathomimetics (decongestants, anorectics)

Diet drugs

Complementary drugs

Erythropoietin licorice (including some chewing tobacco)

Selected over-the-counter dietary supplements and medicines (e.g., ephedra, ma haung, bitter orange)

Note: Adapted from *The Seventh Report of the Joint National Committee on Prevention, Detection, Evaluation, and Treatment of High Blood Pressure. The JNC 7 Report* AMA 2003; **289**, doi: 10.1001/jama.289.19.2560. http://jama.ama-assn.org/cgi/content/full/289.19.2560v1, accessed 3/10/07.

shaker from the table and reducing consumption of high salt foods can reduce the average salt intake from 15 g to 5–7 g daily. In one placebo-controlled RCT, changing regular salt to low sodium, high potassium, high magnesium mineral salt reduced systolic blood pressure (SBP) by an average of 7.6 mm in 100 men and women age 55 to 75.[8]

c. **Weight modification**

There is a definite independent association between hypertension and obesity. The Nurses' Health Study showed that those women with a BMI greater than 31 had a RR of 6.31 for developing high blood pressure. In addition an increase of weight of 1 kg was associated with a 12% increase in risk of developing hypertension.[9]

d. Also, losing weight will lower blood pressure. The risk of hypertension was reduced 15% by a weight loss of 5 to 10 kg.[10]

e. **Exercise**

An active lifestyle may reduce blood pressure in hypertensive individuals. A meta-analysis examining studies in which aerobic exercise

was used in hypertensive patients found that those patients that exercised without drug therapy had a small reduction in resting blood pressure levels.[11,12]

4. Pharmacotherapy (Table 27.5)

a. Not all trials have included women, or if the trials did, the data may not have been analyzed by sex. Most information on hypertensive medications and their side effects are extrapolated from those on men. However, basically, any medication used for treatment of hypertension by men can be used by non-pregnant women. However, there may be differences in side effects and effectiveness.

b. Most experts agree one drug should be started, its effects observed, and the dose of that medicine increased until side effects occur. The last JNC VII, however, observed that most individuals will need more than one drug, often a diuretic is needed, and that treatment should be vigorous to reduce the blood pressure well.

c. There is no one perfect antihypertensive agent for all women. Many drugs can work equally well in many women. One double blind multicentered RCT that included women age 60 to 80 found that atenolol (50–100 mg daily), enalapril (5–20 mg daily) and isradipine (1.25–5.0 mg twice daily) with hydrochlorothiazide as needed all reduced blood pressure adequately. Women on enalapril were more likely to have a cough and those on atenolol dry mouth.[13] Another European RCT of two new drugs examined differences in response to a new ACEI moexipril (15 mg daily) versus a new calcium channel antagonist nitrendipine (20 mg daily). Both medicines were equally effective in lowering blood pressure, but more women on moexipril had a cough and more women on nitrendipine had headaches and flushing.[14]

d. The side effects of beta-blockers have not been as extensively examined in women as in men. The incidence of beta-blocker-induced depression may be more frequent in women. Whether and how beta-blockers affect women's sexual desire and response has not been well investigated.

Table 27.5 Some commonly used medications for treatment of hypertension

Agent	Dose (daily)	Contraindicated in pregnancy
Diurectics		
Thiazide-type		
Chlorothiazide	125–500 mg	Not suggested
Hydro-chlorothiazide	12.5–50 mg	Not suggested
Chlorthalidone	12.5–50 mg	Not suggested
Metolozone	1.25–5 mg	Not suggested
Loop		
Bumetanide	0.5–5 mg in 2–3 doses	
Furosemide	20–320 mg in 2–3 doses	
Potassium-sparing		
Amiloride	5–10 mg	
Spironolactone	12.5–100 mg in 1–2 doses	Not suggested
Triamterene	50–150 mg in 1–2 doses	Not suggested
Beta-blockers		
Atenolol	25–100 mg in 1–2 doses	Not suggested
Metoprolol	50–200 mg in 1–2 doses	Not suggested
Nadolol	20–240 mg in 1–2 doses	Not suggested
Timolol	10–40 mg in 2 doses	Not suggested
ACEIs		
Captopril	12.5–150 mg in 2–3 doses	Contraindicated
Enalapril	2.5–40 mg in 1–2 doses	Contraindicated
Lisinopril	5–40 mg	Contraindicated
Ramipril	1.25–20 mg	Contraindicated
ARBs		
Candesartan	8–32 mg	Not suggested
Losartan	25–100 mg	Not suggested
Valsartan	80–320 mg	Not suggested
Alpha/beta-blockers		
Carvedilol	12.5–50 mg in 2 doses	
Labetalol	200–1200 mg in 2 doses	Not suggested
Calcium channel blockers		
Diltiazem	120–360 mg in 2 doses	
Verapamil	120–400 mg in 2–3 doses	
Nifedipine	30–90 mg	Used in pregnancy
Amlodipine	2.5–10 mg	
Alpha-adrenergic agents		
Prazosin	1–20 mg	
Terazosin	1–20 mg	
Doxazosin	1–16 mg	
Central alpha-adrenergic agents		
Clonidine	0.1–0.6 mg in 2–3 doses	Not suggested
Methyl dopa	250–2000 mg in 2 doses	Used in pregnancy
Direct vasodilators		
Hydralazine	40–200 mg in 2–4 doses	Used in pregnancy
Minoxidil	2.5–40 mg in 1–2 doses	Unknown

e. Women may respond less well on ACEIs than men and they are more likely to develop a cough. However, more women are diabetics, and ACEIs and angiotensin receptor blockers are suggested for use in all diabetics, hypertensive, pre-hypertensive or normotensive. Women of childbearing years who are at risk for pregnancy should not use ACEIs and ACEIs are contraindicated in pregnancy.

f. Whether the use of long acting calcium channel blockers in elderly women is related to an increase in breast cancer is disputed. In a retrospective study of more than 3200 women age 65 or older, the relative risk of developing cancer was 2.57.[15] However, recent studies have not supported this correlation. A more recent large Danish study found no relationship between any hypertensive agents and an increase in breast cancer.[16]

g. Women, as with men, should be started on a diuretic, and/or ACEI or ARB, or beta-blockers as first steps in therapy.

Special populations

Elderly

1. A higher percentage of elderly individuals have high blood pressure. Treating hypertension in the elderly is important and treatment does decrease the risk of mortality and morbidity.[17] Approximately 90% of normotensive elderly adults will develop hypertension.[1]
2. In older individuals, systolic blood pressure (SBP) is a better predictor of severe events including CHD, stroke, and renal disease.
3. As with younger individuals, treatment should begin with lifestyle modifications. The blood pressure levels of older individuals will respond to modest salt reduction and weight loss.
4. In pharmacotherapy, diuretics are effective and inexpensive although may worsen incontinence. Combined with ACEIs, they are very effective and reduce mortality and morbidity, but less so in women.[18] Combined diuretics may be a better choice because they reduce the incidence of hypokalemia and the need for potassium replacement.

Oral contraceptive use

1. Women on combination estrogen containing OCPs usually have a slight increase in SBP and DBP.
2. Hypertension is more common in women on OCPs, especially if they are obese and/or older. Smokers who are older than age 35 should not take OCPs.
3. If women on OCPs develop hypertension, the OCPs should be stopped until the hypertension is controlled. Once the blood pressure is controlled, OCPs, especially low dose estrogen or progesterone only OCPs, may be used, especially

when the risk of pregnancy is higher than the risk of hypertension.

Hypertension in pregnancy

1. Women who are pregnant should not use diurectics or ACEIs. Alpha methyl dopa and hydralazine have been used for a long time. Calcium channel antagonists, especially nifedipine, have also been used. Beta-blockers should not be used.
2. Pre-eclampsia is a clinical syndrome of proteinuria, hypertension and edema occurring after 28 weeks pregnancy. Eclampsia is pre-eclampsia with seizures. The etiology of pre-eclampsia and eclampsia are not known. They are a major cause of maternal mortality in the USA and UK.[19]
3. Pre-eclampsia (PE) occurs in 8–24% of women and is more likely in women whose mother had PE.
4. Eclampsia is unpredictable. More than one-third of eclamptic seizures occur before the classic symptoms of proteinuria and hypertension appear, and up to 44% occur postpartum.
5. Long-term consequences include chronic hypertension. Multiparous women who develop pregnancy induced hypertension or PE are six to seven times more likely to become hypertensive in later life.

Menopause

After menopause, the incidence of hypertension increases until there is equal incidence in both sexes.

Stroke

1. A stroke is a clinical cerebrovascular event that can be caused by ischemia, thrombosis, or hemorrhage. Strokes occur equally in number in men and women, but increase with age.
2. It is a personal catastrophe that can cause death, disability, and/or loss of independence. A stroke has a tremendous cost to the individual and incredible cost to society in rehabilitation and long-term care. Because treatment is seldom possible, primary and secondary prevention is essential. Figure 27.1 shows the one year survival rate after stroke comparing sexes and different ethnic groups.

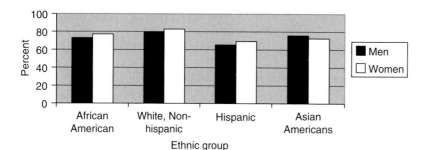

Figure 27.1 One year survival after stroke. Data From Suri M. F., Zhou J., Divani A. A., Qureshi A. I. African American women have poor long-term survival following ischemic stroke. *Neurology* 2006; **67**(9), 1623–1629.

Epidemiology

1. Strokes are the third leading cause of death in the USA, causing more deaths in men and women than chronic lung disease, accidents, pneumonia, diabetes and HIV infections combined.[20]
2. Stroke mortality and incidence increase with age. The frequency of stroke doubles with every decade of life over age 55. Three-quarters of all strokes occur in those older than 65.
3. As women get older, they are more likely than men to have strokes. African American men and women are more likely to die from a stroke than white men and women in the USA and Europe.[21]
4. Women are less likely to suffer ischemic strokes than men before age 65, and more likely after age 65. Women are more likely to have subdural hemorrhage at any age.[22]
5. Strokes are less likely to be lethal, although the first stroke is fatal in 30%. Between 1965 and 1985, there was a rapid and accelerating decline in the mortality of strokes in all areas of the USA and most industrial countries. A retrospective study in Finland found that the changes in cardiovascular risk factors explain the observed changes in mortality. In women the changes in blood pressure levels and decreased incidence of smoking predicted half of the 60% decrease in mortality.[23]
6. Because of increased treatment and control of hypertension, the incidence of stroke has decreased in past years in both men and women.[24]
7. More women than men die from strokes.[25] More African American women are likely to die from strokes than white women.

Primary prevention

1. Six major and four lifestyle risk factors have been identified, which, if treated or modified, should

Table 27.6 Risk factors for stroke

Major
Hypertension
Myocardial infarction
Atrial fibrillation
Diabetes mellitus
Hyperlipidemia
Asymptomatic carotid artery stenosis
Lifestyle factors
Smoking
Alcohol abuse
Physical inactivity
Poor diet

decrease the risk of stroke.[26] These six factors include hypertension, myocardial infarction, atrial fibrillation, diabetes mellitus, hyperlipidemia, and asymptomatic carotid artery stenosis.

2. There are four modifiable lifestyle factors: smoking, alcohol use, physical inactivity and poor diet (Table 27.6).

3. **Hypertension**

 Hypertension is the most important risk factor for stroke in women. RCTs have shown that treatment of hypertension definitely decreases the risk of stroke. Treatment that reduces DBP by an average of 5 mmHg reduces the risk of stroke by 42%.[25]

4. **Atrial fibrillation (AF)**

 a. Atrial fibrillation is a common arrhythmia. If the individual with AF is anticoagulated,

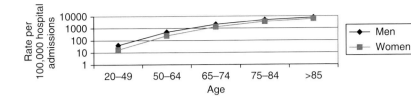

Figure 27.2 Rate of hospitalization for atrial fibrillation by age. Data from Friberg J., Scharling H., Gadsboll N., *et al.* Sex-specific increase in the prevalence of atrial fibrillation (the Copenhagen City Heart Study). *Am J Cardiol* 2003; **92**, 1419–1423.

her risk of stroke is decreased. About 16% of all individuals and one-third of those older than age 75 who suffer an ischemic stroke have had AF.[27]

b. AF can be asymptomatic and discovered by chance on physical examination or the patient can complain of irregular heartbeat, palpitations, congestive heart failure, exercise intolerance, shortness of breath, dyspnea on exertion, and respiratory distress.

c. The Framingham Study found that men were much more likely than women to develop AF, but the absolute number of women with AF exceeded that of men because women live longer.[28] The incidence of AF increases with age; 9% of those individuals older than age 80 have AF[29]. Figure 27.2 shows the rate of hospitalization for AF by age. Approximately 1.8 million individuals in the USA have AF.

d. Although the Framingham study did not find a correlation, several RCTs showed that AF is an independent risk-factor for stroke. AF increases the risk of ischemic stroke fivefold.[30]

e. Treatment for AF is cardioversion, electrically or chemically. Cardioversion is most effective when delivered as soon after AF starts as possible. Elderly individuals have as much chance to cardiovert as younger individuals. Drug therapy with digoxin, quinidine, and/or calcium channel blockers works less often than electrical cardioversion. In addition, studies have shown that reduction of ventricular rate is more important than actual cardioversion to normal sinus rhythm.

f. **Stroke prevention**

   i. Several RCTs have found that anticoagulation with warfarin reduces the risk of stroke by 70% in patients with AF.[31] Warfarin was more effective than aspirin in preventing ischemic stroke but there was an increased incidence in intracranial hemorrhage in the patients treated with warfarin, especially in patients older than 75.[32] RCTs have shown that warfarin reduces the risk of stroke by 84% in women.[33]

   ii. Anticoagulation by warfarin is difficult to maintain, requires frequent visits and blood tests, demands dietary changes, and increases serious risks including gastrointestinal and cerebrovascular hemorrhage. Elderly women are more likely than men to suffer hemorrhage from anticoagulation.

   iii. Contraindications to anticoagulation include any history of bleeding, unexplained liver abnormalities, certain medications, (Table 27.7) use of alcohol, history of balance problems, gait disorders, or seizures, inability to follow-up regularly, or frequent falls. Elderly women are less likely to receive warfarin than men.

   iv. Bleeding can be minimized if warfarin is used only to produce an international normalized ratio (INR) of 2.0 to 3.0 rather than higher. Elderly patients show an increased rate of bleeding with INR>3.0, and younger patients at INR>4.0.

5. **Myocardial infarction**

A woman's risk of stroke is increased 30% in the first month after MI, and then 1 to 2% yearly after MI. Anticoagulation can prevent a stroke, particularly in women who have had a MI, and have AF. Aspirin may reduce the risk.

6. **Hyperlipidemia**

Treatment of hyperlipidemia prevents stroke.

7. **Diabetes**

More women than men have diabetes and diabetes increases the risk of stroke 1.4 to 1.7 times.

313

Table 27.7 Drugs that interfere with the action of warfarin

Increases the levels

Allopurinol

Androgens

Cimetadine

Clofibrate

Disulfiram

Erythromycin

Glucagon

Metronidazole

Omeprazole

Ranitidine

Salicylates

Tamixifen

Thyroid hormones

Trimethoprim/sulfa

Decreases the levels

Antithyroid hormone drugs

Carbamazepine

Cholestyramine

Griseofulvin

Rifampin

Spironolactone

Thiazide diuretics

Tight control of glycemic levels is not yet proven to reduce this risk.

8. Carotid artery stenosis
   a. The risk of stroke is increased in women with carotid artery stenosis, although treatment, which is angioplasty or surgical endarectomy in asymptomatic women, has not been shown to reduce the risk of stroke.
   b. Recent studies have found that although stroke may be better prevented in men with surgical treatment of asymptomatic carotid stenosis, this may not also be true in women. In a meta-analysis of hypertensive elderly women, those who had an endarectomy had

an increased risk of contralateral stroke and death as compared to men.
   c. The treatment of asymptomatic carotid stenosis with endarectomy may be of slight benefit in men, but has not been shown to be of benefit in women.[34]
   d. Secondary prevention, treatment of symptomatic carotid stenosis after a stroke or transient ischemic attack, improves mortality and reduces the risk of future events.
   e. Plaques found in women's carotid arteries may be inherently different than those found in men, less inflammatory and more stable. Asymptomatic women are more likely to have stable plaques. This may be a reason women do less well with treatment of asymptomatic carotid stenosis.[35]

Lifestyle changes

1. Smoking increases the risk of stroke as a function of the number of cigarettes smoked. The Nurses' Health Study found that smokers had two times the risk of stroke and stopping smoking reduced the risk of stroke.[36]
2. Regular alcohol use increases the risk of hypertension and stroke. No studies have proven that reducing alcohol consumption decreases the risk of stroke.
3. Encouraging an active lifestyle may have beneficial effects through a variety of mechanisms.
4. Eating a healthy, low-cholesterol diet has been linked to a decreased risk of stroke.

Secondary prevention of strokes: after a transient ischemic attack or first stroke
Definition

1. Transient ischemic attacks (TIAs) are focal ischemic neurological deficits that resolve within 24 hours. They can present as slurred speech, aphasia, visual problems, blindness, amaurosis fugax ("a curtain came down over my vision"), paresis, hemiparesis, numbness and/or ataxia, but not dizziness or vertigo. Most TIAs last less than 15 minutes, and 60–70% resolve within one hour.

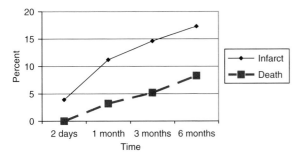

Figure 27.3 Results of TIA in one study over time. Data from Kleindorfer D., Panagos P., Pancioli A., *et al.* Incidence and short-term prognosis of transient ischemic attack in a population-based study. *Stroke* 2005; 36(4), 720–723.

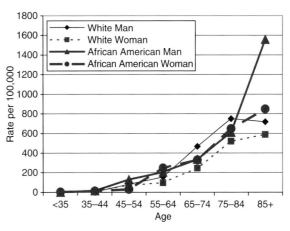

Figure 27.4 Specific incidence rates of TIA per 100,000 by race and gender. Data from Kleindorfer D., Panagos P., Pancioli A., *et al.* Incidence and short-term prognosis of transient ischemic attack in a population-based study. *Stroke* 2005; 36(4), 720–723.

2. TIAs predict strokes. Figure 27.3 shows the results of TIA in one study over time. Only one out of five strokes, however, is preceded by a TIA. One out of three women who have TIA will have a stroke within five years, and one out of five within one month. Overall, approximately 10% of individuals with TIAs will develop a stroke within 90 days.[37]

Diagnosis

1. Other diseases can present like TIAs, including drug toxicity or overdose, metabolic disturbances, seizures, syncope, labyrinthine disorders, tumors, subdural hematomas, small hemorrhages, and migraines. Few individuals with dizziness alone have had TIAs.[38]

2. Men are more likely to have a TIA and African Americans more likely than whites.[39] (Figure 27.4). Delay until diagnosis is higher for women than men.[40]

3. For a woman with a TIA, diagnostic evaluation includes an electrocardiogram and a 24-hour Holter or 30-day event monitor, and echocardiography to detect valvular and cardiac wall disease. An MRI of the head is suggested, because it may show signs of previous infarcts in approximately 40% of patients with TIA.

4. Evaluation for possible significant carotid stenosis is essential. Angiography is the gold standard, but it is invasive and has morbidity and mortality, including acute and chronic renal failure, TIAs, strokes, and cardiovascular problems. An ultrasound or Doppler of the carotids is a safer screening test for detection and characterization of carotid artery stenosis.

Treatment and secondary prevention

1. The primary treatment for TIAs is to modify the risk factors. The patient should quit smoking, should exercise, and eat a low-fat diet. Hypertension, diabetes, and hyperlipidemia should be intensively treated and monitored. One study found that the risk of a stroke increases with the fasting blood glucose over 99 mg/dL (Figure 27.5).[41] Another study found a relative risk of stroke of 1.47 for those patients with triglycerides greater than 200 mg/dL and a decrease with each 5% increase in HDL.[42]

2. All patients should be started on aspirin (85 or 325 mg, depending on the study and day), ticlopidine, clopidogrel (75 mg daily), or other anticoagulants, if not contraindicated.

3. **Choice of anticoagulant**

   Many studies have compared anticoagulants. Recent studies have suggested that ticlopidine or clopidogrel may be no better than aspirin in prevention of strokes in many cases.[43] One meta-analysis found that dipyridamole plus aspirin reduced subsequent risk of stroke, death, and non-fatal cardiac events.[44] Use of aspirin

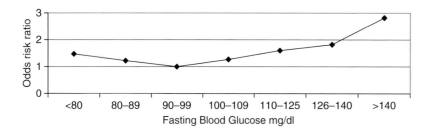

Figure 27.5 Risk of stroke by fasting blood glucose level. Data from Tanne D., Koren-Morag N., Goldbourt U. Fasting plasma glucose and risk of incident ischemic stroke or transient ischemic attacks: a prospective cohort study. *Stroke* 2004; **35**(10), 2351–2355.

after a TIA reduces TIA and strokes in men. Whether aspirin prevents further strokes in women, especially elderly women, is not yet well established. Aspirin intolerant patients may use clopidogrel.

4. Surgical treatment of carotid artery stenosis is suggested in individuals with 70–99% stenosis which will prevent further embolic stroke from that artery. There is a smaller proven benefit for those who have a 50–69% stenosis. The patient undergoing carotid endarectomy should also take aspirin (81 to 325 mg daily).

5. Anticoagulation for patients with a TIA or stroke with AF is necessary. More women than men who have had a stroke present with AF. The rate of stroke was significantly reduced by aspirin or by the use of warfarin, if not contraindicated.

Oral contraceptive pills and thromboembolic disease

1. Although the risk of stroke is very low in women of childbearing age, use of OCPs does increase the risk, especially if the woman has coexistent hypertension, is older than 35 and/or smokes.

2. The risk of thromboembolic disease is higher with higher dose estrogen products, especially those with more than 50 μg/dL ethinyl estradiol. Those women who use 35μg/mL estrogen OCPs had a risk of 2.7 of stoke. Those women who are on OCPs, younger than 35 and do not have high blood pressure have no increased risk of stroke.

3. Once stopped, the relative risk of stroke returns to that of women who did not use OCPs. There is no relation between length of use and risk of stroke.

Summary

As with men, many women who have hypertension do not know it, and many who have the diagnosis do not have their hypertension adequately controlled.

Treating hypertension means vigorously reducing the levels of blood pressure. Most of the studies on medication were performed on men, although all new studies are required to include women. Most information on hypertensive medications and their side effects is extrapolated from that on men. For example, a recent study of the presence of insomnia in patients treated for hypertension found that nearly one-half of treated individuals had insomnia. In addition, women were twice as likely as men to suffer insomnia. The reasons for this were not uncovered.[45] Antihypertensive medications are known to cause sexual dysfunction in men; research on their effects in women is rare. Women are less likely to be treated vigorously for hypertension and less likely to be well controlled.

Since women are more likely to be diabetic and obese, they may do better with an angiotensin converting enzyme or angiotensin receptor blocker as first or second line therapy for hypertension. Diuretics may be less acceptable to women than men, because of increased incidence of urinary incontinence in women; diuretics increase the incidence of incontinence. More women (approximately 50%) than men develop the cough with ACE inhibitors. Other medication choices are likely to be similar in men and women. Women who are still trying to get pregnant should not use beta-blockers or ACE inhibitors.

Conclusion

Many women have hypertension and this is the most common and important risk factor for stroke. Hypertension is often silent and often poorly controlled.

Treatment including lifestyle changes, diet, exercise and medication will prevent morbidity and morality, stroke and heart disease.

References

1. Vasan R. S., Beiser A., Seshadri S., *et al.* Residual lifetime risk for developing hypertension in middle-aged women and men: the Framingham Heart Study. *J Am Med Assoc* 2002; **287**, 1003–1010.

2. *The Seventh Report of the Joint National Committee on Prevention, Detection, Evaluation, and Treatment of High Blood Pressure. The JNC 7 Report AMA,* 2003, **289**, doi:10.1001/jama.289.19.2560. http://jamaama/assn.org/cgi/content/full/289.19.2560v1, accessed 3/10/07.

3. Lewington S., Clarke R., Qizilbash N., Peto R., Collins R. Age-specific relevance of usual blood pressure to vascular mortality. *Lancet* 2002; **360**, 1903–1913.

4. Burt V. L., Whelton P., Roccella E. J., *et al.* Prevalence of hypertension in the US adult population. Results from the Third National Health and Nutrition Examination Survey, 1988–1991. *Hypertension* 1995; **25**, 305–313.

5. Robbins M. A., Elias M. P., Croog S. H., Colton T. Unmediated blood pressure levels and quality of life in elderly hypertensive women. *Psychosoc Med* 1994; **56**, 251–259.

6. Gueyffer F., Bournie F., Boissel J. P., *et al.* Effect of antihypertensive drug treatment on cardiovascular outcomes in men and women. *Ann Intern Med* 1997; **125**, 761–767.

7. Roux O., Chapellier M., Czernichow S., Nisse-Durgeat S., Safar M. E., Blacher J. Determinants of hypertension control in a large French population of treated hypertensive subjects. *Blood Press* 2006; **15**(1), 6–13.

8. Geleijinse J. M., Wetterman J. C., Bak A. A., Breijen J. H., Grobee D. E. Reduction in blood pressure with a low sodium, high potassium, high magnesium salt in older subjects with mild to moderated hypertension. *Br Med J* 1994; **309**, 436–440.

9. Dickinson H. O., Mason J. M., Nicolson. D. J., *et al.* Lifestyle interventions to reduce raised blood pressure: a systematic review of randomized controlled trials. *J Hypertension* 2006; **24**(2), 215–233.

10. Schillaci G., Pasqualini L., Vaudo G. Effect of body weight changes on 24-hour blood pressure and left ventricular mass in hypertension: a 4-year follow-up. *Am J Hypertension* 2003; **16**(8), 634–639.

11. Kelley G. A. Aerobic exercise and resting blood pressure among women: a meta-analysis. *Prev Med* 1999; **28**, 264–275.

12. Fagard R. H. Exercise is good for your blood pressure: effects of endurance training and resistance training *Clin Exp Pharmacol Physiol* 2006; **33**(9), 853–856.

13. Croog S. H., Elias M. F., Coilton T. Effects of antihypertensive medications on quality of life in elderly hypertensive women. *Am J Hypertension* 1994; **7**, 329–339.

14. Agabiti-Rosei E., Ambrosinione E., Pireeli A., Stimpel M., Zanchetti A. Efficacy and tolerability of noexipril and nitrendipine in postmenopausal women with hypertension. MADAM study group. *Eur J Clin Pharmacol* 1999; **545**, 185–189.

15. Fitzpatrick A. I., Daling J. R., Furberg C. D., Kronmal R. A., Weissfeld J. L. Use of calcium channel blockers and breast carcinoma risk in postmenopausal women. *Cancer* 1997; **80**, 1438–1447.

16. Fryzek J. P., Poulsen A. H., Lipworth L., Pedersen L., Norgaard M., McLaughlin J. K., Friis S. A cohort study of antihypertensive medication use and breast cancer among Danish women. *Breast Cancer Res Treat* 2006; **97**(3), 231–236.

17. Gueyffier F., Bulpitt C., Boissel J. P., Schron E., Ekbom T., Fagard R., *et al.* Antihypertensive drugs in very old people: a subgroup meta-analysis of randomised controlled trials. INDIANA Group. *Lancet* 1999; **353**, 793–796.

18. Wing L. M., Reid C. M., Ryan P., Beilin L. J., Brown M. A., Jennings G. L., *et al.* A comparison of outcomes with angiotensin-converting enzyme inhibitors and diuretics for hypertension in the elderly. *N Engl J Med* 2003; **348**, 583–592.

19. Rosenfeld J. A. Hypertension occurring postpartum for the first time postpartum: was it preeclampsia. *Tenn Med J* 1992; **85**, 465–466.

20. Landis S. H., Murray T., Bolden S., Wingo P. A. Cancer statistics 1999. *CA Cancer J Clin* 1999; **49**, 8–31.

21. Agency for Health Care Policy and Research Clinical Practice Guidelines. Post stroke rehabilitations. Assessment, referral and patient management. *Am Fam Physician* 1995; **82**, 461–470.

22. Ayala C., Croft J. B., Greenlund K. J., *et al.* Sex differences in US mortality rates for stroke and stroke subtypes by race/ethnicity and age, 1995–1998. *Stroke* 2002; **33**(5), 1197–1201.

23. Vartianen E., Sarti C., Tuomitehto J., Kuulasmaa K. Do changes in cardiovascular risk factors explain changes in mortality from stroke in Finland? *Br Med J* 1995; **310**, 901–904.

24. Shuaih A., Boyle C. Stroke in the elderly. *Curr Opin Neurol* 1994; **7**, 41–47.

25. Suri M. F., Zhou J., Divani A. A., Qureshi A. I. African American women have poor long-term survival following ischemic stroke. *Neurology* 2006; **67**(9), 1623–1629.

26. Morey S. S. National Stroke Association develops consensus statement on prevention of stroke. *Am Fam Physician* 1999; **99**, 463–467.

27. English K. M., Channer K. S. Managing atrial fibrillation in elderly people. *Br Med J* 1999; **318**, 1088–1089.

28. Benjamin E. J., Levy D., Vaziri S. M., *et al.* Independent risk factors for atrial fibrillation in a population-based cohort: the Framingham Heart Study. *J Am Med Assoc* 1994; **271**, 840–844.

29. Friberg J., Scharling H., Gadsboll N., *et al.* Sex-specific increase in the prevalence of atrial fibrillation (the Copenhagen City Heart Study). *Am J Cardiol* 2003; **92**, 1419–1423.

30. Hart R. G., Sherman D. G., Easton J. D., Cairns J. A. Prevention of stroke in patients with nonvalvular atrial fibrillation. *Neurology* 1998; **51**, 674–681.

31. Albers G. Atrial fibrillation and stroke. Three new studies, three remaining questions. *Arch Intern Med* 1994; **154**, 1443–1457.

32. The Stroke Prevention in Atrial Fibrillation Investigators. Warfarin versus aspirin for prevention of thromboembolism in atrial fibrillation. The stroke Prevention in Atrial Fibrillation Trial II. *Lancet* 1994; **344**, 1383–1389.

33. Stroke Prevention in Atrial Fibrillation Study. Final results. *Circulation* 1991; **84**, 527–539.

34. Redgrave J. N., Rothwell P. M. Asymptomatic carotid stenosis: what to do. *Curr Opin Neurol* 2007; **20**(1), 58–64.

35. Hellings W. E., Pasterkamp G., Verhoeven B. A., *et al.* Gender-associated differences in plaque phenotype of patients undergoing carotid end arterectomy. *J Vasc Surg* 2007; **45**(2), 289–296; discussion 296–297.

36. Colditz G. A., Bonita R., Stampfer M. I., *et al.* Cigarette smoking and risk of stroke in middle aged women. *N Engl J Med* 1988; **318**, 937–941.

37. Hill M. D., Yiannakoulias N., Jeerakathil T., Tu J. V., Svenson L. W., Schopflocher D. P. The high risk of stroke immediately after transient ischemic attack: a population-based study. *Neurology* 2004; **62**, 2015–2020.

38. Kerber K. A., Brown D. L., Lisabeth L. D., Smith M. A., Morgenstern L. B. Stroke among patients with dizziness, vertigo, and imbalance in the emergency department: a population-based study. *Stroke* 2006; **37**(10), 2484–2487.

39. Data from Kleindorfer D., Panagos P., Pancioli A., *et al.* Incidence and short-term prognosis of transient ischemic attack in a population-based study. *Stroke* 2005; **36**(4), 720–723.

40. Barr J., McKinley S., O'Brien E., Herkes G. Patient recognition of and response to symptoms of TIA or stroke. *Neuroepidemiology* 2006; **26**(3), 168–175.

41. Tanne D., Koren-Morag N., Goldbourt U. Fasting plasma glucose and risk of incident ischemic stroke or transient ischemic attacks: a prospective cohort study. *Stroke* 2004; **35**(10), 2351–2355.

42. Tanne D., Koren-Morag N., Graff E., Goldbourt U. Blood lipids and first-ever ischemic stroke/transient ischemic attack in the Bezafibrate Infarction Prevention (BIP) Registry: high triglycerides constitute an independent risk factor. *Circulation* 2001; **104**(24), 2892–2897.

43. Gorelick P., Sechenova O., Hennekens C. H. Evolving perspectives on clopidogrel in the treatment of ischemic stroke. *J Cardiovasc Pharmacol Ther* 2006; **11**(4), 245–248.

44. Leonardi-Bee J., Bath P. M., Bousser M. G., *et al.* Dipyridamole for preventing recurrent ischemic stroke and other vascular events: a meta-analysis of individual patient data from randomized controlled trials. *Stroke* 2005; **36**(1), 162–168.

45. Prejbisz A., Kabat M., Januszewicz A., *et al.* Characterization of insomnia in patients with essential hypertension. *Arch Intern Med* 2006; **15**(4), 213–219.

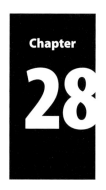

Osteoporosis

Jo Ann Rosenfeld

Introduction

1. More than one-third of postmenopausal women, more than 40 million in the USA, have osteoporosis and more than eight million will have a fracture. Osteoporosis is hastened after menopause and can lead to kyphoscoliosis, pain, respiratory difficulty, vertebral, hip and other fractures.

2. Besides pain and surgery, hip fractures can lead to death, deep venous thrombosis, or pulmonary embolism. When a woman has a hip fracture, she needs extensive rehabilitation, which often necessitates help and dependence, moving into a rehab facility, someone else's home, or a nursing home. Hip fractures often lead to a loss of independence for single or widowed women.

Definition

1. Osteoporosis (OP) occurs when an individual develops a low bone density or mass (BMD, bone mineral density), resulting in an increased risk of fractures. This occurs in both women and men, but there is an increased rate of bone loss in postmenopausal women.

2. OP leads to an increased risk of fractures that result in health complications such as pneumonia, lung disease, thromboembolic disease, chronic pain, disability, and loss of independence.

Epidemiology

1. OP is common and its incidence increases with age. The prevalence of OP in women age 50 to 54 in the UK is between 2 and 3.5%. The prevalence rises to 14–20% in women age 70–74.[1] OP causes more than 150,000 fractures in the UK yearly, including 60,000 hip fractures.

2. With decreasing bone density there is an increasing risk of fractures. A decrease of one standard deviation from the normal of the BMD of a 19-year-old increases the risk of fracture 1.5- to 3-fold.

3. One in six white women will have an OP related hip fracture in her lifetime. Fifty-four percent of 50-year-old women will have an OP related fracture in their lifetimes. The lifetime risk of a hip fracture for a 50-year-old British woman is 14%, a vertebral fracture 11% and a radius fracture 13%. This risk is as great as that of heart disease and six times higher than breast cancer. Figure 28.1 shows the percentage of women in the USA over 50, with osteoporosis by site.

4. Vertebral fractures occur in 25% of white women by age 65 and result in some institutionalization for more than half. There is a mortality rate of 5–25% within the first year after vertebral fracture.[2]

Risk factors

1. Case-controlled and prospective studies have found that the risk factors for OP related hip fractures include being a woman, menopause, being of white or Asian race, cigarette smoking, low body weight, and inactivity (Table 28.1, Figure 28.2).

2. The more risk factors a woman has, the greater is her risk of hip fracture. The risk rises from a rate of 1:1 hip fractures per 1000 woman-years for those women with two or fewer risk factors, to a high of 9.4/1000 woman-years.[3] However, risk factors have a poor specificity and sensitivity in predicting either bone density or risk of fractures in individuals.[4]

Handbook of Women's Health, second edition, ed. Jo Ann Rosenfeld. Published by Cambridge University Press.
© Cambridge University Press 2009.

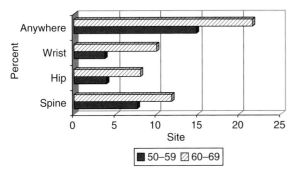

Figure 28.1 Percentage of women in the USA with osteoporosis by site. Data from Osteoporosis prevalence (%) in white women in the U.S. over age 50 by decade. In *AHRQ Evidence Reports*, Number 28, Osteoporosis in Postmenopausal Women: Diagnosis and Monitoring, Table 2, http://www.ncbi.nlm.nih.gov/books/bv.fcgi?rid=hstat1.table.40492, accessed 1/21/07.

3. After menopause, a woman's rate of bone turnover and loss of bone mass increases precipitously.
4. Women who were underweight and those who lose weight are at higher risk for OP.
   A prospective study found that postmenopausal women who lose weight over two years had an increased risk of OP (RR = 1.32/10 lb lost).[5]
5. Whether smoking is a risk factor and how strong is disputed. Several studies correlate active cigarette smoking and OP. However, one study found that smoking was not a risk factor when the data were controlled for weight, health, and difficulty walking. Smokers were in poorer health, had more difficulty rising from a chair, spent fewer hours on their feet, were less likely to walk, and had faster heart rates.
6. Alcohol use was associated with lower risk of hip fractures, but not after adjustment for better self-reported health and ability to stand up from a chair.
7. Fractures occur in 3–6% of individuals who fall. At least one fall occurs in 30% of individuals older than age 70. Individuals with balance and gait disturbances, tremors, difficulty walking or seeing, or on psychotropic medications are at higher risk of falling, and if they have OP, of fracture.

Primary prevention

1. Routine preventive care of women and older men, especially white and Asian women, should include assessment of OP risk. Counseling including diet,

Table 28.1 Risk factors for osteoporosis

Family history and demographics

Older age

History of maternal hip fracture

White or Asian race

Medical history

Postmenopausal

Poor self-rated health

Previous hyperthyroidism

Stroke

Current use of medications, including long-acting benzodiazepines, tricyclic antidepressants, anticonvulsants, steroids

Any fracture since age 50

Social History

Alcohol use

Poor nutrition

On feet less than 4 hours daily

Limited ADLs and physical activity

Physical findings

Resting pulse >80 bpm

Poor memory

Confusion

Disorientation

Poor vision

Low distant depth perception

Poor strength

Absent deep tendon reflexes

Slow rising from sitting

Inability to tandem walk

Note: Data from Cummings S. F., Nevitt M. C., Browner W. S., *et al.* Risk factors for hip fractures in white women. A prospective study. *N Engl J Med* 1995; **332**, 767–771.

physical activity, and consideration of other concurrent medical conditions is important.
2. Most risk factors for osteoporosis are not modifiable. Thin, small women are more likely to have fractures than those with higher BMIs. Chronic diseases, such as renal disease, can cause increased osteoporosis.

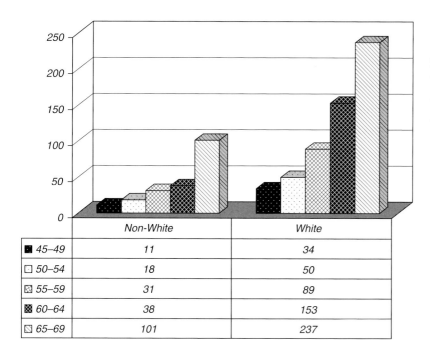

Figure 28.2 Hip fracture incidence in US women by race and age. Data from Hip fracture incidence per 100,000 per year for U.S. women. In *AHRQ Evidence Reports*, Number 28, Osteoporosis in Postmenopausal Women: Diagnosis and Monitoring, Table 4, http://www.ncbi.nlm. nih.gov/books/bv.fcgi?rid=hstat1. table.40494, accessed 1/21/07.

	Non-White	White
■ 45–49	11	34
☐ 50–54	18	50
▨ 55–59	31	89
▩ 60–64	38	153
◱ 65–69	101	237

3. Smoking cigarettes, high caffeine intake, and excessive alcohol use increase the risk of osteoporosis. Long-term use of certain medications such as prednisone can cause osteoporosis (Table 28.1)

4. Excessive athletic training can lead to osteoporosis.

5. Exercise in premenopausal women can increase their total BMD. Thus, when the woman is postmenopausal, she will start with a higher BMD and OP will be prevented or postponed.

6. Similarly, dietary supplementation of calcium (1500 mg daily for teenagers, 1000 mg daily for adult women, 1500 mg daily for postmenopausal women) can increase BMD and prevent OP. Additional use of vitamin D may be needed, if the woman cannot get enough from light exposure or drinking vitamin D enriched milk. The 2006 North American Menopause Society consensus guideline suggests daily calcium and vitamin D supplementation (1200 mg; 400–600 IU daily) "decreases the risk of osteoporosis," and suggested it be given to all perimenopausal and postmenopausal women.[6]

7. However, whether calcium supplementation is appropriate in healthy postmenopausal women in order to decrease the risk of fractures has been very recently disputed. A very large (36,000 women age 50–79) prospective study that followed the women for seven years, found that while calcium supplementation mildly increased hip bone density (RR = 1.06), it did not decrease the hip fracture rate, and did cause a significant increase in kidney stones.[7] The Cochrane review is reexamining the information. A consensus panel found that calcium and vitamin D supplementation could not be shown to reduce fractures in early peri- and postmenopausal women (age 50–63), but was beneficial in reducing bone density loss and reducing incidence of fractures in older women, age 63 and older.[8]

8. Hormone replacement therapy in postmenopausal women is protective against the development of OP, helps reverse the bone loss, treats osteoporosis and prevents fractures. However, with the inadvisability of HRT use, HRT use should be saved for treatment of OP in those women who have no risk factors and who understand the risks and benefits. HRT should not presently be used as primary prevention.

9. Present research does not support the use of selective estrogen receptor modulators (SERMs) such as tamoxifen and raloxifene for primary prevention.

Secondary prevention

1. Secondary prevention of OP is determining which individuals have OP at a preclinical stage and initiating therapy to increase BMD and prevent fractures. Osteopenia may be a late preclinical stage of OP.

2. The diagnosis of OP may be suggested by a new or pathological fracture or noticed incidentally on an X-ray.

3. A history of bone fractures, thinness in older women, kyphoscoliosis or a loss of height may suggest OP. There are few physical findings. In some centers, everyone who has a fracture and is older than 45 receives a DEXA scan.

4. DEXA (dual-energy X-ray absorptiometry) scans are the most precise and common test used to detect bone density. The more sites surveyed, the more likely a diagnosis of osteoporosis occurs. The predictive value of the risk of fractures measured by small DEXA scans that assess only a finger or heel is uncertain. Testing a forearm or heel cannot disprove a diagnosis of osteoporosis; there are too many false-negatives.

5. Osteoporosis is defined as a T-score value of 2.5 below standard deviation for the average bone density of a 19-year-old woman on a bone density DEXA scan. Osteopenia is defined as a T-score value of 1.5–2.5 standard deviation from the same normal.

6. Whether every woman should be screened for osteoporosis, or only those at high risk, is not yet determined by good evidence (Table 28.2). Screening only those with recognized risk factors would miss many who might benefit from treatment. Whether pharmacological treatment for osteopenia is indicated is uncertain. The Cochrane group is presently reevaluating its recommendations for screening and treatment of osteoporosis. In the United States, Medicare will pay for a screening DEXA scan at age 65.

Treatment

1. Treatment includes lifestyle changes and pharmacological therapy.

2. Lifestyle modifications
   a. Exercise can increase BMD, especially with use of other methods including diet, calcium,

Table 28.2 Indications for bone densiometry

Primary prevention

In women with multiple risk factors

  Smoking

  White or Asian race

  Family history

  Hyperthyroidism

  Chronic steroid or anti-metabolite use

  Menopause

  Secondary amenorrhea

  Prolonged use of depot MPA

  Premature ovarian failure

  Anorexia nervosa

Secondary prevention

In women age greater than 50 with any fracture

In women with pathological fractures

Radiological or clinical evidence of vertebral abnormality

Tertiary prevention

Monitoring of therapy

and vitamin D. Estrogen use and exercise together actually increased bone density values in women with low BMD who were followed for two years. Good exercise includes weight-bearing exercise such as walking, jogging, rowing, and weight-lifting.

   b. Moderation in the use of caffeine and alcohol can decrease the bone mass loss rate.

   c. Dietary supplementation of calcium and vitamin D is inexpensive and may increase BMD up to 1% over two years. Postmenopausal women need 1000 to 1500 mg dietary calcium daily. In elderly women, as little as 1000 mg may decrease bone loss. The major side effects are constipation and increased risk of kidney stones.

   d. Cessation of medications
   Many medicines used for comorbid conditions can cause osteoporosis (Table 28.3). Also, medications that affect balance such as psychotropic drugs, sleeping medicines, benzodiazepines, anticholinergic drugs, and

Table 28.3 Medications that can worsen osteoporosis

Diuretics – thiazides, chlorthalidone

Corticosteroids

Antiseizure medications

Cancer chemotherapy drugs

antihistamines, or cause postural hypotension should be modified or stopped to prevent fractures, if possible.

3. **Pharmocological treatment**
    a. Estrogen or HRT used to be the treatment of choice for osteoporosis. Since the evidence of the WHI in 2004, fewer women take HRT because of the risks of breast cancer and thromboembolic disease. The choice to use HRT must be made individually.

    b. **SERMS – tamoxifen and raloxifene**
        i. **Tamoxifen**

            When tamoxifen was used for the treatment of breast cancer, it was noticed that its use increased BMD. However, although it also improves lipid profiles, its use increased the risk of thromboembolic disease and hepatic and endometrial cancer. Thus, it has not been used or approved to treat OP.
        ii. Raloxifen is a SERM that has an antagonistic effect on breast tissue against breast cancer, and an antagonistic effect on the uterus so that it does not increase the risk of endometrial cancer. Its use in a three year RCT trial of more than 6800 women decreased the risk of vertebral fractures by half at 60 or 120 mg/day. The risk of non-vertebral fractures was unchanged. Raloxifen also improves the lipid profile, and increases the risk of DVT (RR = 3.3) It can cause stomach upset.[9]

    c. Biphosphonates include etidronate (Didromel), alendrodate (Fosamax), and Boniva.
        i. When compared to placebo in a RCT, alendronate resulted in a BMD increase of 8.8% in vertebrae and 6.9% in the femoral neck, and reduced all fractures from 18% to 13%.[2]
        ii. These drugs are effective in decreasing the rate of fractures. A RCT compared women using calcium plus alendronate (5 or 10 mg daily for three years or 20 mg daily for two years) to those using just calcium and placebo. Use of alendronate was associeated with a 48% decrease in new vertebral fractures, a decrease in progression in vertebral deformities and significant reduction in height loss.[10]
        iii. These drugs also increase bone density. Another multicentered RCT studying more than 2000 white women for three years found that alendronate increased average BMD, while decreasing by half the rate of vertebral fractures.[11]
        iv. Gastrointestinal side effects are significant and include nausea, constipation, pain and diarrhea. These drugs must be taken on an empty stomach with more than 8 oz of water on awakening, at least half an hour before food, drink, and other medication. They are expensive.

    d. **Calcitonin**

        The usual dose is 100 IU calcitonin salmon preparation or 0.5 mg recombinant form subcutaneously three times a week. Nausea is a side effect. Intranasal salmon calcitonin given once daily (200 IU), in alternating nostrils is another form that is used.

    e. Parathyroid hormone (PTH) has been suggested in an intermittent low dose form. PTH can increase bone formation while high doses cause bone resorption.

Follow-up and further evaluation

1. Normal postmenopausal bone loss is 2% per year. A woman with OP should be started on lifestyle changes and pharmacotherapy. After 18–24 months, a repeat DEXA scan can be obtained to assess for improvement. Decreasing bone loss to less than 4% bone loss over two years or an increase in bone density is acceptable.
2. This is a slowly progressive disease with long-term treatment necessary.

3. What should be done if the bone loss is greater than 4% over two years with treatment is not yet well established. No studies have investigated whether the use of another drug or two drugs together should then be used.

Treatment for osteopenia, defined as a T-score of 1.5–2.5 times below standard deviation of young 19-year-old density, has not been proven to reduce the risk of osteoporosis and bone fracture. Treatment should include calcium supplementation, vitamin D supplementation and weight-bearing exercise. Whether pharmocological treatment for osteopenia reduces the risk of osteoporosis and fractures is not yet known.

References

1. Compston J. E., Cooper C., Kanis J. A. Bone densitometry in clinical practice. *Br Med J* 1995; **310**, 507–510.

2. Bellatoni M. F. Osteoporosis and treatment. *Am Fam Physician* 1996; **54**, 986–996.

3. Cummings S. F., Nevitt M. C., Browner W. S., *et al.* Risk factors for hip fractures in white women. A prospective study. *N Engl J Med* 1995; **332**, 767–771.

4. Compston J. E. Risk factors for osteoporosis. *Clin Endocrinol* 1992; **36**, 223–224.

5. Ensrud K. E., Cauley J., Lipschutz R., Cummings S. R. Weight change and fractures in older women. *Ann Intern Med* 1997; **157**, 857–861.

6. North American Menopause Society. The role of calcium in peri- and postmenopausal women: 2006 position statement of the North American Menopause Society. *Menopause* 2006; **13**(6), 862–877; quiz 878–880.

7. Jackson R. D., LaCroix A. Z., Gass M. Women's Health Initiative Investigators. Effects of calcium supplementation on clinical fracture and bone structure: results of a 5-year, double-blind, placebo-controlled trial in elderly women. *N Engl J Med* 2006; **354**(7), 669–683.

8. Malabanan A. O., Holick M. F. Vitamin D and bone health in postmenopausal women. *J Womens Health (Larchmt)* 2003; **12**(2), 151–156.

9. Ettinger B., Black D. M., Midal B. H., *et al.* Reduction of vertebral fracture risk in postmenopausal women with osteoporosis treated with raloxifene. Results from a 3 year randomized clinical trial. *J Am Med Assoc* 1999; **282**, 637–642.

10. Liberman U. A., Weiss S. R., Broll J. *et al.* Effect of oral alendronate on bone mineral density and the incidence of fractures in postmenopausal osteoporosis. *N Engl J Med* 1995; **333**, 1437–1443.

11. Black D. M., Cummings S. R., Karpf D. B., *et al.* Randomized trial of effect of alendronate on risk of fracture in women with existing vertebral fractures. *Lancet* 1996; **348**, 1535–1541.

Chapter

29

Arthritis

Jo Ann Rosenfeld

Osteoarthritis

1. Arthritis is very prevalent and the most common cause of disability (Figure 29.1). Both osteoarthritis and rheumatoid arthritis are more common in women and more women are disabled from arthritis.
2. Osteoarthritis (OA) is the degenerative disease of cartilage and joints with a slow progressive non-deforming course. The joints most affected are usually the hands and large weight-bearing joints.

Incidence

1. Arthritic changes are very common. Twenty-four percent of women age 54–75 and more than half of women age 75 and older report symptomatic OA. In 2003, in the USA approximately 46 million individuals reported arthritis, costing approximately $81 billion in health care and lost work.[1]
2. In the Third National Health and Nutrition Examination Survey (NHANES III), women had more carpal deformities than men. Almost one-quarter of women reported first carpal-metacarpal deformities, compared to 10% of men. Fifty-eight percent reported Heberden's nodes, 29.9% had Bouchard's nodes, and 18.2% had first carpal-metacarpal deformities.[2] Painful hand arthritis incidence increased with age and caused difficulty dressing, lifting, and eating.
3. In the NHANES III, knee arthritis was also very common. Thirty-seven percent of adults reported knee osteoarthritis. Significantly more women reported knee arthritis than men. Knee replacement occurred in 1.5%. Adults with symptomatic knee OA were more likely to use

non-steroidal anti-inflammatory agents, use canes, and have slower gaits.[3] A survey in the UK showed that approximately 9% of all individuals reported knee OA.
4. Hip arthritis is prevalent but reported more by men than women. Approximately 15% of survey participants older than age 60 reported hip pain. More minority women reported hip pain than men.[4]
5. Risk factors for knee osteoarthritis included obesity, elevated BMI, older age, African Americans, and in men, manual labor occupations.
6. Disability from OA was more likely in older populations, non-whites, African Americans, and Mexican American. Minority women reported more disability than men.[5]
7. Arthritis can lead to disability, social isolation, staying at home, and lead to nursing home placement.
8. The knee is the most common join affected. Those with knee OA are more than two times as likely to report difficulty walking, most likely to complain of difficulty with activities of daily living, and five times more likely to have difficulty going up and down stairs.

Primary prevention

1. The risk factors for osteoarthritis may be modifiable, but there is no proof that changing them will reduce the risk for developing OA (Table 29.1).
2. Increased weight, BMI, and obesity increase the risk of developing OA. Each 10 lb increase in weight increases the relative risk by 1.4. Obesity

---

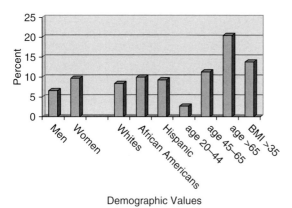

Demographic Values

Figure 29.1 Reported disability from arthritis. Data from Centers for Disease Control and Prevention (CDC). Prevalence of doctor-diagnosed arthritis and arthritis-attributable activity limitation – United States, 2003–2005. *MMWR Morb Mortal Wkly Rep.* 2006; **55**(40), 1089–1092, Erratum 2006; **55**(41), 1129. *MMWR Morb Mortal Wkly Rep.* 2007; **56**(3), 55, PMID 17035926.

Table 29.1 Risk factors for osteoarthritis

	Relative risk
Obesity	8.0
Physical activity	3.2
High BMI	1.7
Occupational injury	1.5
Smoking	0.5

increases the risk of knee, hip, and hand arthritis. However, whether this increased risk is caused by wear and tear or has a metabolic cause is not yet determined. Women with a BMI greater than 27 have an increased age-adjusted risk of arthritis.[6,7]

3. Increased physical activity is associated with an increased risk of osteoarthritis. However, older individuals who engage in vigorous running and aerobic activity had lower mortality and slower development of disability, fewer chronic joint pains, but the same risk of bone fractures.

4. Women with OA have less incidence of osteoporosis (OP). This inverse relationship may be linked, first to obesity, and increased BMI, and secondly, to the development of osteophytes.

5. Women increased the incidence of OA, with a more rapid rise in occurrence with age, particularly of the small joint hand OA.[8]

   a. An increase in symptoms with menopause has been documented for nearly 200 years, although there is no relation between a woman's age at menarche or at menopause, or parity and the development of OA. Some studies have suggested this may be caused by weight gain after menopause.

   b. The course of OA in women may be different. Older women may be more likely to report joint symptoms at the same level of radiographic severity of knee OA, and OA of

the hip progresses more rapidly in women than men.

   c. Many studies show an inverse relationship between the use of HRT and development of OA, while a few show no difference.[9] Never having used estrogen was associated with an increased risk of OA in the Melbourne Longitudinal Women's Midlife Health Project.[10] Estrogen exposure and OA may be unrelated.

Clinical presentation and diagnosis

1. Women present with joint pain and stiffness. After months, usually, the pain and disease burn out in one joint.

2. The disease is migratory and waxes and wanes. The course of the disease varies widely from person to person. The joints are usually not deformed.

3. There is "gelling," pain that occurs after rest or sitting, that is reduced with movement. The pain is often worse after physical activity or in the evening.

4. OA is a clinical diagnosis, established in the presence of joint stiffness, pain, warmth, and the absence of systemic features. The affected joints are usually warm and often swollen, but not hot and red (Table 29.2).

5. Examination will reveal enlarged joints with crepitus with movement. Joint tenderness, warmth, and reduction in movement occurs first, and later decreased muscle strength, reduced range of motion and contractures can occur.

6. Radiological findings do not correlate with the severity of the clinical disease or with the amount or degree of pain. However, osteophytes are the radiographic feature associated best with knee

Table 29.2 Criteria for diagnosis of osteoarthritis of hip and knees: data from the American College of Rheumatology Classification Criteria

Hip osteoarthritis

Hip pain

At least two of the following three items:

   Erythrocyte sedimentation rate <20 mm/hr

   Radiographic femoral or acetabular osteophytes

   Radiographic finding of joint narrowing

Knee osteoarthritis

Knee pain

Radiological osteophytes

At least one of the following three items:

   Age >50

   Morning stiffness less than 30 minutes each morning

   Crepitus on motion

pain. Joint space narrowing and subchondral sclerosis can occur.

7. The differential diagnosis includes several forms of arthritis (Table 29.3).

Treatment and secondary prevention

1. The goals of treatment are to maintain function, protect the joint, reduce pain and prevent complications and disabilities. Treatment must be individualized and includes exercise, education, and pain control. Treatment should include:

   a. stabilization of existing disease,
   b. social and psychological support,
   c. education and reassurance,
   d. physiotherapy and occupational therapy,
   e. pain control that does not include chronic narcotics,
   f. reduction of body weight to closer to ideal,
   g. use of assistive devices,
   h. self-management programs.

2. No screening tests to detect the disease are available and there is no treatment that started early will change the course of OA.

3. Exercise can affect the course of disease and reduce the subsequent disability. Individuals should receive an exercise prescription from their physicians. Arthritis can lead to deconditioning

Table 29.3 Clinical differential diagnosis of osteoarthritis

Crystalline arthritis

Calcium pyrophosphate disease (CPP) has increasing incidence with age, occurring in the same joints as OA; approximately 30 to 60% of individuals age 65 to 75 can have this. It usually presents as an acute monoarticular synovitis of the knee, wrist or shoulder. Associated with hyperparathyroidism, hypothyroidism, gout, hypophosphatemia and hypermagnesemia. Treatment of primary cause does not affect the arthopathy.

Gout, usually sudden excrutiating red swollen joint, often the first metatarsal-phalangeal joint (podagra). Can also occur as a chronic arthritis with hyperuricemia and renal disease.

Connective tissue arthritides

Rheumatoid arthritis, usually a migratory polyarthritis affecting the small joints of the hands, and knees, shoulder and hips. Women usually have systemic symptoms. Joints are often very swollen, hot, red, and tender. Deforming with time.

Psoriatic arthritis, associated with psoriasis, it often appears like RA.

Other connective tissue disease

Infective arthritis

Septic arthritis, usually a single, very swollen, tender, red, hot joint in patient with fever, high white blood count, and systemic symptoms. Often associated with a break in the skin or abrasion. May be caused by *Staphylococcus*, gonorrhea, or other organisms.

Lyme arthritis, usually starts as a single, warm, red joint, usually knees or elbows. Associated with a tick bite (which may not be remembered) in an endemic area and sometimes with a rash.

Traumatic arthritis

and prolonged inactivity that further causes muscle weakness, decreased flexibility, poor endurance, osteoporosis, fatigue, depression, and social isolation. Individuals with OA who walk decrease their pain and use of pain medication.

4. **Education**

   Patients should learn about OA. A study of a self-management program that followed more than 100 women for 12 months found that using education and behavioral and cognitive modification techniques improved physical and psychological health and reduced pain.[11]

5. Pain control

    a. Acetaminophen (up to 1000 mg every 6 hours) is the preferred analgesia. NSAIDs can be used if acetaminophen does not work.

    b. NSAIDs should be used for short periods and for as low doses as possible. Nearly 1.5 million person-years of NSAIDs are prescribed yearly in the UK. Ibuprofen has been suggested as the most appropriate alternative to acetaminophen.

    c. Side effects of NSAIDs include upper gastrointestinal bleeding. Gastric ulcer occurs in approximately 15% of those on chronic use. Edema, hyponatremia, hyperklalemia, bleeding problems, and renal and hepatic toxicity can occur. The role of topical NSAIDs is unclear.

    d. Intra-articular steroid injections for single-joint arthritis can be used.

    e. Bracing the painful limb may help.

    f. There is no place for systemic steroids or narcotics.

    g. Glucosamine with and without chondroitin sulfate has been suggested for chronic treatment and pain relief of OA. Double blind RCTs found that a once-daily dose of glucosamine (1500 mg) relieved pain better than acetaminophen or placebo with few side effects.[12] A multi-centered double blind placebo controlled study of more than 1500 participants found that more pain relief occurred with glucosamine combined with chondroitin sulfate that with glucosamine alone.[13]

6. Surgery is indicated in patients with severe disease. Either arthroscopy with debridement of cartilage and washout of joint space or joint replacement may be indicated.

7. Replacement is indicated for individuals with chronic pain, considerable impairment, joint failure, moderate to severe persistent pain, and/or severe disability not relieved by an extended course of non-surgical management.

Rheumatoid arthritis

Rheumatoid Arthritis (RA) is one of a group of connective tissue diseases that is systemic and affects multiple joints. Usually progressive, disabling, and deforming, treatment of RA now uses disease modifying therapy to prevent further destruction of the joints.

Epidemiology

1. The prevalence of RA is 2% rising to a high of 5% in women older than age 55. The incidence in the USA is approximately 70 per 100,000.[14]

2. RA is a disease of women. There is some proof that estrogen use may affect its course. Noticing that RA improved during pregnancy led to the discovery of steroid hormones. How estrogen affects RA is complex and not completely understood.

3. OCP use may protect against RA or reduce the severity of the disease. A retrospective study found that women who used OCPs for more than five years had a RR of 0.1 of developing RA.[15] Disease symptoms are less severe in the second half of the menstrual cycle.[16]

4. Women with RA on average had more children. A retrospective study found that having more than three children increased the risk of developing RA by 4.8 times and increased the risk of poorer prognosis.[14] Women who breast fed their infants had twice the rate of RA.

5. The treatment goal for early rheumatoid arthritis is remission of symptoms. In a study of more than 600 patients with early RA, being a woman was the only factor that predicted poor remission of symptoms over two years.[17] Women had fewer remission and more severe disease.

Clinical course

1. RA is a disabling disease that deforms and destroys joints, causes a loss of function and decreases the lifespan by an average of 13–18 years.[18]

2. The course of the disease is variable. RA occurs at any age but its peak incidence is at age 30 to 50. The women-to-men ratio is 3:1.

3. The disease waxes and wanes from weeks to years, with remissions and exacerbations occurring spontaneously. There is usually a remission in the first year.

4. The disease ranges from mild to disabling and destructive. There is some evidence that individuals who develop the disease after age 60 have a more severe course, greater damage in the

joints, greater disease activity and worse damage seen on X-rays.

5. Individuals with high rheumatoid factor titers and high C-reactive protein titers have a worse prognosis.

6. Predictors of a more severe course include being a man, younger age at onset, use of prednisone, being single, and not having social supports or a job.

7. Any synovial joint can be affected. Most commonly, RA starts as a bilateral symmetrical disease. The joints most frequently affected are the small joints of the hands and feet, wrists, knees, elbows, and acromioclavicular joints.

8. It is a systemic disease. It usually occurs in one of two forms – an acute arthritis involving single or multiple joints or a subacute form with multiple systemic manifestations. The systemic symptoms can include fatigue, fever, weight loss, anorexia, malaise, night sweats, parasthesias, and myalgias, all of which can precede the development of arthritis.

Diagnosis

1. The diagnosis is clinical and usually gathered over a period of months to years (Table 29.4). The criteria in Table 29.4 have a 91% sensitivity and 89% specificity for the diagnosis of RA

2. Extra-articular manifestations include the following.

   a. Fever.

   b. Rheumatoid nodules occur in 20–30% of individuals usually on extensor surfaces, but can occur anywhere.

   c. Vasculitis can affect any system and is usually seen in individuals with high rheumatoid factor titers. This can cause polyneuropathy, gangrene, ulcers, and rarely visceral infarctions.

   d. Muscle weakness and atrophy of skeletal muscles.

   e. Lung and pleural symptoms including fibroisis, nodules, pneumonitis, arteritis.

3. **Radiological diagnosis**

   a. Early in the course of the disease, the radiological changes may not be symmetrical.

   b. There are usually both osseous and soft tissue manifestations. Findings include marginal

Table 29.4 Criteria for rheumatoid arthritis

Four of seven of the following criteria are necessary for diagnosis.

1. Radiographic changes: typical changes of posteroanterior hand and wrist erosions or bony decalcifications

2. Morning stiffness lasting one hour or more

3. Arthritis of three or more joints at the same time, consisting of swelling or joint effusions. Joints include proximal interphalangeal, metacarpophalangeal, wrist, elbow, knee, ankle and metarsophalangeal joints

4. Rheumatoid nodules

5. Arthritis of hand joints

6. Symmetrical arthritis

7. Serum rheumatoid factor positive

erosions, uniform joint space loss, fusiform periarticular soft tissue swelling, and juxta-articular osteoporosis.

   c. The MRI scan is a good diagnostic test finding early joint changes.

4. **Serological diagnosis**

   a. **Anemia**

      This is usually a normocytic normochromic anemia present in active RA.

   b. The erythrocyte sedimentation rate and C-reactive protein level are usually elevated.

   c. The rheumatoid factor comprises auto-antibodies that occur in two-thirds of individuals with the disease. However, rheumatoid factor also occurs in 5% of normal individuals and in patients with lupus or mixed connective tissue disease, chronic liver disease, sarcoidosis, tuberculosis, syphilis, and other disease.

   d. Joint fluid analysis is not specific but is usually turbid, with decreased or normal glucose, increased protein and a white blood count of 5000 to 50,000, mostly polymorphonuclear lymphocytes.

Treatment

1. The goals of therapy are relief of pain, reduction of inflammation, reduced disability of joints and

relief of systemic symptoms. Treatment includes behavioral and pharmacological therapy, patient education and assistive devices.

2. Life-altering therapy includes moderate exercise. Those individuals with RA who did exercise for more than five hours weekly for more than five years had less progression of joint damage, fewer hospitalizations and less work disability.[19] Non-weight-bearing exercise such as swimming may help considerably. Long-term, high-intensity activity may reduce disability.[20]

3. **Pharmocological treatment**

   There are five main therapies including aspirin and NSAIDs, oral steroids, disease modifying drugs (DMDs), including Embrel[R] and its relatives, and intra-articular steroid injections.

   a. In the past, DMDs were reserved for individuals who failed on NSAIDs and oral steroids or who had severe rapidly progressive disease. Recently, DMDs have been started early in the course of the illness. Predictor of remission was a good response to initial DMD. Studies have found that delay from diagnosis to treatment with DMD of as little as four months can decrease the likelihood of remission.[21]

   b. Aspirin and NSAIDS are used both for pain relief and control of inflammation. They work well but do not affect the progression of the disease. As well, they have potentially serious side effects, including gastric ulcers in up to 25%, renal side effects, and blood disorders.

   c. Low dose systemic oral steroids will reduce pain and inflammation, and may slow progression of bone erosions. In a general practice in the UK, more than 1% of the patients were using chronic steroids and one-fourth of these were for RA.[22] Oral steroids have been used as short-term medication, a bridge until DMDs work, and as chronic medication. Steroids have significant side effects including gastrointestinal upset and ulcer, bone density loss, immunosuppression, and other problems.

   d. Disease modifying drugs include methotrexate, d-penicillamine, plaquinyl

and Embrel. These do not relieve pain and usually an NSAIDs must be given in addition. They take weeks to show effect. However, they do produce significant improvement in approximately two-thirds of individuals.

   e. Etanercept (Embrel) has had good success. In a meta-analysis of many studies, etanercept showed significant improvement within three months of initiation of treatment of both elderly and young patients, with early or late RA, and maintained the improvement over six years of treatment. The open-label extension trials for up to a total of six years of etanercept therapy.[23] Etanercept has been shown to produce significant improvement in patients with early RA, and in those that had failed other DMD or late RA. However, it was more effective early in the disease.[24]

   f. Studies have shown some improvement with gamma-linolenic acid.[25]

   g. Tai Chi has long been shown to be an effective exercise program to help RA.[26]

   h. Intra-articular steroid injections can be used for severe pain or inflammation of one joint.

4. Surgical replacement is used for severe intractable pain or disability.

Disability

More than half of women who have RA become disabled and unable to work. Women who can modify their pace at work are less likely to become disabled.

References

1. Centers for Disease Control and Prevention (CDC). National and state medical expenditures and lost earnings attributable to arthritis and other rheumatic conditions – United States, 2003. *MMWR Morb Mortal Wkly Rep* 2007; **56**(1), 4–7.

2. Dillon C. F., Hirsch R., Rasch E. K., Gu Q. Symptomatic hand osteoarthritis in the United States: prevalence and functional impairment estimates from the third U.S. National Health and Nutrition Examination Survey, 1991–1994. *Am J Phys Med Rehabil* 2007; **86**(1), 12–21.

3. Dillon C. F., Rasch E. K., Gu Q., Hirsch R. Prevalence of knee osteoarthritis in the United States: arthritis data from the Third National Health and Nutrition

Examination Survey 1991–94. *J Rheumatol* 2006; **33**(11), 2271–2279.

4. Christmas C., Crespo C. J., Franckowiak S. C., Bathon J. M., Bartlett S. J., Andersen R. E. How common is hip pain among older adults? Results from the Third National Health and Nutrition Examination Survey. *J Fam Pract* 2002; **51**(4), 345–348.

5. Ostchega Y., Harris T. B., Hirsch R., Parsons V. L., Kington R. The prevalence of functional limitations and disability in older persons in the US: data from the National Health and Nutrition Examination Survey III. *J Am Geriatr Soc* 2000; **48**(9), 1132–1135.

6. Felson D. T., Zhang Y., Anthony I. M., Nimark A., Anderson H. Weight loss reduces the risk of symptomatic knee osteoarthritis in women: The Framingham Study. *Ann Intern Med* 1992; **116**, 535–539.

7. Szoeke C., Dennerstein L., Guthrie J., Clark M., Cicuttini F. The relationship between prospectively assessed body weight and physical activity and prevalence of radiological knee osteoarthritis in postmenopausal women. *J Rheumatol* 2006; **33**(9), 1835–1840.

8. Silman A. J., Newman J. Obstetric and gynecological factors in susceptibility to peripheral joint osteoarthritis. *Ann Rheum Dis* 1996; **55**, 671–673.

9. Nevitt M. C., Felson D. T. Sex hormones and the risk of osteoarthritis in women. Epidemiologic evidence. *Ann Rheum Dis* 1996; **55**, 673–676.

10. Szoeke C. E., Cicuttini F. M., Guthrie J. R., Clark M. S., Dennerstein L. Factors affecting the prevalence of osteoarthritis in healthy middle-aged women: data from the longitudinal Melbourne Women's Midlife Health Project. *Bone* 2006; **39**(5), 1149–1155.

11. Barlow J. H., Turner A. P., Wrighty C. C. Long term outcomes of an arthritis self-management programme. *Br J Rheumatol* 1998; **37**, 1315–1319.

12. Herrero-Beaumont G., Ivorra J. A., Del Carmen Trabado M., *et al.* Glucosamine sulfate in the treatment of knee osteoarthritis symptoms: a randomized, double-blind, placebo-controlled study using acetaminophen as a side comparator. *Arthritis Rheum* 2007; **56**(2), 555–567.

13. Clegg D. O., Reda D. J., Harris C. L., *et al.* Glucosamine, chondroitin sulfate, and the two in combination for painful knee osteoarthritis. *N Engl J Med* 2006; **354**(8), 795–808.

14. Matsumoto A. K. *Rheumatoid Arthritis Clinical Presentation*. Johns Hopkins Arthritis, http://www.hopkinsarthritis.org/rheumatoid/rheum_clin_pres.html, accessed 3/15/07.

15. Jorgensen C., Picot M. C., Bologna C., Sany J. Oral contraception, parity, breast feeding, and severity of rheumatoid arthritis. *Ann Rheum Dis* 1996; **55**, 94–98.

16. Van der Bink H. R., Van Everdingen A. A., Van Wijk M. J. G., Jacobs J. W. G., Bijlsma J. W. Adjuvant oestrogen therapy does not improve disease activity in postmenopausal patients with rheumatoid arthritis. *Ann Rheum Dis* 1993; **52**, 862–865.

17. Forslind K., Hafstrom I., Ahlmen M., Svensson B. The BARFOT Study Group. Sex: a major predictor of remission in early rheumatoid arthritis. *Ann Rheum Dis* 2007; **66**(1), 46–52.

18. Abyad A., Boyer J. T. Arthritis and aging. *Curr Opin Rheum* 1992; **4**, 153–156.

19. Nordermar R., Ekblom B., Zachrisson I., Lundquist K. Physical training in rheumatoid arthritis: a long term study. *Scan J Rheumatol* 1981; **10**, 25–30.

20. de Jong Z., Munneke M., Zwinderman A. H., *et al.* Is a long-term high-intensity exercise program effective and safe in patients with rheumatoid arthritis? Results of a randomized controlled trial. *Arthritis Rheum* 2003; **48**(9), 2415–2424.

21. Mottonen T., Hannonen P., Korpela M., *et al.* Delay to institution of therapy and induction of remission using single-drug or combination-disease-modifying antirheumatic drug therapy in early rheumatoid arthritis. *Arthritis Rheum* 2002; **46**(4), 894–898.

22. Callahan L. F., Rao J., Boutaugh M. Arthritis and women's health. Prevalence, impact and prevention. *Am J Prev Med* 1996; **12**, 400–407.

23. Schiff M. H., Yu E. B., Weinblatt M: E., *et al.* Long-term experience with etanercept in the treatment of rheumatoid arthritis in elderly and younger patients: patient-reported outcomes from multiple controlled and open-label extension studies. *Drugs Aging* 2006; **23**(2), 167–178.

24. Baumgartner S. W., Fleischmann R. M., Moreland L. W., Schiff M. H., Markenson J., Whitmore J. B. Etanercept (Enbrel) in patients with rheumatoid arthritis with recent onset versus established disease: improvement in disability. *J Rheumatol* 2004; **31**(8), 1532–1537.

25. Little C. V., Parsons T. Herbal therapy for treating rheumatoid arthritis. *Cochrane Database Syst Rev* 2007; 1.

26. Han A., Judd M. G., Robinson V. A., Taixiang W., Tugwell P., Wells G. Tai chi for treating rheumatoid arthritis. *Cochrane Database Syst Rev* 2007; 1.

Index